IDIOPATHIC INFLAMMATORY MYOPATHIES – RECENT DEVELOPMENTS

Edited by **Jan Tore Gran**

Idiopathic Inflammatory Myopathies – Recent Developments
Edited by Jan Tore Gran

Published by InTech

Janeza Trdine 9, 51000 Rijeka, Croatia

Publishing Process Manager Alenka Urbancic

Technical Editor Teodora Smiljanic

Cover Designer InTech Design Team

Additional hard copies can be obtained from orders@intechopen.com

Idiopathic Inflammatory Myopathies – Recent Developments, Edited by Jan Tore Gran
p. cm.
ISBN 978-953-307-694-2

For EU product safety concerns:
IN TECH d.o.o., Prolaz Marije Krucifikse Kozulić 3, 51000 Rijeka, Croatia,
info@intechopen.com or visit our website at intechopen.com.

Meet the editor

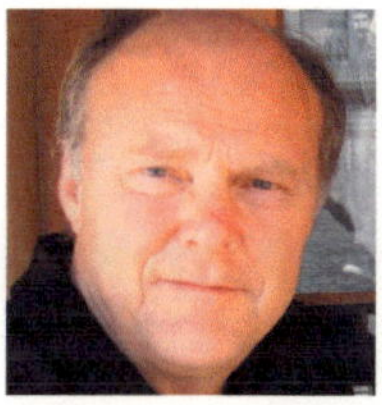

Dr. Jan Tore Gran was born on April 29, 1949 in Oslo, Norway. He studied at the Medical school of University of Oslo, where he graduated in 1977. Dr. Tore Gran specialized in rheumatology in 1985, and presented his Doctoral thesis on Ankylosing spondylitis at the University of Tromsø in 1985. He was the Head of Department of Rheumatology at the University Hospital of Tromsø 1996-1997, Professor at the University of Tromsø 1996-1999, and the Head of the Department of Rheumatology at the Oslo University Hospital, Rikshospitalet, Oslo 2001-2011. Other Dr. Tore Gran's appointments include: Chairman of Govermental Committee on climatic treatment in 2001, member of the Editorial board for the Scandinavian Journal of Rheumatology, and the Journal of the Norwegian Medical Association. He was also the Chairman of the Norwegian Rheumatologist Association 2002-2003, as well as the Chairman of Nordic Research Group for Arthritis mutilans 2005-2011. Dr. Tore Gran has published about 185 full length articles, covering aspects of rheumatic diseases, with particular emphasis on systemic connective tissue diseases. His current main scientific interests are clinical and immunological aspects of the Antisynthetase syndrome. He is currently a professor of rheumatology at the University of Oslo, and a consultant at the Department of Rheumatology, Oslo University Hospital, Rikshospitalet.

Contents

Preface

The idiopathic inflammatory myopathies present some of the most challenging clinical problems in medicine. For many years, these myopathies were simply classified into polymyositis, dermatomyositis and myositis associated with other connective tissue diseases. The treatment relied solely on administration of glucocorticosteroids. Fortunately, our understanding of the immunology, pathology, genetics and clinical aspects of the idiopathic inflammatory myopathies has increased enormously in recent years. The discovery of the myositis specific autoantibodies is of particular imporance, linking specific immunological reactions to distinct clinical subsets of myositis. These advances will most likely contribute to improved definitions and classification of the myopathies, and in due time better treatment and care for the patients. The clinicians involved will be equipped with better tools for predicting disease outcome and final prognosis.

As new important findings are continously published, reliable and up-to-date reviews are strongly warranted. The emphasis of this book is to provide the reader with recent developments in etiopathogenesis, diagnostics and treatment of the idiopathic inflammatory myopathies.

The purpose has not been to present comprehensive descriptions of all myopathic disorders, which can be found in most traditional textbooks. Our goal was to have chapters written by authors with the most expertice. The contributors to this book represent some of the most competent and dedicated workers in the field of myopathies today. I am confident that the book will provide physicians of varied medical specialities with new information, which will be of great value to their research and patient care.

Jan Tore Gran
Consultant, Professor dr. med.
Departement of Rheumatology
Oslo University Hospital, Rikshospitalet
Sognsvannsveien 200026, Oslo
Norway

1

Idiopathic Inflammatory Myopathies: A Review of Immunopathological Features and Current Models of Pathogenesis

Cristina Cappelletti, Lucia Morandi, Marina Mora, Franco Salerno, Paolo Confalonieri, Renato Mantegazza and Pia Bernasconi
Department of Neurology IV – Neuromuscular Diseases and Neuroimmunology, Fondazione Istituto Neurologico "Carlo Besta", Milan, Italy

1. Introduction

The idiopathic inflammatory myopathies (IIMs) are a heterogeneous group of chronic systemic disorders characterized by muscle inflammation and progressive muscle weakness. The major clinical variants are dermatomyositis (DM) including a distinct juvenile (JDM) subtype, polymyositis (PM), and inclusion body myositis (IBM) (Engel & Hohlfeld, 2004). IBM is divided into sporadic IBM (sIBM), the most common muscle disease starting after age 50 years, occurring mainly in men and leading to severe disability, and hereditary inclusion body myopathy, characterized by pathologic alterations resembling those of sIBM except for a lack of muscle inflammation (hence "myopathy" instead of "myositis") (Askanas & Engel, 1998). DM may occur in children or adults and is considered a humorally-mediated microangiopathy, while PM occurs mainly after the second decade of life and is a T cell-mediated disease characterized by cytotoxic attack against non-necrotic muscle fibers (Dalakas, 2011c). For all IIM forms, both target antigens and triggering factors for autoimmune response remain unknown. A growing body of evidence suggests that genetically susceptible individuals probably develop an idiopathic inflammatory myopathy in response to particular environmental stimuli (Feldman et al., 2008; Needham & Mastaglia, 2007; O'Hanlon et al., 2006; O'Hanlon & Miller, 2009; Rider et al., 2010; Sarkar et al., 2005; Vegosen et al., 2007).

2. Clinical aspects

2.1 Dermatomyositis

DM is a rare multisystemic autoimmune disease that affects children and adults of both sexes (with females more commonly affected than males) and all ethnic groups (Amato & Barohn, 2009; Mantegazza & Bernasconi, 2005; Mantegazza et al., 1997). It is characterized clinically by progressive symmetrical proximal muscle weakness and specific skin manifestations, including Gottron's papules, heliotrope rash, and macular erythema. The skin manifestations may precede myositis onset by months or years and can be worsened by exposure to ultraviolet light (UVA or UVB) (Hengstman et al., 2000; Love et al., 2009). This photosensitivity appears associated with the TNF-α-308A allele of the tumor necrosis factor-α (TNF-α) gene, present at high frequency in adult and juvenile Caucasian DM patients (Santmyire-Rosenberger & Dugan, 2003).

Major differences between juvenile and adult DM include the presence of subcutaneous calcinosis affecting the elbows and knees with or without ulceration, vasculopathy affecting various regions of the gastrointestinal tract, acquired lipodystrophy and related metabolic abnormalities (insulin resistance, acanthosis nigricans and type 2 diabetes), and lung disease (Kao et al., 2011). Extramuscular manifestations comprise joint contractures, dysphagia, cardiopathy, arthralgia, Raynaud's phenomenon and pulmonary symptoms. Furthermore, DM is associated with an underlying malignancy in about 24% of cases, in particular with an adenocarcinoma of the ovary, lung, or gastrointestinal tract, as well as with other systemic autoimmune, viral or connective tissue diseases (Dalakas & Hohlfeld, 2003).

2.2 Polymyositis

The diagnosis of PM is often delayed because of lack of distinguishing clinical features (Amato & Barohn, 1997; Dimachkie, 2011). The diagnosis is mainly one of exclusion: absence of skin rash, no extraocular or (generally) facial muscle involvement, no family history of neuromuscular disease, no history of exposure to myotoxic drugs/toxins, no endocrinopathy, no neurogenic disorder, no muscular dystrophy, and no biochemical muscle disease (such as muscle enzyme deficiency) (Dalakas, 2007b). Patients present neck flexor and symmetric proximal arm and leg weakness that typically develops sub-acutely over weeks to months (Amato & Barohn, 1997). Distal muscles may become involved but to a lesser degree than proximal muscles. Dysphagia occurs in a third of patients, and mild facial weakness is occasionally present. The extraocular muscles are spared, sensation is normal and muscle stretch reflexes are usually preserved. PM on its own is rare; it is usually seen in association with interstitial lung disease or polyarthritis. The risk of malignancy with PM is lower than DM, but may be slightly higher than in the general population (Amato & Barohn, 1997; Dimachkie, 2011).

2.3 Inclusion body myositis

Sporadic IBM (sIBM) is the most common IIM in patients over 50 years old, although symptoms can start up to 20 years earlier (Dalakas, 2007b; Needham & Mastaglia, 2007). Because onset is insidious and disease course slow, disease onset and disease incidence are difficult to establish. IBM is more common in males (male to female ratio 3:1) and in Caucasians than Afro-Americans (Needham & Mastaglia, 2007).

Characteristic features of sIBM are atrophy and weakness of wrist and finger flexors and quadriceps. Dysphagia is common, occurring in up to 60% of cases and can be severe enough to interfere with nutrition or give rise to episodes of choking. Although most patients have no sensory symptoms, evidence of generalized peripheral neuropathy is present in up to 30% of patients on clinical examination and electrophysiological testing. As many as 15% of sIBM patients have an underlying autoimmune disorder (systemic lupus erythematosus, Sjögren syndrome, scleroderma, sarcoidosis, variable immunoglobulin deficiency or thrombocytopenia). However, unlike DM and PM, sIBM is not associated with myocarditis, lung disease or increased risk of malignancy (Amato & Barohn, 2009).

Although IBM is considered acquired, familial cases have been described, some associated with leukoencephalopathy. Lack of responsive to immunosuppressive therapy in suspected PM patients gives rise to the suspicion of IBM (Mantegazza & Bernasconi, 2005).

3. Autoantibodies

High titers of autoantibodies are present in the serum of 60-80% of IIM patients (Suber et al., 2008; Ghirardello et al., 2010). These may be myositis-specific (MSAs) - highly specific for particular IIM subtypes - or myositis-associated. Myositis-associated autoantibodies may also by present in patients with other autoimmune diseases and overlap syndromes (Suber et al., 2008). Most MSAs target ubiquitously expressed cytoplasmic or nuclear molecules (Ghirardello et al., 2010) with autoantibodies against cytoplasmic aminoacyl-tRNA synthetases being particularly common (Mammen, 2010). Autoantibodies against histidyl-tRNA synthetase are found in 25-30% of IIM patients (Mammen, 2010) and autoantibodies against the synthetases of threonyl-tRNA, alanyl-tRNA, glycyl-tRNA, isoleucyl-tRNA, asparaginyl-tRNA, tyrosyl-tRNA, and phenylalanyl-tRNA have all been documented (Mathews et al., 1984; Bunn et al., 1986; Targoff, 1990; Hirakata et al., 1999; Betteridge et al., 2007; Targoff, 2008; Zong & Lundberg, 2011).

Anti-Mi-2 antibodies (Mammen, 2010) are a specific marker for DM, being present in 20-30% of adult and juvenile patients. Mi-2 is a major component of the nucleosome-remodeling deacetylase (NuRD) complex, which regulates transcription by modifying chromatin structure. DM patients with anti-Mi-2 autoantibodies tend to have severe cutaneous manifestations, including heliotrope rashes, shawl rashes on the upper back and neck, and cuticle overgrowth, but also have a more favourable prognosis, with good response to steroid therapy, and low incidence of malignancy compared to DM patients without anti-Mi-2 antibodies (Mammen, 2010). Anti-Mi-2 antibody positivity seems to occur more frequently at lower latitudes, and it has been found that in human keratinocyte cell lines exposed to UV Mi-2 protein expression is upregulated. It has therefore been proposed that UV drives the autoimmune response against Mi-2. This suggestion is in line with the observation that increased Mi-2 protein levels are often found in DM muscle biopsies, while in normal and PM muscle biopsies, Mi-2 protein levels are relatively low (Casciola-Rosen et al., 2005).

Autoantibodies against components of the signal recognition particle (SRP) are reported in 4-6% of patients with PM/DM. The SRP is a highly conserved constitutively expressed cytoplasmic ribonucleoprotein, consisting of six polypeptides and a single 7SL RNA (Ghirardello et al., 2010). The SRP complex is involved in the translocation of nascent secretory or membrane proteins across the endoplasmic reticulum. Histopathological features of patients with antibodies against SRP are prominent muscle fibre necrosis and regeneration, without significant inflammatory cell infiltration, and, as in DM, a reduced number of capillaries, that are enlarged, and show deposits of membrane attack complex (MAC) (Targoff, 2008).

Anti-p155/140 antibodies are found in 20-30% of DM and JDM patients; these recognize nuclear transcriptional intermediary factor 1-gamma (TIF1-γ) and are associated with severe skin involvement and high risk of developing cancer (Ghirardello et al., 2010). Anti-small ubiquitin-like modifier activating enzyme (SAE) antibodies are found in about 8% of DM patients (Ghirardello et al., 2010). A novel MSA - anti-CADM-140 antibody - was identified recently in a Japanese cohort of DM patients (Nakashima et al., 2010). These antibodies seem particularly associated with clinically amyopathic DM who also have acute progressive interstitial lung disease. The antigen target of anti-CADM-140 antibody was found to be RNA helicase C domain-containing protein 1 (IFIH1), also known as melanoma differentiation associated protein-5 (MDA-5), one of the RIG-I-like receptors involved in the recognition of viral RNAs during the innate immune responses. RIG-I and IFIH1 interact with viral RNA and mediate signalling pathways leading to the transcription of type I interferons (IFNs) and inflammatory cytokines (Takeuchi & Akira, 2008). The finding that IFIH1 provokes MSA reinforces the idea of an association between myositis and viral infection: self-tolerance might be broken when IFIH1 interacts with certain viral RNAs and generates cryptic epitopes or when elevated IFN-β levels up-regulate IFIH1 synthesis, resulting in over-expression and release from damaged cells (Nakashima, 2010).

It is not well understood how a self-molecule can be singled out as target for autoantibody response. It may occur as a consequence of the proinflammatory properties of molecule itself or as a result of modifications to autoantigen structure occurring during cell damage or cell death (Suber et al., 2008). Structural changes in self-molecules generally result in modification of antigen processing and presentation and also to activate immune responses against epitopes not generated during tolerance induction. In myositis tissues, a common alteration in molecular structure is that induced when cells are killed by the release of cytotoxic enzymes by CD8+ T cells, especially granzyme B (Casciola-Rosen et al., 1999).

4. Treatments

The main concerns about drug treatment for IIMs are that controlled trials are few and there are no standardized outcome measures to reflect changes in disability or quality of life (Distad et al., 2011). The main treatments for PM and DM are drugs that suppress or modify the immune system (Distad et al., 2011). Oral corticosteroids (in particular a high dose of prednisone) represent the first-line medications used to manage these conditions. When the treatment with these drugs is prolonged for a long period, or when the disease reveals refractory to therapy, a second-line agent, usually a chronic, steroid-sparing immunosuppressive drug such as azathioprine, methotrexate, cyclosporine, cyclophosphamide, and mycophenolate mofetil is added. Such medications often allow corticosteroid dosages to be reduced, but monitoring is required for their own side effects, such as bone marrow suppression, kidney dysfunction, and respiratory concerns. Intravenous immunoglobulin has also been reported effective by some controlled studies (Basta & Dalakas, 1994; Saadeh et al., 1995; Cherin et al., 1994; Sansome & Dubowitz, 1995, as cited in Choy & Isenberg, 2002), producing clinical improvement together with reduction in complement deposition, membrane attack complex formation, inflammation, fibrosis, cytokines, chemokines and adhesion molecules, especially in DM patients (Dalakas, 2011a).

Rituximab, a monoclonal antibody that depletes B cells, has also shown efficacy in uncontrolled studies on DM patients and is a promising treatment for the disease (Noss et al., 2006; Levine, 2005). Other treatments currently under study include new agents targeting intracellular T-cell signalling pathways (associated with antigen recognition and costimulation), B cells or B cell growth factors. Monoclonal antibodies against components of the complement pathway, inhibitors of TNF-α and IFN-α, and antagonists of the IL-1 receptor are also under study.

5. Pathology

PM and sIBM are characterized by the presence of an endomysial mononuclear cell infiltrate mainly consisting of activated (HLA-DR+, LFA-1+) cytotoxic CD8+ T lymphocytes with a memory phenotype (CD45RO+). The infiltrate surrounds and eventually invades non-necrotic muscle fibers. When CD8+ T cells are in close contact with muscle fibers, perforin and granzyme containing granules accumulate within the T cells close to the point of contact (polarization), and are eventually released at the immunological synapse that forms between the T cell and the fiber. Sporadic IBM is also characterized by abnormal accumulation of proteins within the muscle fibers.

The muscle pathology of DM is characterized by presence of infiltrates consisting of both B cells, T cells and plasmacytoid dendritic cells, together with perifascicular muscle fiber atrophy. CD4+ T cells are prominent perivascularly; CD4+ plasmacytoid dendritic cells spread through the endomysial, perimysial, and perivascular regions (Greenberg et al., 2005a). Membrane attack complex (MAC) deposition can be observed on capillaries where it is thought to induce capillary depletion, leading to muscle fiber necrosis and the perifascicular atrophy pathognomic for DM even in the absence of inflammation. It has been proposed that in DM perifascicular myofiber damage mainly occurs as a result of chronic overproduction of α/β-interferon-inducible proteins (Greenberg et al., 2005a; Greenberg, 2007b & 2008). However this seems unlikely as the damaged fibers display all the markers of regeneration and tissue remodeling (Dalakas, 2011c), suggesting that the expression of these proteins is a consequence and not the cause of the regeneration process. The chronic overproduction of α/β-interferon-inducible proteins hypothesis is also difficult to reconcile with the reduction in number of capillaries and early activation and deposition of MACs on capillaries before perifascicular atrophy is evident (Dalakas, 2011c). Furthermore up-regulation of α/β-interferon-inducible genes is not specific to DM: it also occurs in PM and other connective tissue diseases (Cappelletti et al., 2011; Walsh et al., 2007).

6. Immunopathogenesis

6.1 Dermatomyositis

The etiology of DM is not clearly understood. It has been suggested that DM develops as a result of a combination of autoimmune reactions in genetically susceptible individuals in response to environmental triggers such as infectious agents (Batthish & Feldman, 2011).

6.1.1 Complement activation and vascular endothelial damage

The most striking characteristic of DM is early and persisting damage to the vascular endothelium of endomysial capillaries, and, to a lesser extent, of larger blood vessels (Greenberg & Amato, 2004; Dalakas, 2011c) (Fig. 1). The earliest observed anomaly is deposition of MAC on small arterioles and capillaries supplying the muscle fibers. This may be observed before inflammatory or structural changes. Thus, microscopic blood vessel damage appears to be complement-mediated; however the mechanism of complement activation remains unclear. It has been suggested that the presence of antibodies against endothelial cells (Dalakas, 2011c) activates C3 leading to the formation of C3b and C4b fragments and subsequently C5b-9. Deposition of the membranolytic C5b-9 complex on the walls of intramuscular arterioles and capillaries and increased expression of intercellular adhesion molecules by capillary endothelial cells have been reported in several studies (Kissel et al., 1986; Whitaker & Engel, 1972, as cited in Greenberg & Amato, 2004), although data are conflicting regarding the frequency of these occurrences and their specificity for DM (Greenberg & Amato, 2004). Other suggestions are that complement activation is secondary to injury to the vascular endothelium or, alternatively, that the membrane attack complexes derive from plasma where they circulate in the form of immune complexes.

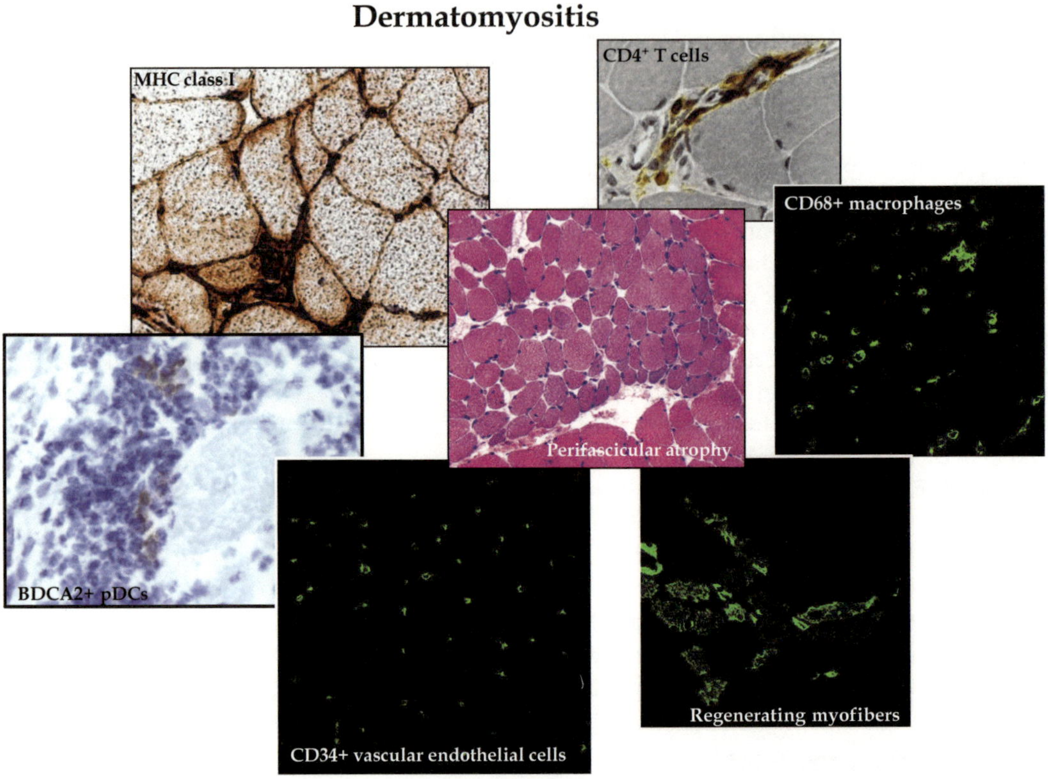

Fig. 1. Major pathological features of DM muscle. Muscle biopsy shows upregulation of major histocompatibility complex class I (MHC-I) on the surface of the majority of fibers, and perivascular invasion by CD4+ T cells and CD68+ macrophages. BDCA2+ plasmacytoid dendritic cells (pDCs) - natural interferon-producing cells - are present in endomysial regions. Regenerating myofibers are often present in perifascicular regions.

Irrespective of where complement activation occurs in the chain of pathological events, the result is a marked reduction in the number of capillaries per muscle fiber followed by the compensatory dilatation of the lumen of the remaining capillaries (Dalakas, 2006a) (Fig. 1). The endothelial cells become swollen and necrotic, and develop tubuloreticular inclusions and microvacuoles. These alterations result in perivascular inflammation, muscle ischemia and the characteristic perifascicular atrophy (Fig. 1). It is frequently stated that the perifascicular atrophy is a direct consequence of hypoperfusion of the vulnerable perifascicular regions of the muscle fascicles (Dalakas, 2006a), implying that DM is a true microvasculopathy (Hohlfeld & Dornmair, 2007; Probst-Cousin et al., 2010). Gene expression studies have demonstrated that both angiogenic and angiostatic genes are expressed in juvenile and adult DM muscle. In particular, angiostatic factors, including inducible protein 10 kDa (IP-10 or CXCL10), monokine induced by IFNγ (MIG/CXCL9), and IFNγ-inducible T-cell α chemoattractant (I-TAC/CXCL11), have been detected in peripheral blood during active disease and at high levels in muscle biopsies from untreated patients. In untreated patients they correlate with the extent of capillary loss and mononuclear cell infiltration (Baechler et al., 2007; Bilgic et al., 2009; Fall et al., 2005). Neovascularization (αVβ3-positive capillaries) is suggested to occur later in the disease and is more prevalent in

JDM than adult DM (Nagaraju et al., 2006). Transcript levels of genes involved in endothelial cell adhesion (cathepsin B, CD146), proliferation (cyclin D1), differentiation (jagged protein), migration (hepatocyte growth factor) and angiogenesis (ITPR1, HIF1A, angiogenic inducer 61) are up-regulated in DM patients compared to controls, suggesting that affected muscle possesses all the molecules required for the initiation of angiogenic response (Nagaraju et al., 2006). Notwithstanding increased expression of pro-angiogenic factors in DM, the vascular network does not recover and symptoms persist. To explain this it has been suggested that the capillary damage is so great that microvascular neogenesis is unable to effect a restoration of the microvasculature, or that the potency of the angiogenesis inhibitors exceeds that of the angiogenic factors. Alternatively the angiogenic stimuli may not be sufficiently co-coordinated to exert an overall positive effect. It is also possible that the anti-endothelial immune response and toxicity damage the endothelial cells to such an extent that they are unable to respond to the angiogenic stimuli (Konttinen et al., 2004).

6.1.2 Type I interferons

Type I IFNs have only recently been recognized to play a role in DM, particularly JDM, pathogenesis (Feldman et al., 2008). Gene expression profiling of muscle samples from untreated juvenile and adult DM patients showed that almost half of the most differentially expressed genes were associated with immune responses, and most of these were inducible by type I IFNs (Tezak et al., 2002; Greenberg et al., 2002; Greenberg et al., 2005a; Salajegheh et al., 2010a; Cappelletti et al., 2011). Among these, transcript levels of 15 kDa interferon-stimulated ubiquitin-like modifier protein (ISG15), interferon-induced protein with tetratricopeptide repeats 3 (IFIT3), and myxovirus resistance protein A (MxA) - three important mediators of biological and therapeutic effects of type I IFNs - were significantly higher in affected muscle than controls (Greenberg et al., 2002; Greenberg et al., 2005a; Salajegheh et al., 2010a; Cappelletti et al., 2011), and these higher levels were directly associated with muscle weakness, but not with the extent or severity of inflammatory skin involvement, suggesting muscle-specific pathophysiology (O'Connor et al., 2006).
Increased serum levels of type I IFN-inducible α-type CXC chemokines (IP-10, MIG, and I-TAC) and monocyte chemoattractant proteins (MCP-1, MCP-2, MIP-1α, MIP-1β) have been found in a number of patients with severe forms of DM (Bilgic et al., 2009; Khanna & Reed, 2010). These proinflammatory molecules appear to result in angiostasis in affected tissues by acting as chemoattractants to recruit CXCR3-bearing lymphocytes to sites of inflammation in muscle and skin (Fall et al., 2005; De Paepe et al., 2005).
Although type I IFNs are critical for the host immune response, several lines of evidence suggest that these cytokines are directly involved in the onset of autoimmunity, as demonstrated by the appearance of autoimmune phenomena following high-dose IFN therapy (Hall & Rosen, 2010). Type I IFNs are able to influence the induction of an adaptive immune response through the activation and maturation of dendritic cells (DCs) and the subsequent production of high levels of proinflammatory cytokines and chemokines, such as IL-8, IL-6, IL-1β, CCL3 and CCL4 (Hall & Rosen, 2010). IFN-α/β are also involved in the expression of MHC class I and II molecules, as well as of costimulatory molecules on DCs, promoting an efficiently activation of T cells.

6.1.3 Innate immunity and Toll-like receptors

The innate immune system is the first line of defense against invading organisms. In addition to cellular and humoral components, the innate immune system has also anatomical structures that act as barriers to pathogen infection (Mayer, 2006). Unlike adaptive immunity, which is antigen specific and requires some time to react to an invading organism, the innate immune response is not antigen specific and it is activated within a few hours of exposure to almost any microbe. The main characteristic of innate immunity is that it recognizes pathogen molecules that contain specific molecular patterns - pathogen-associated molecular patterns (PAMPs). Molecules thus recognized include lipopolysaccharide (LPS) from the Gram-negative bacteria cell wall, peptidoglycan and lipoteichoic acids from the cell wall of Gram-positive bacteria, mannose, bacterial and viral unmethylated CpG DNA, bacterial flagellin, the amino acid N-formylmethionine found in bacterial proteins, double and single stranded RNA from viruses, and glucan from fungal cell wall.

Recognition of PAMPs depends on a series of soluble pattern-recognition receptors (PRRs) that circulate in blood or are associated with the membrane of various cell types, including macrophages, mast cells, lymphocytes and DCs. The most important PRRs that activate the innate immune response are cytoplasmic RNA helicases, including RIG-I, Mda-5 and LGP2, and Toll-like receptors (TLRs) (Kumar et al., 2011). TLR3, TLR7 and TLR9 - a subfamily of TLRs localized in endolysosomes - have been found to be the most potent promoters of type I IFN production. TLR3 is expressed by DCs and macrophages, as well as non-immune cells including fibroblasts, epithelial and skeletal muscle cells (Schreiner et al., 2006); TLR7 and TLR9 are expressed by mDCs and pDCs (Kawai & Akira, 2010).

A recent study on endosomal TLR involvement in IIM pathogenesis (Cappelletti et al., 2011) found that the pattern of expression of TLR3, TLR7 and TLR9 differed between DM and PM, suggesting distinct disease mechanisms in these two forms of myopathy. In DM, numerous TLR3-expressing mDCs were identified among immune infiltrating cells in the endomysial space and around blood vessels; these cells are probably associated with IFN-β overproduction, which is a peculiar feature of DM. It was also found that TLR3 was prominently expressed on the vascular endothelial cells of capillaries in DM, plausibly as a primary response to capillary injury caused by a still unknown factor. It was suggested that TLR3 production was responsible for the chronic overexpression of type I IFNs in DM, reinforcing the older idea that this form of myopathy is a microvasculopathy. It was also suggested that TLR3 is actively involved in the neoangiogenic process, since it was observed on pathological and neovascular structures in both DM and JDM. Moreover, in JDM, where muscle fiber regeneration is prominent, as revealed by antibody against developmental myosin heavy chain antibody (MHCdev), numerous TLR3+ MHCdev+ fibers were identified, particularly in atrophic perifascicular areas (Cappelletti et al., 2011). This finding confirms ongoing regeneration in these muscle regions and supports the idea of TLR3 involvement in the regeneration or differentiation of damaged muscle. In this view, TLR3 could be responsible for the induction of several immune mediators, which would be in turn involved in the remodelling of the area and not just in the atrophic process as previously suggested.

6.2 Polymyositis

Polymyositis is an autoimmune disease principally characterized by T-cell-mediated injury (Fig. 2). While factors responsible for inducing such damage have been identified in some autoimmune conditions, the mechanisms of the immune reaction in PM remain poorly understood (Liang et al., 2000).

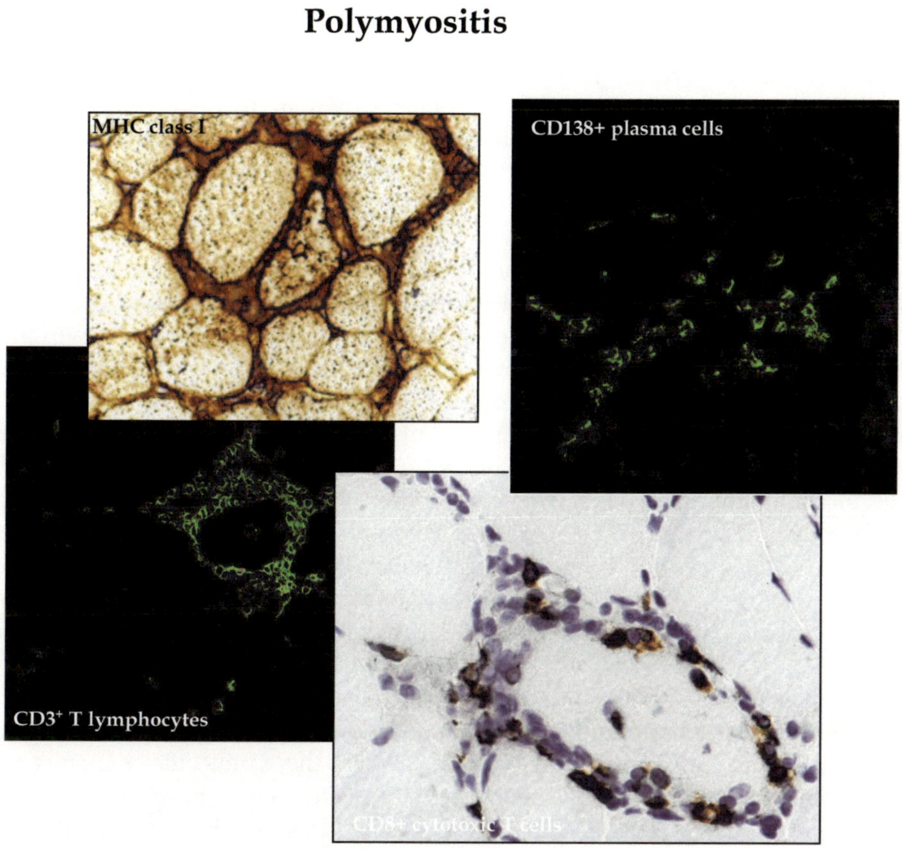

Fig. 2. Polymyositis is a T-cell-mediated autoimmune disease. The main pathological features are the presence of perimysial and endomysial mononuclear cell infiltrates (mainly cytotoxic CD8+ T lymphocytes) surrounding or invading non-necrotic MHC-I and MHC-II-positive muscle fibers. CD138-positive plasma cells are also abundant in endomysial areas and are probably the main source of autoantibodies in PM muscle.

6.2.1 Immunological synapse between T cells and muscle fibers

The immunological synapse is a specialized cell-cell junction between T cell and antigen-presenting cell surfaces. The specificity of T cell recognition is determined by engagement of the T cell receptor (TCR) on T cells with the cognate peptide-MHC complex presented by the antigen-presenting cells (Dustin et al., 2010b; Dustin & Long, 2010a; Jenkins & Griffiths, 2010). The contact point between the TCR and the antigen-MHC complex lies in complementarity-determining region 3 (CDR3), consisting of the V-(D)-J combination. If the TCR recognizes a presented antigen, the amino acid sequence of the CDR3 region is conserved in the activated T cells (García et al., 1999 and Davis et al., 1998, as cited in Mantegazza & Bernasconi, 2005).

The TCR repertoire in IIM patients has been investigated by various methods, including CDR3 spectratyping, laser microdissection combined with single-cell PCR of individual myocytotoxic T cells, and immunohistochemistry (Hofbauer et al., 2003; Benveniste et al., 2004; Bender et al., 1995; Mantegazza et al., 1993). These studies have shown that, in IBM and PM in particular, distinct clones of T cells expand in muscle (Hofbauer et al., 2003; Bender et al., 1995; Mantegazza et al., 1993) after exposure to specific local antigens and persist there for long periods (Benveniste et al., 2004). TCR gene usage has also been investigated in other organs involved by inflammation in IIMs: T cell expansion was demonstrated in CD4+ and CD8+ cells obtained by bronchoalveolar lavage fluid but not in peripheral blood cells. This finding, together with the finding of a biased TCR V-gene usage in muscle, seems to suggest a shared specific, antigen-induced response in these target organs (Englund et al., 2007).

Class I and II MHC upregulation is an early and consistent finding in the skeletal muscle of IIM patients and is an essential prerequisite for the interaction of muscle with infiltrating CD8+ and CD4+ T cells, and for the formation of an immunological synapse (Fig. 2). In order for an antigen-specific T-cell response to be activated, the MHC I- and II-expressing muscle fibers also need to express costimulatory molecules. In PM and IBM, BB-1 but not B7-1 or B7-2 have been found in the cytoplasm of N-CAM-positive regenerating fibers and also in areas remote from inflammation (Murata & Dalakas, 1999; Bernasconi et al., 1998); at the same time autoinvasive CD8+ T cells have been found to present CD28 and CTLA-4 counter receptors. CD28 and CTLA-4 counter receptors are similar to each other in overall structure, but are expressed differently and have different functions. CD28 is usually expressed on resting T cells and when it binds to B7 promotes T cell activation and the subsequent production of cytokines, cytokine receptors and genes for cell survival (Reiser & Stadecker, 1996). By contrast, CTLA-4 is expressed only on activated T cells and its binding to B7 results in an inhibitory signal that blocks further T cell activation (Reiser & Stadecker, 1996). The implication of simultaneous CD28 and CTLA-4 expression of T cells in IIMs is not well understood. It is possible that the balance between these molecules depends on many factors including disease stage, and type or length of treatment (Nagaraju et al., 1999).

Recently, however, CD4+ and CD8+ $CD28^{null}$ T cells have also been reported in muscle-infiltrating cells of DM and PM patients (Fasth et al., 2009). In addition to releasing cytotoxic granules and inducing MHC I and II upregulation in muscle fibers, these cells are considered to be potent inducers of TNF and IFN-γ – proinflammatory cytokines that exert myotoxic effects and interfere with the contractile properties of muscle fibers (Fasth et al., 2009). It has been suggested that the differentiation of T cells into $CD28^{null}$ occurs in the inflamed muscle as a result of the local production of IFN-α by resident pDCs.

The fact that muscle fibers also express the CD40 costimulatory molecule constitutes additional evidence that these fibers act as non-professional antigen presenting cells (APCs) in PM. Interaction of CD40 with its ligand CD40L on infiltrating T cells has been shown to induce leukocyte adhesion and cytokine production: VCAM, ICAM, thrombospondins, MMP-9 and MMP-2 metalloproteinases, interleukin(IL)-6, IL-8 and IL-15, are all produced and serve to enhance T cell activation and differentiation (Dalakas, 2001 & 2011b).

Immunological synapse formation and T cell polarization toward professional or non-professional APC requires cytoskeletal reorganization and microtubule-organizing centers (Lasserre & Alcover, 2010; Billadeau et al., 2007). F-actin and actin-associated proteins are also recruited to establish the interaction between the T cell and target cell. Secretory vesicles are transported along microtubules to dock with the T cell membrane during maturation of immunological synapse – a process involving dyneins and kinesins (Stinchcombe et al., 2006; Dustin, 2010a). The kinesin motor protein KIF4 was recently shown to play a role in the interaction between muscle fiber and T cell infiltrates in IIM

(Bernasconi et al., 2008). In particular, KIF4 was upregulated in IIM muscle biopsies and KIF4-positive cells were abundant in mononuclear cells surrounding individual muscle fibers. Furthermore, KIF4 involvement in lytic granule delivery to the muscle cell-T cell interaction site is suggested by the finding that, in activated PBLs in vitro, KIF4 colocalized with lysosome-associated membrane protein 1 (marker of lytic vesicles) and also to a considerable extent with the perforin normally present in these vesicles (Bernasconi et al., 2008).

6.2.2 Cytokines, chemokines and activation of the innate immune response

Cytokines and chemokines, soluble chemical messengers communicating between immune cells and tissue cells, are essential players in leukocyte activation and migration (Borish & Steinke, 2003). A wide range of these inflammatory molecules (e.g. IL-1α and 1β, IL-2, IL-4, IL-6, IL-10, IL-17, TNF-α, IFN-α/β, IFN-γ, and TGF-β) is expressed at elevated levels in the muscle and blood of IIM patients (De Paepe et al., 2009; Mantegazza & Bernasconi, 2005). IL-1α, IL-1β and IFNs seem to play a critical role in IIM pathogenesis. IL-1α is localized on the endothelial cells of capillaries and on some infiltrating inflammatory cells in PM and DM muscle. IL-1β transcripts are highly up-regulated in IBM and PM muscle, and IL-1β protein localizes to myofibers in areas of severe inflammation and also in endomysial infiltrates. IFNs are a large family of regulators of innate and adaptive immunity, with documented antiviral properties (De Paepe et al., 2009). Type I IFNs (comprising IFN-α, IFN-β, IFN-ω, IFN-ε and IFN-κ) and type III IFNs (also known as IFN-λs) are produced by almost all nucleated cells and mediate potent antiviral effects. Type II IFN (i.e. IFN-γ) is produced only by natural killer cells, natural killer T cells and T cell populations, which is involved in the modulation of the adaptive immune response.

IFN-γ transcript expression has been shown up-regulated in PM muscle compared to other IIM and also control muscle (Cappelletti et al., 2011), emphasizing the involvement of IFN-γ in the induction of MHC class II molecules present on muscle fibers in PM muscle. IFN-γ is also involved in the synthesis of important chemotactic cytokines that govern leukocyte migration from blood to sites of inflammation (CCL2, CXCL9 and CXCL10) and sustain the active invasion of nonnecrotic myofibers by inflammatory cells (Confalonieri et al., 2000; De Bleecker et al., 2002; Raju et al., 2003, as mentioned in Mantegazza & Bernasconi, 2005).

The high levels of IFN-γ, as well as of IL-4 and IL-17, present in PM muscle, suggest involvement of activated CD4+ T cells in the pathophysiology of this disorder. A recent study (Kim et al., 2010) demonstrated a significant direct correlation between the expression of these proinflammatory cytokines and the expression of TLR2, TLR4 and TLR9 in IIMs. TLR2 activation is involved in induction of the Th2 immune response; while TLR4 induces Th1 and Th17 immune responses; TLR9 is also involved in the Th1 immune response (Re & Strominger, 2001; Agrawal et al., 2003; Dillon et al., 2004; Redecke et al., 2004; Abdollahi-Roodsaz et al., 2008, as cited in Kim et al., 2010). Thus, the TLR overexpression found in IIM muscle points to involvement of innate immunity in the pathogenesis of these diseases and is likely to be a link between innate and adaptive immunity in IIMs.

Immunohistochemical and molecular studies have shown that transcriptionally active CD138+ plasma cells – that have undergone affinity maturation and switched their isotype from IgM to IgG or IgA – are abundant in PM muscle (Greenberg, 2007a; Salajegheh et al., 2010b; Cappelletti et al., 2011). In view of the recently demonstrated ability of TLR9 to induce B cells to mature to plasma cell in vitro (Giordani et al., 2009), together with the observed upregulation of TLR9 in this form of myopathy (Cappelletti et al., 2011), it is reasonable to hypothesize a role for this receptor in immunoglobulin production in PM.

6.3 Sporadic inclusion body myositis

Sporadic IBM is the most common muscle disease in older persons. Triggering factors for this form of myopathy are not well understood and no enduringly effective treatment has been found.

Factors pointing an immunopathogenic mechanism in sIBM include association with other autoimmune diseases (Koffman et al., 1998), association with common variable immunodeficiency and increased levels of natural killer cells (Dalakas et al., 1995), and occurrence of autoantibodies at similar levels to those seen in classic autoimmune disorders (Badrising et al., 2004) (Fig. 3). sIBM is also often seen in same generation family members, as occurs with other autoimmune disorders, and there is a strong association with certain human leukocyte antigen (HLA) genes (Badrising et al., 2004).

Furthermore, sIBM is characterized by strong up-regulation of cytokines, chemokines and their receptors both as transcripts and proteins in muscle (Figarella-Branger et al., 2003),

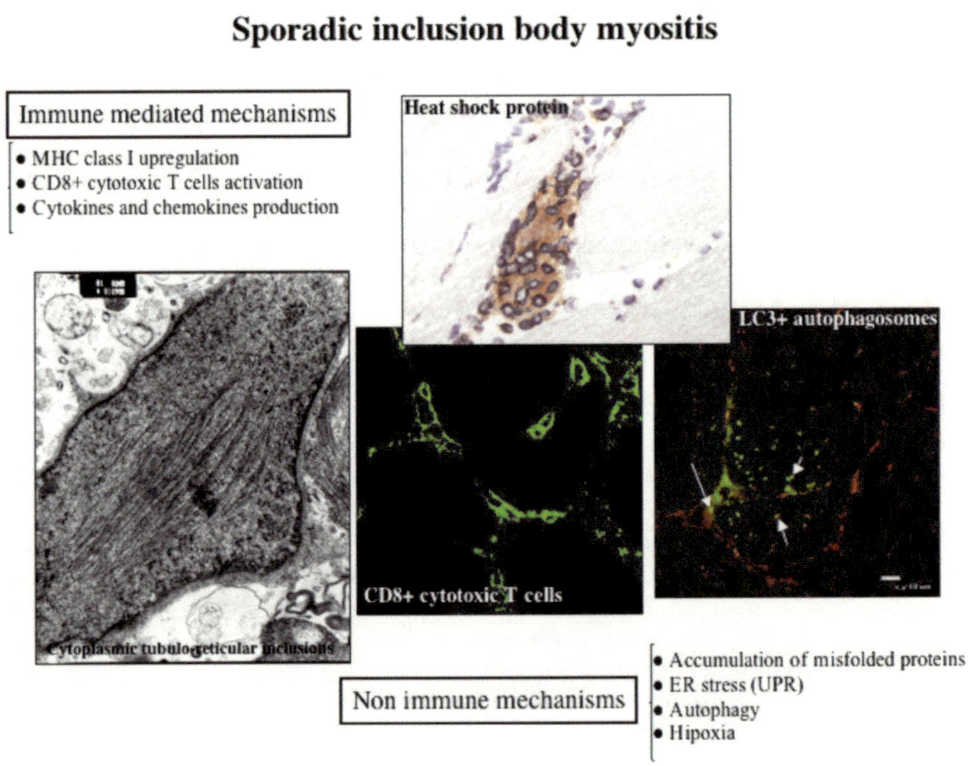

Fig. 3. Pathophysiology of sIBM. sIBM is a multifactorial disease presenting autoimmune and degenerative features. Mononuclear cell inflammation (CD8+ cytotoxic T cells), endoplasmic reticulum stress, dysregulation of protein folding mechanisms (heat shock protein upregulation), mitochondrial abnormalities and possibly inhibition of the autophagic pathway (LC3 upregulation), are salient features of this myopathy.

together with ubiquitous overexpression of MHC class I antigen and costimulatory molecules on muscle fibers, even those not invaded by inflammatory infiltrating cells (Dalakas, 2006b). Immunological synapses between muscle fibers and clonally expanded autoinvasive CD8+ T cells are also present in sIBM muscle (Fig. 3). These CD8+ T cells express perforin and other lytic enzymes. Dendritic cells (mainly mDCs) and CD138+ plasma cells are also abundant in the endomysium of sIBM muscle (Greenberg et al., 2005b; Cappelletti et al., 2011). Finally, it is worth noting that IBM-like myopathy can be associated with HIV and HTLV-1 infection (Dalakas et al., 2007a) and also with post-polio syndrome (Parissis et al., 2003) suggesting the possibility of a viral trigger to the autoimmunity of sIBM.

sIBM also shows several features typical of degenerative diseases (Fig. 3). These include presence of vacuoles (mainly in muscle fibers not invaded by T cells) and intracellular deposition of ubiquitinated, multiprotein aggregates in vacuole-free regions of muscle cytoplasm (Askanas et al., 2009). These aggregates contain amyloid-β, phosphorylated tau, several proteins (α-synuclein, presenilin-1 and cellular prion protein) that tend to

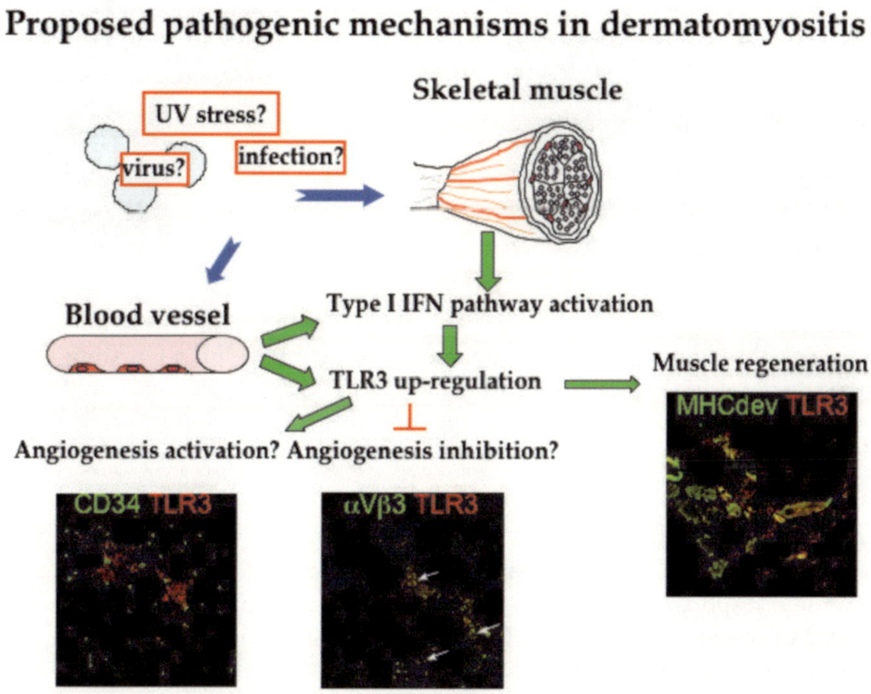

Fig. 4. Proposed immunopathogenetic mechanisms in DM. Activation of type I interferon pathway, together with overexpression of endosomal Toll-like receptors (TLRs), suggests the possibility of a viral or bacterial trigger to onset. In DM, the primary site of infection seems to be the microvascular endothelium, reinforcing the idea that the disease is primarily a microvasculopathy. The presence of TLR3 on neovascular structures and regenerating myofibers in adult and juvenile DM muscle tissue suggests a possible protective role for this receptor or its involvement in the regeneration or differentiation of damaged muscle tissue. Over-expression of type I IFNs might be involved in muscle fiber atrophy.

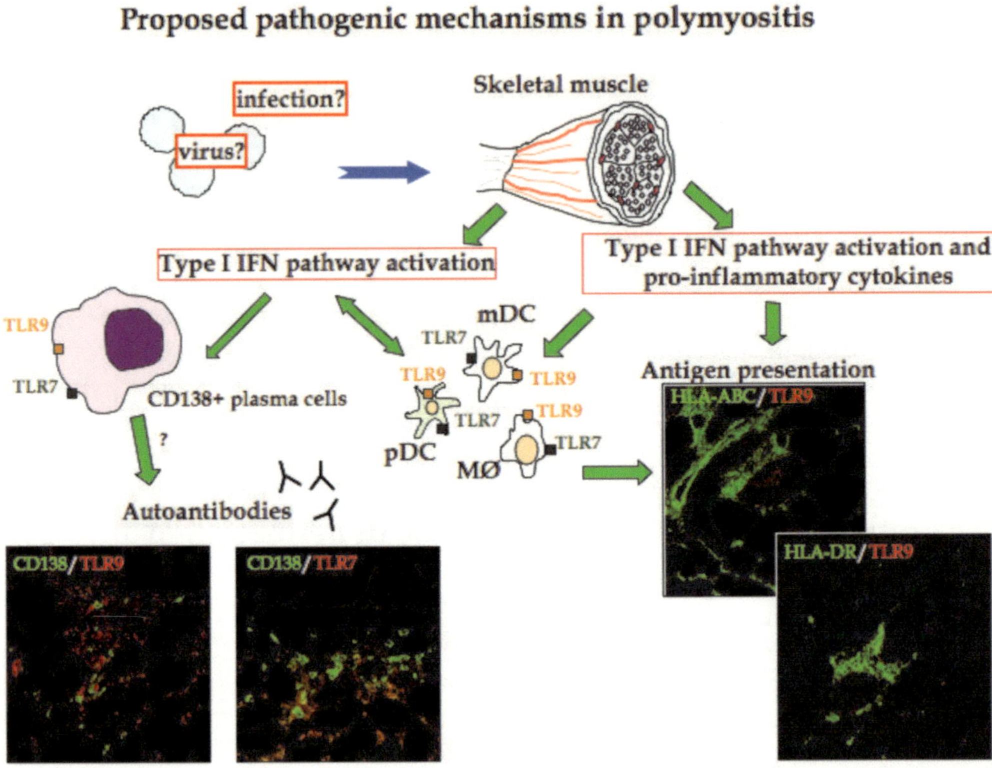

Fig. 5. Proposed immunopathogenetic mechanisms in PM. In PM upregulation of type I and type II IFNs, possibly caused by a pathogenic agent or by intracellular autoantigens released during myocyte damage, may be responsible for TLR7 and TLR9 activation in dendritic cells (both myeloid and plasmacytoid), macrophages and plasma cells. Induction of TLR9 may sustain the autoimmune process by increasing immunoglobulin production as well as contributing to antigen presentation.

unfold/misfold to form β-pleated sheet and a number of other proteins of varying function, including: (i) markers of oxidative stress; (ii) endoplasmic reticulum chaperones, signs of the unfolded protein response (UPR); (iii) 26S proteasome components and proteasome shuttle protein p62; (iv) mutated ubiquitin (UBB+1); (v) heat shock proteins; (vi) nuclear-related proteins such as TDP-43, and other transduction and transcription factors.
It is unknown whether the autoimmune or protein dysregulation process constitutes the primary event; a plausible hypothesis is that both develop as a consequence of still unknown causative agent or agents (Karpati & O'Ferrall, 2009).

7. Conclusion

The principal clinical and pathological features of the three main types of IIM have been described together with evidence regarding pathogenetic mechanisms. Dermatomyositis is considered a microvasculopathy, characterized by injury to the capillary endothelium leading to depletion of capillaries in muscle; the damage to muscle manifests as perifascicular atrophy and is accompanied by inflammatory cell stress. In DM the findings that type I interferon-associated genes are up-regulated and TLR3 overexpressed suggest that a pathogen infection may be a triggering factor for this myopathy (Fig. 4). In PM recent findings that plasma cells are abundant in the endomysium and that immunoglobulin genes are up-regulated suggest that a humoral immune response to tissue injury is important in this disorder and that the ideas that PM as an exclusively T cell-mediated myopathy requires revision (Fig. 5). Sporadic IBM is a degenerative muscle disease, with no effective treatment, characterized by the coexistence of autoimmune and protein conformation abnormalities. New investigations in the protein dysregulation processes of this disease hold the hope that effective treatments may soon be found (Henriques-Pons & Nagaraju, 2009).

8. Acknowledgments

The authors wish to thank their research and clinical colleagues for their participation in various aspects of these studies, and Donald Ward for help with the English.

9. References

Amato, A.A. & Barohn, R.J. (1997). Idiopathic inflammatory myopathies. *Neurologic Clinics*, Vol. 15, No. 3, (Aug., 1997), pp. (615-648), ISSN: 0733-8619

Amato, A.A. & Barohn, R.J. (2009). Inclusion body myositis: old and new concepts. *Journal Neurology, Neurosurgery and Psychiatry*, Vol. 80, No. 11, (Nov., 2009), pp. (1186-1193), ISSN: 0022-3050

Askanas, V. & Engel, W.K. (1998). Sporadic inclusion-body myositis and hereditary inclusion-body myopathies: current concepts of diagnosis and pathogenesis. *Current Opinion in Rheumatology*, Vol.10, No.6, (Nov., 1998), pp. (530-542), ISSN: 1040-8711

Askanas, V.; Engel, W.K. & Nogalska, A. (2009). Inclusion body myositis: a degenerative muscle disease associated with intra-muscle fiber multi-protein aggregates, proteasome inhibition, endoplasmic reticulum stress and decreased lysosomal degradation. *Brain Pathology*, Vol. 19, No. 3, (Jul., 2009), pp. (493-506), ISSN: 1015-6305

Badrising, U.A.; Schreuder, G.M.; Giphart, M.J.; Geleijns, K.; Verschuuren, J.J.; Wintzen, A.R.; Maat-Schieman, M.L.; van Doorn, P.; van Engelen, B.G.; Faber, C.G.; Hoogendijk, J.E.; de Jager, A.E.; Koehler, P.J.; de Visser, M.; van Duinen, S.G.; Dutch, S.G. & Dutch IBM Study Group. (2004). Associations with autoimmune disorders and HLA class I and II antigens in inclusion body myositis. *Neurology*, Vol. 63, No. 12, (Dec., 2004), pp. (2396-2398), ISSN: 0028-3878

Baechler, E.C.; Bauer, J.W.; Slattery, C.A.; Ortmann, W.A.; Espe, K,J,; Novitzke, J.; Ytterberg, S.R.; Gregersen, P.K.; Behrens, T.W. & Reed, A.M. (2007). An interferon signature in the peripheral blood of dermatomyositis patients is associated with disease activity. *Molecular Medicine*, Vol. 13, No. 1-2, (Jan-Feb., 2007), pp. (59-68), ISSN: 1076-1551

Basta, M. & Dalakas, M.C. (1994). High-dose intravenous immunoglobulin exerts its beneficial effect in patients with dermatomyositis by blocking endomysial deposition of activated complement fragments. *The Journal of Clinical Investigation,* Vol. 94, No. 5, (Nov., 1994), pp. (1729-1735), ISSN: 0021-9738

Batthish, M. & Feldman, B.M. (2011). Juvenile dermatomyositis. *Current Rheumatology Reports,* Feb., 2011, epub ahead of print

Bender, A.; Ernst, N.; Iglesias, A.; Dornmair, K.; Wekerle, H. & Hohlfeld, R. (1995). T cell receptor repertoire in polymyositis: clonal expansion of autoaggressive CD8+ T cells. *The Journal of Experimental Medicine,* Vol. 181, No. 5, (May, 1995), pp. (1863-1868), ISSN: 0022-1007

Benveniste, O.; Herson, S.; Salomon, B.; Dimitri, D.; Trébeden-Nègre, H.; Jean, L.; Bon-Durand, V.; Antonelli, D.; Klatzmann, D. & Boyer, O. (2004). Long-term persistence of clonally expanded T cells in patients with polymyositis. *Annals of Neurology,* Vol. 56, No. 6, (Dec., 2004), pp. (867-872), ISSN: 0364-5134

Bernasconi, P.; Confalonieri, P.; Andreetta, F.; Baggi, F.; Cornelio, F. & Mantegazza, R. (1998). The expression of co-stimulatory and accessory molecules on cultured human muscle cells is not dependent on stimulus by pro-inflammatory cytokines: relevance for the pathogenesis of inflammatory myopathy. *Journal of Neuroimmunology,* Vol. 85, No. 1, (May, 1998), pp. (52-58), ISSN: 0165-5728

Bernasconi, P.; Cappelletti, C.; Navone, F.; Nessi, V.; Baggi, F.; Vernos, I.; Romaggi, S.; Confalonieri, P.; Mora, M.; Morandi, L. & Mantegazza, R. (2008). *Journal of Neuropathology & Experimental Neurology,* Vol. 67, No. 6, (Jun., 2008), pp. (624-632), ISSN: 0022-3069

Betteridge, Z.; Gunawardena, H.; North, J.; Slinn, J. & McHugh, N. (2007). Anti-synthetase syndrome: a new autoantibody to phenylalanyl transfer RNA synthetase (anti-Zo) associated with polymyositis and interstitial pneumonia. *Rheumatology,* Vol. 46, No. 6, (Jun., 2007), pp. (1005-1008), ISSN: 1462-0324

Bilgic, H.; Ytterberg, S.R.; Amin, S.; McNallan, K.T.; Wilson, J.C.; Koeuth, T.; Ellingson, S.; Newman, B.; Bauer, J.W.; Peterson, E.J.; Baechler, E.C. & Reed, A.M. (2009). Interleukin-6 and type I interferon-regulated genes and chemokines mark disease activity in dermatomyositis. *Arthritis & Rheumatism,* Vol. 60, No. 11, (Nov., 2009), pp. (3436-3446), ISSN: 0004-3591

Billadeau, D.D.; Nolz, J.C. & Gomez, T.S. (2007). Regulation of T-cell activation by the cytoskeleton. *Nature Reviews. Immunology,* Vol. 7, No. 2, (Feb., 2007), pp. (131-143), ISSN: 1474-1733

Borish, L.C. & Steinke, J.W. (2003). Cytokines and chemokines. *The Journal of Allergy and Clinical Immunology,* Vol. 111, No. 2 Suppl., (Feb., 2003), pp. (S460-475), ISSN: 0091-6749

Bunn, C.C.; Bernstein, R.M. & Mathews, M.B. (1986). Autoantibodies against alanyl-tRNA synthetase and tRNAAla coexist and are associated with myositis. *Journal of Experimental Medicine,* Vol. 163, No. 5, (May, 1986), pp. (1281-1291), ISSN: 0022-1007

Cappelletti, C.; Baggi, F.; Zolezzi, F.; Biancolini, D.; Beretta, O.; Severa, M.; Coccia, E.; Confalonieri, P.; Morandi, L.; Mora, M.; Mantegazza, R. & Bernasconi, P. (2011). Type I interferon and Toll-like receptor expression characterizes inflammatory myopathies. *Neurology*, Vol. 76, No. 24, (Jun., 2011), pp. (2079-2088), ISSN: 0028-3878

Casciola-Rosen, L.; Andrade, F.; Ulanet, D.; Wong, W.B. & Rosen A. (1999). Cleavage by granzyme B is strongly predictive of autoantigen status: implications for initiation of autoimmunity. *Journal of Experimental Medicine,* Vol. 190, No. 6, (Sept., 1999), pp (815-826), ISSN: 0022-1007

Casciola-Rosen, L.; Nagaraju, K.; Plotz, P.; Wang, K.; Levine, S.; Gabrielson, E.; Corse, A. & Rosen, A. (2005). Enhanced autoantigen expression in regenerating muscle cells in idiopathic inflammatory myopathy. *Journal of Experimental Medicine,* Vol. 201, No. 4, (Feb., 2005), pp. (591-601), ISSN: 0022-1007

Choy, E.H.S. & Isenberg, D.A. (2002). Treatment of dermatomyositis and polymyositis. *Rheumatology,* Vol. 41, No. 1, (Jan., 2002), pp. (7-13), ISSN: 1462-0324

Dalakas, M.C. & Illa, I. (1995). Common variable immunodeficiency and inclusion body myositis: a distinct myopathy mediated by natural killer cells. *Annals of Neurology,* Vol. 37, No. 6, (Jun., 1995), pp. (806-810), ISSN: 0364-5134

Dalakas, M.C. (2001). The molecular and cellular pathology of inflammatory muscle diseases. *Current Opinion in Pharmacology,* Vol. 1, No. 3, (Jun., 2001), pp. (300-306), ISSN: 1471-4892

Dalakas, M.C. & Hohlfeld, R. (2003). Polymyositis and dermatomyositis. *The Lancet,* Vol. 362, No. 9388, (Sep., 2003), pp. (971-982), ISSN: 0140-6736

Dalakas, M.C. (2006a). Mechanisms of disease: signalling pathways and immunobiology of inflammatory myopathies. *Nature Clinical Practice. Rheumatology,* Vol. 2, No. 4, (Jul., 2006), pp. (219-227), ISSN: 1745-8382

Dalakas, M.C. (2006b). Sporadic inclusion body myositis-diagnosis, pathogenesis and therapeutic strategies. *Nature Clinical Practice. Neurology,* Vol. 2, No. 8, (Aug., 2006), pp. (437-447), ISSN: 1745-834X

Dalakas, M.C.; Rakocevic, G.; Shatunov, A.; Goldfarb, L.; Raju, R. & Salajegheh, M. (2007a). Inclusion body myositis with human immunodeficiency virus infection: four cases with clonal expansion of viral-specific T cells. *Annals of Neurology,* Vol. 61, No. 5, (May, 2007), pp. (466-475), ISSN: 0364-5134

Dalakas, M.C. (2007b). Advances in the immunobiology and treatment of inflammatory myopathies. *Current Rheumatology Reports,* Vol. 9, No. 4, (Aug., 2007), pp. (291-297), ISSN: 1523-3774

Dalakas, M.C. (2011a). Immunotherapy of inflammatory myopathies: practical approach and future prospects. *Current Treatment Options in Neurology,* Published online (Mar., 2011), ISSN: 1092-8480

Dalakas, M.C. (2011b). Pathophysiology of inflammatory and autoimmune myopathies. *Presse Medicale,* Vol. 40, No. 4 Pt 2, (Mar., 2011), pp. (e237-247), ISSN: 0755-4982

Dalakas, M.C. (2011c). Review: an update on inflammatory and autoimmune myopathies. *Neuropathology and Applied Neurobiology,* Vol. 37, No. 3, (Apr., 2011), pp. (226-242), ISSN: 0305-1846

De Paepe, B.; De Keyzer, K.; Martin, J.J. & De Bleecker, J.L. (2005). Alpha-chemokine receptors CXCR1-3 and their ligands in idiopathic inflammatory myopathies. *Acta Neuropathologica,* Vol. 109, No. 6, (Jun., 2005), pp. (576-582), ISSN: 0001-6322

De Paepe, B.; Creus, K.K & De Bleecker, J.L. (2009). Role of cytokines and chemokines in idiopathic inflammatory myopathies. *Current Opinion in Rheumatology,* Vol. 21, No. 6, (Nov., 2009), pp. (610-616), ISSN: 1040-8711

Dimachkie, M.M. (2011). Idiopathic inflammatory myopathies. *Journal of Neuroimmunology,* Vol. 231, No. 1-2, (Nov., 2010), pp. (32-42), ISSN: 0165-5728

Distad, B.J.; Amato, A.A. & Weiss, M.D. (2011). Inflammatory myopathies. *Current Treatment Options in Neurology,* Vol. 13, No. 2, (Jan., 2011), pp. (119-130), ISSN: 1092-8480

Dustin, M.L. & Long, E.O. (2010a). Cytotoxic immunological synapses. *Immunological Reviews,* Vol. 235, No. 1, (May, 2010), pp. (24-34), ISSN: 0105-2896

Dustin, M.L.; Chakraborty, A.K. & Shaw, A.S. (2010b). Understanding the structure and function of the immunological synapse. *Cold Spring Harbor Perspectives in Biology,* Vol. 2, No. 10, (Sep., 2010), (a002311), ISSN:1943-0264

Engel, A.G. & Hohlfeld, R. (2004). The polymyositis and dermatomyositis syndromes, In: *Myology – Basic and Clinical,* Engel, A.G. & Franzini-Armstrong, C., pp. (1321-1366), Mc Graw Hill, ISBN: 0-07-137180-X, New York

Englund, P.; Wahlström, J.; Fathi, M.; Rasmussen, E.; Grunewald, J.; Tornling, G. & Lundberg, I.E. (2007). Restricted T cell receptor BV gene usage in the lungs and muscles of patients with idiopathic inflammatory myopathies. *Arthritis & Rheumatism,* Vol. 56, No. 1, (Jan., 2007), pp. (372-383), ISSN: 0004-3591

Fall, N.; Bove, K.E.; Stringer, K.; Lovell, D.J.; Brunner, H.I.; Weiss, J.; Higgins, G.C.; Bowyer, S.L.; Graham, T.B.; Thornton, S. & Grom, A.A. (2005). Association between lack of angiogenic response in muscle tissue and high expression of angiostatic ELR-negative CXC chemokines in patients with juvenile dermatomyositis: possible link to vasculopathy. *Arthritis & Rheumatism,* Vol. 52, No. 10, (Oct., 2005), pp. (3175-3180), ISSN: 0004-3591

Fasth, A.E.R.; Dastmalchi, M.; Rahbar, A.; Salomonsson, S.; Pandya, J.M.; Lindroos, E.; Nennesmo, I.; Malmberg, K.J.; Söderberg-Nauclér, C.; Trollmo, C.; Lundberg, I.E. & Malmström, V. (2009). T cell infiltrates in the muscles of patients with dermatomyositis and polymyositis are dominated by CD28 ^{null} T cells. *The Journal of Immunology,* Vol. 183, No. 7, (Oct., 2009), pp. (4792-4799), ISSN: 0022-1767

Feldman, B.M.; Rider, L.G.; Reed, A.M. & Pachman, L.M. (2008). Juvenile dermatomyositis and other idiopathic inflammatory myopathies of childhood. *The Lancet,* Vol. 371, No. 9631, (Jun., 2008), pp. (2201-2212), ISSN: 0140-6736

Figarella-Branger, D.; Civatte, M.; Bartoli, C. & Pellissier, J.F. (2003). Cytokines, chemokines, and cell adhesion molecole in inflammatory myopathies. *Muscle & Nerve,* Vol. 28, No. 6, (Dec., 2003), pp. (659-682), ISSN: 0148-639X

Ghirardello, A.; Zampieri, S.;Tarricone E.; Iaccarino, L.; Gorza, L. & Doria, A. (2010). Cutting edge issues in polymyositis. *Clinical Reviews in Allergy and Immunology,* Published online (Dec., 2010)

Giordani, L; Sanchez, M.; Libri, I.; Quaranta, M.G.; Mattioli, B. & Viora, M. (2009). IFN-α amplifies human naïve B cell TLR-9-mediated activation and Ig production. *Journal of Leukocyte Biology,* Vol. 86, No. 2, (Apr., 2009), pp. (261-271), ISSN: 0741-5400

Greenberg, S.A.; Sanoudou, D.; Haslett, J.N.; Kohane, I.S.; Kunkel, L.M.; Beggs, A.H. & Amato, A.A. (2002). Molecular Profiles of inflammatory myopathies. *Neurology,* Vol. 59, No. 8, (Oct., 2002), pp. (1170-1182), ISSN: 0028-3878

Greenberg, S.A. & Amato, A.A. (2004). Uncertainties in the pathogenesis of adult dermatomyositis. *Current Opinion in Neurology,* Vol. 17, No. 3, (Jun., 2004), pp. (359-364), ISSN: 1350-7540

Greenberg, S.A.; Pinkus, J.L.; Pinkus, G.S.; Burleson, T.; Sanoudou, D.; Tawil, R.; Barohn, R.J.; Saperstein, D.S.; Briemberg, H.R.; Ericsson, M; Park, P. & Amato, A.A. (2005a). Interferon-alpha/beta-mediated innate immune mechanisms in dermatomyositis. *Annals of Neurology,* Vol. 57, No. 5, (May, 2005), pp. (664-678), ISSN: 0364-5134

Greenberg, S.A.; Bradshaw, E.M.; Pinkus, J.L.; Pinkus, G.S.; Burleson, T.; Due, B.; Bregoli, L.S.; O'Connor, K.C. & Amato, A.A. (2005b). Plasma cells in muscle in inclusion body myositis and polymyositis. *Neurology,* Vol. 65, No. 11, (Dec., 2005), pp. (1782-1787), ISSN: 0028-3878

Greenberg, S.A.; Pinkus, G.S.; Amato, A.A. & Pinkus, J.L. (2007a). Myeloid dendritic cells in inclusion-body myositis and polymyositis. *Muscle & Nerve,* Vol. 35, No. 1, (Jan., 2007), pp. (17-23), ISSN: 0148-639X

Greenberg, S.A. (2007b). Proposed immunologic models of the inflammatory myopathies and potential therapeutic implications. *Neurology,* Vol. 69, No. 21, (Nov., 2007), pp. (2008-2019), ISSN: 0028-3878

Greenberg, S.A. (2008). Inflammatory myopathies: evaluation and management. *Seminars in Neurology,* Vol. 28, No. 2, (Apr., 2008), pp. (241-249), ISSN: 0271-8235

Hall, J.C. & Rosen, A. (2010). Type I interferons: crucial participants in disease amplification in autoimmunity. *Nature Reviews. Rheumatology,* Vol. 6, No. 1, (Jan., 2010), pp. (40-49), ISSN: 1759-4790

Hengstman, G.J.; van Venrooij, W.J.; Vencovsky, J.; Moutsopoulos, H. & van Engelen, B.G.M. (2000). The relative prevalence of dermatomyositis and polymyositis in Europe exhibits a latitudinal gradient. *Annals of the Rheumatic Diseases,* Vol. 59, No. 2, (Feb., 2000), pp. (141-142), ISSN: 0003-4967

Henriques-Pons, A. & Nagaraju, K. (2009). Nonimmune mechanisms of muscle damage in myositis: role of the endoplasmic reticulum stress response and autophagy in the disease pathogenesis. *Current Opinion in Rheumatology,* Vol. 21, No. 6, (Nov., 2009), pp. (581-587), ISSN: 1040-8711

Hirakata, M.; Suwa, A.; Nagai, S.; Kron, M.A.; Trieu, E.P.; Mimori, T.; Akizuki, M. & Targoff, I.N. (1999). Anti-KS: identification of autoantibodies to asparaginyl-transfer RNA synthetase associated with interstitial lung disease. *Journal of Immunology*, Vol. 162, No. 4, (Feb., 1999), pp. (2315-2320), ISSN: 0022-1767

Hofbauer, M.; Wiesener, S.; Babbe, H.; Roers, A.; Wekerle, H.; Dornmair, K.; Hohlfeld, R. & Goebels, N. (2003). Clonal tracking of autoaggressive T cells in polymyositis by combining laser microdissection, single-cell PCR, and CDR3-spectratype analysis. *Proceedings of the National Academy of Sciences of the United States of America*, Vol. 100, No. 7, (Apr., 2003), pp. (4090-4095), ISSN: 0027-8424

Hohlfeld, R. & Dornmair, K. (2007). Revisiting the immunopathogenesis of the inflammatory myopathies. *Neurology*, Vol. 69, No. 21, (Nov., 2007), pp. (1966-1967), ISSN 0028-3878

Jenkis, M.R. & Griffiths, G.M. (2010). The synapse and cytolytic machinery of cytotoxic T cells. *Current Opinion in Immunology*, Vol. 22, No. 3, (Jun., 2010), pp. (308-313), ISSN: 0952-7915

Kao, L.; Chung, L. & Fiorentino, D.F. (2011). Pathogenesis of dermatomyositis: role of cytokines and interferon. *Current Rheumatology Reports*, (Feb., 2011), ISSN: 1523-3774

Karpati, G. & O'Ferrall, E.K. (2009). Sporadic inclusion body myositis: pathogenic considerations. *Annals of Neurology*, Vol. 65, No. 1, (Jan., 2009), pp. (7-11), ISSN: 0364-5134

Kawai, T. & Akira, S. (2010). The role of pattern-recognition receptors in innate immunity: update on Toll-like receptors. *Nature Immunology*, Vol. 11, No. 5, (May, 2010), pp. (373-384), ISSN: 1529-2908

Khanna, S. & Reed, A.M. (2010). Immunopathogenesis of juvenile dermatomyositis. *Muscle & Nerve*, Vol. 41, No. 5, (Apr., 2010), pp. (581-592), ISSN: 0148-639X

Kim, G.T.; Cho, M.L.; Park, Y.E.; Yoo, W.H.; Kim, J.H.; Oh, H.J.; Kim, D.S.; Baek, S.H.; Lee, S.H.; Lee, J.H.; Kim, H.Y. & Kim, S.I. (2010). Expression of TLR2, TLR4, and TLR9 in dermatomyositis and polymyositis. *Clinical Rheumatology*, Vol. 29, No. 3, (Mar., 2010), pp. (273-279), ISSN:0770-3198

Koffman, B.M.; Rugiero, M. & Dalakas, M.C. (1998). Immune-mediated conditions and antibodies associated with sporadic inclusion body myositis. *Muscle & Nerve*, Vol. 21, No. 1, (Jan., 1998), pp. (115-117), ISSN: 0148-639X

Konttinen, Y.T.; Mackiewicz, Z.; Povilenaite, D.; Sukura, A.; Hukkanen, M. & Virtanen, I. (2004). Disease-associated increased HIF-1, alphavbeta3 integrin, and Flt-1 do not suffice to compensate the damage-inducing loss of blood vessels in inflammatory myopathies. *Rheumatology International*, Vol. 24, No. 6, (Nov., 2004), pp. (333-339), ISSN: 0172-8172

Kumar, H.; Kawai, T. & Akira, S. (2011). Pathogen recognition by the innate immune system. *International Review of Immunology*, Vol. 30, No. 1, (Feb., 2011), pp. (16-34), ISSN: 0883-0185

Lasserre, R. & Alcover, A. (2010). Cytoskeletal cross-talk in the control of T cell antigen receptor signaling. *FEBS Letters*, Vol. 584, No. 24, (Dec., 2010), pp. (4845-4850), ISSN: 0014-5793

Levine, T.D. (2005). Rituximab in the treatment of dermatomyositis: an open-label pilot study. *Arthritis & Rheumatism,* Vol. 52, No. 2, (Feb., 2005), pp. (601-607), ISSN: 0004-3591

Liang, Y.; Inukai, A.; Kuru, S.; Kato, T.; Doyu, M. & Sobue, G. (2000). The role of lymphotoxin in pathogenesis of polymyositis. *Acta Neuropathologica,* Vol. 100, No. 5, (Nov., 2000), pp. (521-527), ISSN: 0001-6322

Love, L.A.; Weinberg, C.R.; McConnaughey, D.R.; Oddis, C.V.; Medsger, T.A.; Reveille, J.D.; Amett, F.C.; Targoff, I.N. & Miller, F.W. (2009). Ultraviolet radiation intensity predicts the relative distribution of dermatomyositis and anti-Mi-2 autoantibodies in women. *Arthritis & Rheumatism,* Vol.60, No.8, (Aug., 2009), pp. (2499-2504), ISSN: 0004-3591

Mammen, A.L. (2010). Dermatomyositis and polymyositis - Clinical presentation, autoantibodies, and pathogenesis. *Annals of the New York Academy of Sciences,* Vol.1184, (Nov., 2009), pp. (134-153), ISSN: 0077-8923

Mantegazza, R.; Andreetta, F.; Bernasconi, P.; Baggi, F.; Oksenberg, J.R.; Simoncini, O.; Mora, M.; Cornelio, F. & Steinman, L. (1993). Analysis of T cell receptor reperto ire of muscle-infiltrating T lymphocytes in polymyositis. Restricted V alpha/beta rearrangements may indicate antigen-driven selection. *The Journal of Clinical Investigations,* Vol. 91, No. 6, (Jun., 1993), pp. (2880-2886), ISSN: 0021-9738

Mantegazza, R.; Bernasconi, P.; Confalonieri, P. & Cornelio, F. (1997). Inflammatory myopathies and systemic disorders: a review of immunopathogenetic mechanisms and clinical features. *Journal of Neurology,* Vol. 244, No. 5, (May, 1997), pp. (277-287), ISSN: 0340-5354

Mantegazza, R. & Bernasconi, P. (2005). Inflammatory myopathies: dermatomyositis, polymyositis and inclusion body myositis, In: *Immunogenetics of Autoimmune Disease,* Oksenberg J.R. & Brassat, D., pp. (119-135), Springer-Landes Bioscience, ISBN: 0-387-36004-2, New York (USA)

Mathews, M.B.; Reichlin, M.; Hughes, G.R. & Bernstein, R.M. (1984). Anti-threonyl-tRNA synthetase, a second myositis-related autoantibody. *Journal of Experimental Medicine,* Vol. 160, No. 2, (Aug., 1984), pp. (420-434), ISSN: 0022-1007

Mayer, G. (2006). Innate (non-specific) immunity, In: *Immunology,* Male, D.; Brostoff, J.; Roth, D.B. & Roitt, I., pp. (19-28), Mosby - Elsevier, ISBN: 978-0-323-03399-2, London

Murata, K. & Dalakas, M.C. (1999). Expression of the costimulatory molecule BB-1, the ligands CTLA-4 and CD28, and their mRNA in inflammatory myopathies. *American Journal of Pathology,* Vol. 155, No. 2, (Aug., 1999), pp. (453-460), ISSN: 0002-9440

Nagaraju, K.; Raben, N.; Villalba, M.L.; Danning, C.; Loeffler, L.A.; Lee, E.; Tresser, N.; Abati, A.; Fetsch, P. & Plotz, P.H. (1999). Costimulatory markers in muscle of patients with idiopathic inflammatory myopathies and cultured muscle cells. *Clinical Immunology,* Vol. 92, No. 2, (Aug., 1999), pp. (161-169), ISSN: 1521-6616

Nagaraju, K.; Rider, L.G.; Fan, C.; Chen, Y.W.; Mitsak, M.; Rawat, R.; Patterson, K.; Grundtman, C.; Miller, F.W.; Plotz, P.H.; Hoffman, E. & Lundberg, I.E. (2006).

Endothelial cell activation and neovascularisation are prominent in dermatomyositis. *Journal of Autoimmune Diseases,* Vol. 3, pp. (2-9), ISSN: 1740-2557

Nakashima, R.; Imura, Y.; Kobayashi, S.; Yukawa, N.; Yoshifuji, H.; Nojima, T.; Kawabata, D.; Ohmura, K.; Usui, T.; Fujii, T.; Okawa, K. & Mimori, T. (2010). The RIG-I-like receptor IFIH1/MDA5 is a dermatomyositis-specific autoantigen identified by the anti-CADM-140 antibody. *Rheumatology,* Vol. 49, No. 3, (Dec., 2009), pp. (433-440), ISSN: 1462-0324

Needham, M. & Mastaglia, F.L. (2007). Inclusion body myositis: current pathogenetic concepts and diagnostic and therapeutic approaches. *Lancet Neurology,* Vol. 6, No. 7, (Jul., 2007), pp. (620-631), ISSN: 1474-4422

Noss, E.H.; Hausner-Sypek, D.L. & Weinblatt, M.E. (2006). Rituximab as therapy for refractory polymyositis and dermatomyositis. *The Journal of Rheumatology,* Vol. 33, No. 5, (May, 2006), pp. (1021-1026), ISSN: 0315-162X

O'Connor, K.A.; Abbott, K.A.; Sabin, B.; Kuroda, M. & Pachman, L.M. (2006). MxA gene expression in juvenile dermatomyositis peripheral blood mononuclear cells: association with muscle involvement. *Clinical Immunology,* Vol. 120, No. 3, (Sep., 2006), pp. (319-325), ISSN: 1521-6616

O'Hanlon, T.P.; Rider, L.G.; Mamyrova, G.; Targoff, I.N.; Arnett, F.C.; Reveille, J.D.; Carrington, M.; Gao, X.; Oddis, C.V.; Morel, P.A.; Malley, J.D.; Malley, K.; Shamim, E.A.; Chanock, S.J.; Foster, C.B.; Bunch, T.; Reed, A.M.; Love, L.A. & Miller, F.W. (2006). HLA polymorphisms in African Americans with idiopathic inflammatory myopathy: allelic profiles distinguish patients with different clinical phenotypes and myositis autoantibodies. *Arthritis & Rheumatism,* Vol. 54, No. 11, (Nov., 2006), pp. (3670-3681), ISSN: 0004-3591

O'Hanlon, T.P. & Miller, F.W. (2009). Genetic risk and protective factors for the idiopathic inflammatory myopathies. *Current Rheumatology Reports,* Vol. 11, No. 4, (Aug., 2009), pp. (287-294), ISSN: 1523-3774

Parissis, D.; Karkavelas, G.; Taskos, N. & Milonas, I. (2003). Inclusion body myositis in a patient with a presumed diagnosis of post-polio syndrome. *Journal of Neurology,* Vol. 250, No. 5, (May, 2003), pp. (619-621), ISSN: 0340-5354

Probst-Cousin, S.; Neundörfer, B. & Heuss, D. (2010). Microvasculopathic neuromuscular diseases: lessons from hypoxia-inducible factors. *Neuromuscular Disorders,* Vol. 20, No. 3, (Feb., 2010), pp. (192-197), ISSN: 0960-8966

Reiser, H. & Stadecker, M.J. (1996). Costimulatory B7 molecules in the pathogenesis of infectious and autoimmune diseases. *New England Journal of Medicine,* Vol. 335, No. 18, (Oct., 1996), pp. (1369-1377), ISSN: 0028-4793

Rider, L.G.; Wu, L.; Mamyrova, G.; Targoff, I.N.; Miller, F.W. & Childhood Myositis Heterogeneity Collaborative Study Group. (2010). Environmental factors preceding illness onset differ in phenotypes of the juvenile idiopathic inflammatory myopathies. *Rheumatology,* Vol. 49, No. 12, (Dec., 2010), pp. (2381-2390), ISSN: 1462-0324

Salajegheh, M.; Kong, S.W.; Pinkus, J.L.; Walsh, R.J.; Liao, A.; Nazareno, R.; Amato, A.A.; Krastins, B.; Morehouse, C.; Higgs, B.W.; Jallal, B.; Yao, Y.; Sarracino, D.A.; Parker,

K.C. & Greenberg, S.A. (2010a). Interferon-stimulated gene 15 (ISG15) conjugates proteins in dermatomyositis muscle with perifascicular atrophy. *Annals of Neurology,* Vol. 67, No. 1, (Jan., 2010), pp. (53-63), ISSN:0364-5134

Salajegheh, M.; Pinkus, J.L.; Amato, A.A.; Morehouse, C.; Jallal, B.; Yao, Y. & Greenberg, S.A. (2010b). Permissive environment for B-cell maturation in myositis muscle in the absence of B-cell follicles. *Muscle & Nerve,* Vol. 42, No. 4, (Oct., 2010), pp. (576-583), ISSN: 0148-639X

Santmyire-Rosenberger, B. & Dugan, E.M. (2003). Skin involvement in dermatomyositis. *Current Opinion in Rheumatology,* Vol.15, No.6, (Nov., 2003), pp. (714-722), ISSN: 1040-8711

Sarkar, K.S.; Weinberg, C.R.; Oddis, C.V.; Medsger, T.A.; Plotz, P.H.; Reveille, J.D.; Arnett, F.C.; Targoff, I.N.; Genth, E.; Love, L.A. & Miller, F.W. (2005). Seasonal influence on the onset of idiopathic inflammatory myopathies in serologically defined groups. *Arthritis & Rheumatism,* Vol. 52, No. 8, (Aug., 2005), pp. (2433-2438), ISSN: 0004-3591

Schreiner, B.; Voss, J.; Wischhusen, J.; Dombrowski, Y.; Steinle, A.; Lochmüller, H.; Dalakas, M.; Melms, A. & Wiendl, H. (2006). Expression of toll-like receptors by human muscle cells in vitro and in vivo: TLR3 is highly expressed in inflammatory and HIV myopathies, mediates IL-8 release and up-regulation of NKG2D-ligands. *FASEB Journal,* Vol. 20, No. 1 (Jan., 2006), pp. (118-120), ISSN: 0892-6638

Stinchcombe, J.C.; Majorovits, E.; Bossi, G.; Fuller, S. & Griffiths, G.M. (2006). Centrosome polarization delivers secretory granules to the immunological synapse. *Nature,* Vol. 443, No. 7110, (Sep., 2006), pp. (462-465), ISSN: 0028-0836

Suber, T.L.; Casciola-Rosen, L. & Rosen, A. (2008). Mechanisms of disease: autoantigens as clues to the pathogenesis of myositis. *Nature Clinical Practice. Rheumatology,* Vol. 4, No. 4, (Apr., 2008), pp. (333-340), ISSN: 1523-3774

Takeuchi, O. & Akira, S. (2008). MDA5/RIG-I and virus recognition. *Current Opinion in Immunology,* Vol. 20, No. 1, (Feb., 2008), pp (17-22), ISSN: 0952-7915

Targoff, I.N. (1990). Autoantibodies to aminoacyl-transfer RNA synthetases for isoleucine and glycine. Two additional synthetases are antigenic in myositis. *Journal of Immunology,* Vol. 144, No. 5, (Mar, 1990), pp. (1737-1743), ISSN: 0022-1767

Targoff, I.N. (2008). Autoantibodies and their significance in myositis. *Current Rheumatology Reports,* Vol. 10, No. 4, (Aug., 2008), pp. (333-340), ISSN: 1523-3774

Tezak, Z.; Hoffman, E.P.; Lutz, J.L.; Fedczyna, T.O.; Stephan, D.; Bremer, E.G.; Krasnoselska-Riz, I.; Kumar, A. & Pachman, L.M. (2002). Gene expression profiling in DQA1*0501+ children with untreated dermatomyositis: a novel model of pathogenesis. *Journal of Immunology,* Vol. 168, No. 8, (Apr., 2002), pp. (4154-4163), ISSN: 0022-1767

Vegosen, L.J.; Weinberg, C.R.; O'Hanlon, T.P.; Targoff, I.N.; Miller, F.W. & Rider, L.G. (2007). Seasonal birth patterns in subgroups of myositis suggest a role for early environmental exposures in etiology. *Arthritis & Rheumatism,* Vol. 56, No. 8, (Aug., 2007), pp. (2719–2728), ISSN: 0004-3591

Walsh, R.J.; Kong, S.W.; Yao, Y.; Jallal, B.; Kiener, P.A.; Pinkus, J.L.; Beggs, A.H.; Amato, A.A. & Greenberg, S.A. (2007). Type I interferon-inducible gene expression in blood is present and reflects disease activity in dermatomyositis and polymyositis. *Arthritis & Rheumatism,* Vol. 56, No. 11, (Nov., 2007), pp. (3784-3792), ISSN: 0004-3591

Zong, M. & Lundberg, I.E. (2011). Pathogenesis, classification and treatment of inflammatory myopathies. *Nature Reviews Rheumatology,* Vol. 7, No. 5, (May, 2011), pp. (297-306), ISSN: 1759-4790

2

Serological Aspects of Myositis

Johannes Schulte-Pelkum
Dr. Fooke Laboratorien GmbH, Neuss
Germany

1. Introduction

Idiopathic polymyositis is a chronic inflammatory systemic disease with preponderant infestation of the musculature. Dermatomyositis also involves skin participation (Conrad et al., 2001c; Kalovidouris, 1992; Mimori, 1996). Idiopathic, secondary and paraneoplastic forms of the disease can also be observed. The first report about myositis was given in 1863 by Wagner (Wagner, 1863). Also Unverricht (Unverricht, 1887) reported in 1887 about a case about Myositis, and introduced the concept of dermatomyositis in 1891.

In addition, distinct forms of interstitial myositis, marked by an appearing from foci of inflammation in the muscular interstitium and causative organism conditioned Myositis can be observed. The cause-conditioned myositis can be driven by Toxoplasma gondii or Trichinella spiralis infections (parasitcal myositis) and by Clostridium perfringens or staphylococcal infections (bacterial myositis).

Although myositis is a rather rare disease with an annual incidence of 1:100 000- 280.000 inhabitants, this illness belonging to the collagenosis group is, on account of the therapeutic consequences (Glucocorticoides and Immunsuppressiva) and the clinically often observed muscle discomfort, of considerable differential-diagnostic meaning.

Women are more frequently affected than men, the relation being about 2:1. The age distribution is marked by two maxima, for the juvenile form between the 5th and 15th year and the adult form beyond the 5th decade (2004).

The aetiology is unknown. A toxic infectious genesis is discussed among other causes and, in particular with juvenile dermatomyositis, Coxsackie viruses are considered as the cause, an allergic genesis on account of the appearance of a dermatomyositis after taking of antibiotics or sulphonamides and an immunologic genesis on account of the proof of autoantibodies. The illnesses relation with cancer could originate on the base of immunological cross reactions between tumour antigens and skin-muscle antigens or by a myotoxical substance secreted by the tumour tissue (Burmester et al., 2001). A causal connection between malignant and autoimmune disease could be seen in the disappearance or the decline of myositis symptoms after successful treatment of the tumour (in more than 10 % of the observed cases). Various studies show a raised appearance of cancer of the most different kind with patients with diagnosed Myositis (Manchul et al., 1985; Maoz et al., 1998; Zantos et al., 1994).

2. Serological aspects

Myositis can be serologically diagnosed by autoreactivity against a distinct pattern of autoantibodies. Different subsets of autoantibodies targeting distinct groups of antigens facilitate a differential diagnosis of the subforms of myositis and discrimination to other autoimmune diseases. Many myositis specific antibodies (MSA) and myositis associated antibodies (MAA) have been found and described, as shown in Table 1 and Table 2.

Antibody	**Nature of antigen**	**prevalence [% of IIM]**	**Clinical relevance**
Myositis specific			
a-Jo1	Histidyl-tRNA synthetase(50 kDa)	30 PM 18-46	antisynthetase syndrom
a-PL7	Threonyl-tRNA synthetase(80 kDa)	<5	
a-PL12	Alanyl-tRNA synthetase(110 kDa)	<5	
a-OJ	Isoleucyl-tRNA synthetase(multienzyme)	<5	
a-EJ	Glycyl-tRNA synthetase(75 kDa)	<5	
a-Ks	Asparaginyl-tRNA-Synthetase	<1	Intersititial lung manifestation
a-YRS	Tyrosyl-tRNA Synthetase	<1	
a-Zo	Phenylalanyl tRNA synthetase	<1	Nonspec interstitial lung disesae
a-SRP	Signal Recognition particle	<5	severe PM
a-Mi-2	218 kDa DNA helicase	15-31	DM
a-KJ	Translation factor	<1	PM
a-Fer	Elongation factor 1 α (48 kDa)	<1	Nodular myositis
a-Mas		<1	
a-MDA 5 a-CADM140	melanoma differentiation-associated gene 5	~ 25% in DM	Interstital lung disease with amyopathic DM
a-TIF1-gamma	transcriptional intermediary factor 1-gamma	~ 15% in DM	DM and malignancy
a-p100/p200	unknown	unknown	Necrotising myopathy w/o other specificities

Table 1. Myositis specific antigens (MSA) targeted by the immune system in myositis.

3. Synthetases

T-RNA-synthetases are the most prominent group of autoantigens targeted in myositis. The antibodies here target a group of proteins all having a similar function in the cell: the binding of an aminoacid to its determined tRNA molecule to form the aminoacyl tRNA which afterwards is used by a ribosome in the protein biosynthesis. There are two classes of tRNA synthetases, class 1 and class 2. Aminoacyl tRNA synthetase molecules are differentiated via the different ways of tRNA binding and characteristically structural motives. Class 1 tRNA synthetases have two highly conserved structural motives while class 2 synthetases have three characteristical motives.

Myositis associated			
a-Ku	DNA PK regulating subunit	5-25	PM SSc overlap
a-PmScl	Nuclear protein complex 110-20 kDa	24	PM SSc overlap
a-U2RNP	U2 small RNP(mRNA splicing factor)	<5	PM SSc overlap
a-DNA PKcs	DNA PK katalytic subunit	<5	PM, PM-SSC overlap
a-Ro52	(RBCC) tripartite motif protein ubiquitin-ligase	5-10	antisynthetase syndrom PM/DM
a-U1RNP	U1 small RNP(mRNA splicing factor)	4-17	PM 100% MCTD
Anti Calpastatin	Calpain Inhibitor	24	Often ass.with RA
Anti Annexin	Ca dep. Phospholipid binding protein	10	-

Table 2. Myositis associated antigens (MAA) targeted by the immune system in myositis.

3.1 Jo-1 histidyl-tRNA-synthetase

Antibodies against the Jo-1 antigen are the most frequent antibodies to be found in Polymyositis/Dermatomyositis (PM/DM). They occur with a prevalence of 20-30%, independent of ethnic and geographical population (Nishikai and Reichlin, 1980). The characterisation of Jo-1 as histidyl-tRNA-synthetase was achieved using immunoprecipitation of $tRNA_{HIS}$ together with a 50 kDa protein by Hirkata et al. in 1992 (Hirakata et al., 1992). Patients with serological reactivity against Jo-1 often suffer from Myositis, Polyarthritis, mechanics hands and Raynaud´s phenomenon (Nishikai and Reichlin, 1980). Like mentioned, tRNA-synthetases can be classed into two subgroups, class 1 and class 2 synthetases. Most synthetases targeted by the immune system in myositis belong two the class 2 group of enzymes. The epitope often is the synthetase enzyme itself, not the tRNA. Therefore myositis with reactivities against Jo-1, PL12, PL7, EJ and OJ is often called the synthetase syndrome. Figure 1 shows the three dimensional structure of the Jo-1 Antigen in a monomeric form (Guex and Peitsch, 1997; Peitsch et al., 2000; Schwede et al., 2003; Aberg et al., 1997), figure 2 shows the tetrameric form as the protein occurs in the cell. Structures have been taken from the protein databank (www.pdb.org). The figure shows how the four subunits interdigitate to form an H-like structure. For visualisation the subunits are shown in different colours. Jo-1 can be easily produced recombinantly using the Baculovirus expression system (Hentschel et al., 2002; Schulte-Pelkum, 2005).

3.2 PL7 threonyl-tRNA-synthetase

Anti PL7 autoantibodies, also called TRS-antibodies, bind the tRNA for threonine and an 80 kDa protein of the threonyl-tRNA-synthetase complex. In indirect immunofluorescence microscopy(IIF) a diffuse fine granular cytoplasmic fluorescence can be seen (Conrad et al., 2001a). The clinical manifestations of patients with anti-TRS- antibodies are similar to the clinical manifestations of patients with anti Jo-1 antibodies, but the prevalence of these reactivities is much lower (2-5 %).

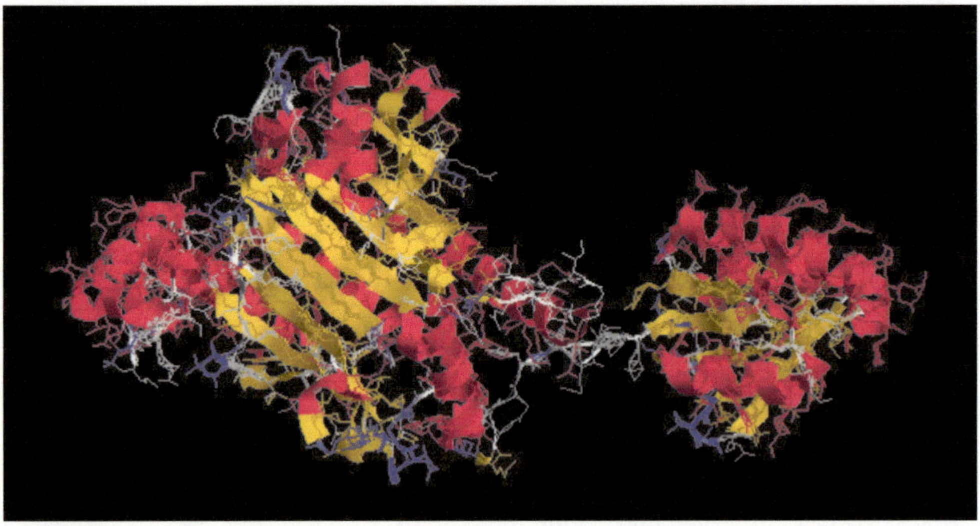

Fig. 1. Histidyl tRNA Ligase monomer, according Aberg et al. (Aberg et al., 1997).

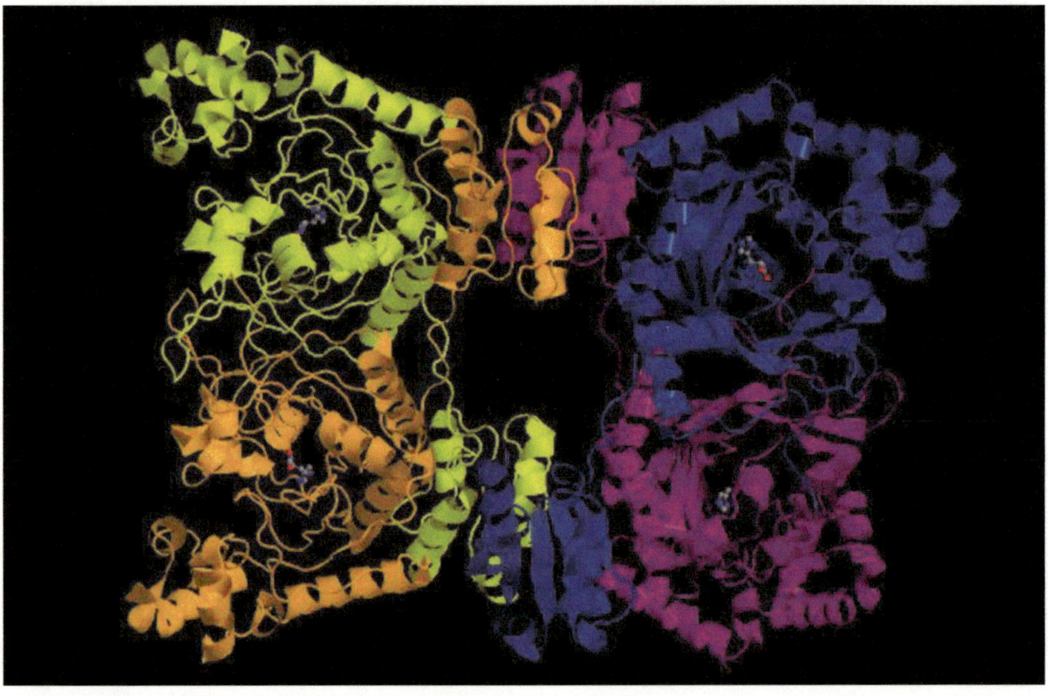

Fig. 2. Histidyl tRNA Ligase tetramer (Aberg et al., 1997).

3.3 PL12 alanyl-tRNA synthetase

Anti-Pl 12-antibodies react with a 110 kDa protein, the alanyl-tRNA synthetase. Sera having this reactivity also contain antibodies directly binding the alanyl aminoacyl tRNA. Next to the relative low prevalence of less than 5 % in myositis, these antibodies are also found in interstitial lung diseases without myositis manifestation (Hirakata et al., 1995).

3.4 EJ glycyl-tRNA synthetase

Anti-EJ-Antibodies bind a 75 kDa-protein of glycyl-tRNA synthetase together with four of the glycyl-tRNAs. This parameter is also of a low frequence. Of interest may be, that anti-EJ antibodies can, like anti Jo-1 antibodies precede the clinical symptoms of myositis (Targoff, 2000). Anti-EJ-antibodies have a prevalence of less than 5 % in myositis patients.

3.5 OJ- isoleucyl-tRNA synthetase

Anti OJ antibodies have Isoleucyl-tRNA synthetases as a main target, but also bind to other synthetases. The main epitope of anti OJ antibodies seems to be directed against a multienzyme complex, containing aminoacyl-tRNA synthetase activity for up to nine different amino acid systems. Anti OJ-antibodies have a prevalence of less than 5 % in myositis

3.6 KS- asparaginyl tRNA-synthetase

Anti KS antibodies bind Asparaginyl tRNA-synthetase. An anti KS-reactivity is not a clear marker for myositis, the majority of patients showing anti KS-reactivity suffers from interstitial lung disease and not from myositis (Hirakata et al., 1999).

3.7 ZO phenylalanyl tRNA synthetase

First described by Betterige (Betteridge et al., 2007) in a patient showing clinical symptoms of an antisynthetase syndrome, but showing no positive serological reaction to the previously identified anti-synthetase autoantibodies. Up to now only one patient has been found with this reactivity.

4. Mi2 antigen: nucleosome remodeling deacetylase

Anti Mi2 Antibodies are well known markers for dermatomyositis with an apparent prevalence of 15-30 % in patients with DM (Conrad et al., 2001b), although the biological function of the Mi2 protein in the cell remained elusive for a long time (Targoff, 2000). Anti Mi2 Antibodies can be found in ca. 20 % of patients suffering from the adult form of dermatomyositis. The function of this protein seems to be to catalyze the unwinding of chromatin structures in chromosomal DNA. The protein possesses one DNA binding domain and one helicase domain (Targoff, 2000; Woodage et al., 1997). It is assumed that the Mi2 complex catalyses an ATP dependand mechanism of Nucleosome remodelling, which makes activated genes accessible on the chromosome. This complex, called Nucleosome Remodeling Deacetylase (NuRD) seems to play a central role in one previously unknown way of gene activation (Zhang et al., 1998). Due to the size of the protein (240 kDa), attempts were made to identify the epitope sequences and to produce a smaller protein for diagnostic purposes. Independently, Mi2 alpha and Mi2 beta were described in 1995 by Ge et al. (Ge et al., 1995) and Seelig et al. (Seelig et al., 1995) wich share a sequential homology of 68 % and have parts of high similarity (Seelig et al., 1996). Sera reacting with the natural form of the Mi2 autoantigen also react with the two different recombinant forms in a highly similar matter. First attempts to solve the three dimensional structure were made by Kwan et al. in 2003 seen in figure 3 (Kwan et al., 2003). The structure of the complex was revealed only lately by Lejon et al. (Lejon et al., 2011a), as shown in figure 4. Mi2 can be easily produced recombinantly using the Baculovirus expression system (Hentschel et al., 2002; Schulte-Pelkum, 2005).

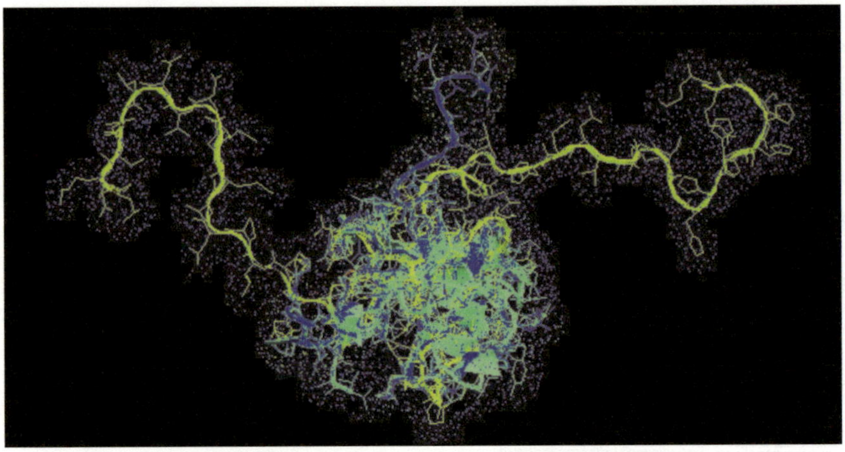

Fig. 3. Chromodomain helicase-DNA-binding protein Mi2 subunit (Kwan et al., 2003).

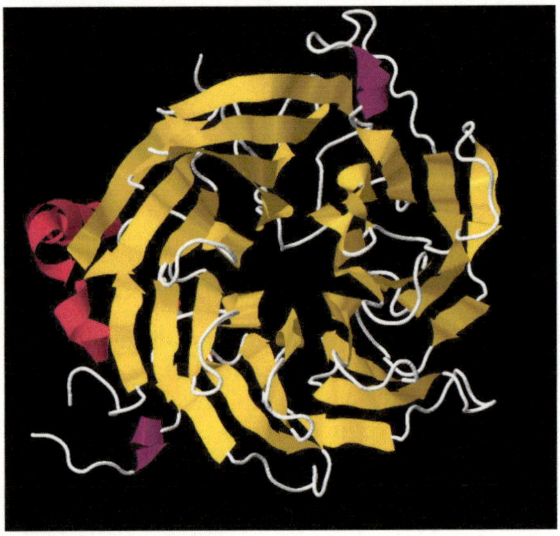

Fig. 4. The NURD complex (Lejon et al., 2011b).

5. PM-Scl- and PM1 Alpha

Although found in high frequency in patients with myositis, autoantibodies against the PM/Scl Antigen are rather myositis associated antibodies (maa) than myositis specific antibodies (msa) (Targoff, 2000). The main antigen, targeted by nearly all anti-PM/Scl positive sera is the PM/Scl 100 protein, which is part of a major protein complex of 11 proteins. Many sera also react with a 75 kDa protein referred to as PM/Scl 75. This protein migrates with an apparent size of 75 kDa in SDS PAGE, but has a calculated size of about 40 kDa, a phenomenon which can be explained by the highly charged carboxyterminal half of the protein. The other proteins of this complex are not targeted by autoantibodies associated with polymyositis. The biological function of the protein complex containing PM/Scl 100 and PM/Scl 75 seems to be analogous to the exosome complex of yeast, in which RNA is processed. Within this complex the degradation of RNA, the maturation of 5,8 S rRNA and the processing of small nuclear RNAs and AU-rich mRNAs (Raijmakers et al., 2003) is processed. Allmang et al. found out, that size and structure of the yeast exosome complex are the same as the PM/Scl complex in a human cell (Allmang et al., 1999). This complex can be found in the granular parts of the nucleoli and within the nucleoplasma. The PM/Scl 100 protein is the analogue to the yeast Rrp6p-protein, the PM/Scl 75 protein the analogue to the Rrp4p- protein (Van Eenennaam et al., 2002). As there was no three dimensional structure available, Parker and Song published a theoretical structure showing a ring-like structure of the proteins of the exosome complex (Parker and Song, 2004), shown in figure 5.

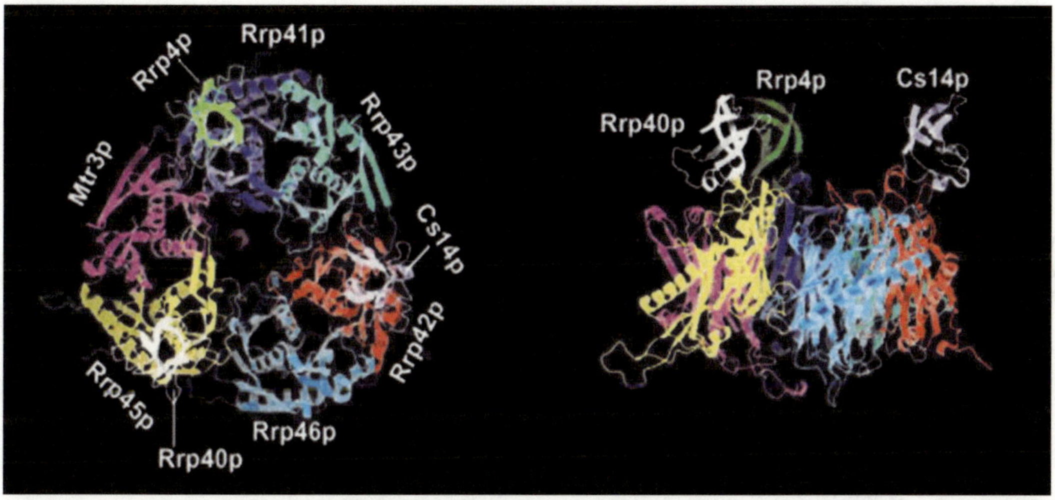

Fig. 5. The hypothetical exosome complex according to Parker et al. (Parker and Song, 2004).

Brouwer et al. (Brouwer et al., 2002) described reactivities towards the exosome complex for patients with idiopathic inflammatory myopathies, overlap syndromes and scleroderma. These reactivities were only found in a combination with reactivity against PM/Scl 100. Initial use of the PM/Scl 100 antigen showed good sensitivity and specificity using a full length 100 kDa antigen (Hentschel et al., 2002). While a debate was going on whether the PM/Scl 75 or the PM/Scl 100 antigen should be used as the preferred antigen for IVD testing (Raijmakers et al., 2004; Mahler and Raijmakers, 2007a; Brouwer et al., 2002), a peptide sequence between amino acids 231 and 245 was found which could be proven as the main site of autoantibody binding in the PM/Scl autoantigen (Bluthner et al., 2000a; Mahler et al., 2003; Mahler and Raijmakers, 2007b). The major epitope of PM/Scl referred to as PM1 alpha, consists of a local alpha helical structure. When an PM1 Alpha ELISA was recently compared to ELISA tests using the recombinant antigens with 75 and 100 kDa respectively, the best discrimination between preselected PM/Scl positive Sera (defined by Immunoblot, indirect immunofluorescence and Immunodiffusion) and control sera was observed with the PM1-Alpha ELISA with an area under the curve, AUC =1.0 compared to the PM/Scl-100 (AUC = 0.98) and PM/Scl-75 ELISA (AUC = 0.85) as revealed by receiver operating characteristics (ROC) analysis. This observation shows an interesting aspect: due to the higher local density of the immunodominant sequence, a peptide can even be the better antigen than the protein sequence it was derived from.

6. Ku –DNA-PK

Antibodies against the Ku-Complex can be found in 1-7 % of myositis patients and in 5 to 25 % of patients suffering from the polymyositis scleroderma overlap syndrome. The Ku autoantigen in its natural form is the regulatory subunit of the DNA phosphokinase complex (DNA-PK). This complex catalyses the non-homologous-end-joining (NHEJ), a repair mechanism for DNA double strand breaks. The complex consists of three subunits: Ku70, Ku80, and the much bigger catalysing subunit. If DNA-double strand breaks occur, e.g. due to ionizing radiation, the Ku-proteins form a dimer around the broken DNA and form a binding site for the 460 kDa catalysing subunit of the DNA-PK complex. The three units form the DNA-PK holoenzyme (Mimori, 1996; Dynan and Yoo, 1998; Wang et al., 1998). This complex also seems to play a central role in the genetic recombination of the different genetic subsequences of antibodies, facilitating the recombination of the different light and heavy chain- coding sequences (VDJ-joining). Here the 75-100 V-genes, the 10-20 D-genes and the 6 J-genes are recombinated freely to form ~12000 different forms of heavy chain genes, which, combined with the 1000 different forms of light (L) chains form up to 10^7 to 10^8 different antibody specificities that form the human immune system. The recombination is catalyzed by enzyme complexes called RAG-1 and RAG-2, the ligation of the DNA strands by the DNA-PK-complex containing the KU-proteins (Manis et al., 1998; Stryer et al., 2002). A defect in the catalytic or regulatory subunit of DNA-PK causes for the severe combined immunodeficiency syndrome as known from SCID-mice. The three dimensional structure of the Ku70/80-DNA binding mechanism was identified in 2001 by Walker et al. (Walker et al., 2001) and shows the spacial interaction of the two Ku-proteins, which, both binding the DNA, mate to form a complex structure, as shown in figure 6. The figure shows the two units in different colours to ease differentiation. The interdigitating structures of the two protein subunits can be clearly seen forming a complex structure surrounding the DNA.

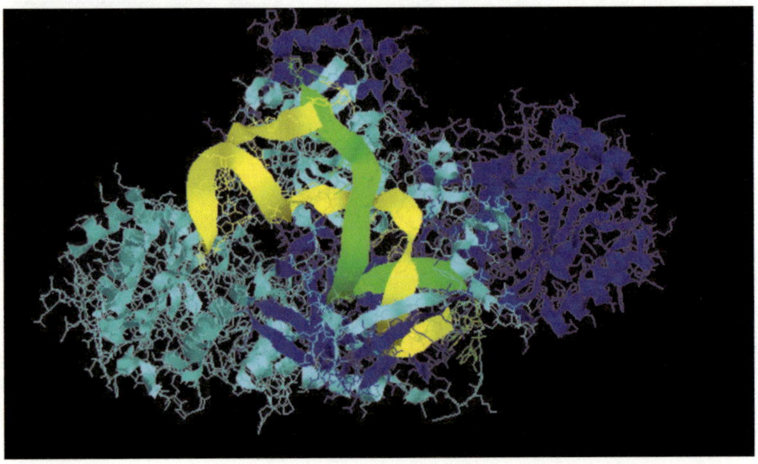

Fig. 6. Ku 70/80 Heterodimer, bound to a DNA molecule (Walker et al., 2001).

The name Ku is derived from the initials of a myositis patient. Anti Ku70/80 antibodies were firstly described by Mimori et al. (Mimori et al., 1981) in a Japanese patient suffering from the polymyositis/scleroderma overlap syndrome. Even in this early stage it was shown, that sometimes autoantibodies against only one of the subunits, but sometimes autoantibodies against both subunits occurred. Antibodies were also detectable against the whole complex of both regulatory subunits and the catalyzing subunit of DNA-PK. This so called particle antigen was assembled from highly purified native components. Antibodies were found against subunits but also against three dimensional structures of the complete particle antigen (Jafri et al., 2001). The question which one of the two subunits of the Ku antigen offers the higher sensitivity and specificity for myositis diagnosis was raised and Wang et al. (Wang et al., 1997) published a study with showed that about 50 % of the patients showed reactivity against both subunits, 30 % reacted only with the 80 kDa subunit whereas only 3 % showed exclusive reactivity against the 70 kDa Subunit alone. Also of interest in this study was the observation that 18 % of the screened myositis patients had no reactivity against the one or the other subunit, but instead showed antibodies against the heterodimeric form of Ku70/80. For diagnostic purposes a native form of the heterodimeric Ku70/80 complex is the antigen of choice. Experiments showed a far better discrimination using the heterodimeric naitve antigen compared to separately purified subunits, which later were co-coated on an ELISA plate (Schulte-Pelkum, 2005)

7. SRP –Signal recognition particle

Anti Signal recognition particle (SRP, SRP 54) antibodies are rare autoantibodies in myositis with a prevalence of only 5 %, but the anti SRP reactivity coincides with a severe onset of polymyositis (Targoff et al., 1990). Normal corticosteroid treatment usually shows no positive effect on the disease progress on aSRP 54 pos patients. Newer data as described by Hengstman (Hengstman et al., 2006), after conducting an international study with 23 aSRP positive patient samples found anti SRP 54 reactivity as a marker for a necrotising myopathy rather than a classical myositis. The patients symptoms differed only in some cases from the symptoms of the anti-SRP negative myositis control group, but anti SRP pos patients suffered significantly more often from dysphagia and muscle atropy. Also the biopsy samples differed significantly, as there were no myositis specific histological features like inflammatory infiltrates, making anti SRP antibody positive patients a distinct group next to the more classical myositis. Firstly described as an autoantibody by Reeves et al. (Reeves et al., 1986), the SRP is the primary tool for the targeting of the nascent polypeptide chain. proteins which have to be folded and/or glycosylated within the endoplasmatic reticulum have to have a signal peptide sequence on the aminoterminus. The exact structure of this signal sequence seems to be of lesser importance, although all signal-sequences contain repeating motives of hydrophobic aminoacids alternating with serine and threonine residues, which can be found in many different signal sequences moderating the protein targeting. The complex which catalyzes the targeting of the de-novo sequences is the SRP. This complex contains the 7SL-RNA and six proteins of 9, 14, 19, 54, 68 and 72 kDa. The SRP 54 kDa is the protein which directly binds to the signal sequence of the nascent protein. The complex containing ribosome, nascent protein and SRP then binds to the SRP-receptor and to a translocon, a protein on the outside of the rough ER, which then forms a channel inside the ER-lumen. Inside the ER the signal sequence is cleaved by a signal peptidase, while the rest of the protein is now synthesized directly into the lumen of the ER. The three dimensional structure of SRP 54 as shown in figure 7, was determined by Gowda et al. (Gowda et al., 1998; Gowda et al., 1999). The epitopes of SRP 54 showed to be structural epitopes, which is easily understood looking at the structure of the protein, consisting nearly only from Helix-turn-Helix motives. Interestingly Beneviste et al. observed that the aSRP54 antibody titer in a cohort of 8 longitudinally followed patients correlated (Benveniste et al.,

2011) to a high degree with disease activity as measured e.g. by serum creatine kinase activity.

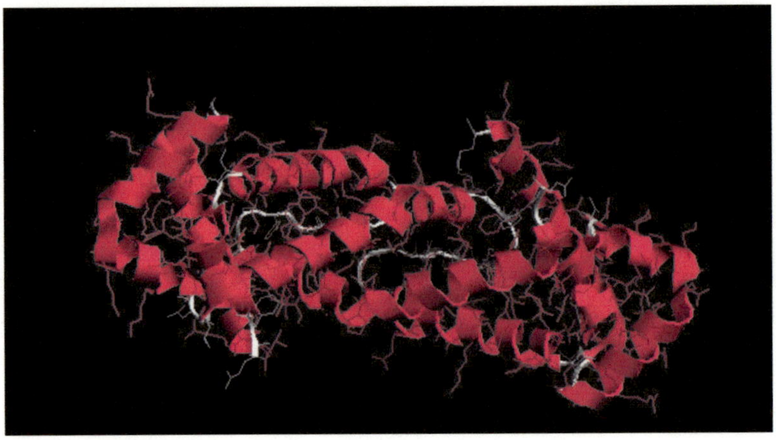

Fig. 7. Structure of SRP 54 (Gowda et al., 1998).

8. CADM140 / MDA 5

Newly shown by Nakashima (Nakashima et al., 2010) the antibody firstly described as a-CADM140 autoantibody recognises the melanoma differentiation-associated Gene 5 protein (MDA 5) which plays a role in innate immune responses. Patients with this reactivity suffer from clinically amyopathic Dermatomyositis (CADM) and have a high risk for life-threatening complications in DM, namely due to the rapidly progressing interstitial lung involvement. After the antibodies were first reported in Japan with a prevalence of around 25 % in DM cohorts (Hoshino et al., 2010), retrospective testing of dermatomyositis groups revealed also in Europe that up to 13 % of DM patients have antibodies against MDA 5, with a clear correlation for severe forms of rapidly progressing ILD and poor prognosis (Labirua and Lundberg, 2010; Fiorentino et al., 2011).

9. TIF1 gamma

First described as the anti P155 antibody the antigen bound by this antibody was revealed to be the TIF1 gamma protein of the tripartite motive family (TRIM 33) like other autoantigens, a zinc finger protein (Targoff et al., 2006a). It is (at the moment) thought to be a transcriptional corepressor. It was described first by Targoff et al. (Targoff et al., 2006b). The clinical manifestations of this reactivity involve high prevalences in dermatomyositis, as reported by Targoff et al., but with a high specificity the occurrence of this MSA correlates with a risk of malignancies as (Kaji et al., 2007). This observation was statistically underlined when Selva O´Canaghan et al. performed a meta analysis for anti TIF 1 gamma antibodies and predictive values for malignancies (Selva-O'Callaghan et al., 2010) and found that anti p155/TIF1 y antibodies have a 70 % sensitivity and a 90 % specificity to detect occult malignancies in DM. The TIF1 gamma protein as described by Venturini et al. shows a strong silencing activity towards gentic promoter sequences. In this promoter sequences, binding affinity of TIF1 gamma is dependant of a single motive (Venturini et al., 1999).

10. U1-snRNP

Antibodies against the U1-RNP complex are, like anti-Ku and anti-PM/Scl antibodies MAA. An association with PM can be found in 4-17 % of myositis cases, whereas these autoantibodies have a prevalence of 100 % in mixed connective tissue disease (MCTD). Absence of this antibodies rules out the diagnosis of MCTD (Conrad et al., 2001a). The U1 RNP consists of three small nuclear ribonuclear proteins (snRNP-"SNURPS") A (34 kDa); C (22 kDa) and the 68 kDa protein. Most prominent is reactivity against the 68 kDa protein. Considering this reactivity the coincidence of an autoimmune disease and a cytomegalo virus infection was discussed (Newkirk et al., 2001), after high rates of coinciding SLE after CMV infections were reported (Newkirk et al., 2001). The U1-snRNP complex belongs to the snRNP protein and is involved in the splicing process of the pre-messenger RNA. In mammalian cells the U1-snRNP binds the 5´splicing site of an intron with a 15 nucleotide consensus sequence of its 165 base long snRNA sequence; the subunits of the U1-RNP then bind to this snRNA. Not all proteins bind directly to the snRNA, RNP-C for example binds with a zinc finger motive to the complex of RNA and the other RNP-proteins (Nelissen et al., 1991). The sequences were published by Sillekens et al (U1-RNP-A), Yamamoto et al. (U1-RNP-C) and by Theissen et al. (U1-RNP-68) (Sillekens et al., 1987; Yamamoto et al., 1988; Theissen et al., 1986). Figure 8 shows the structure of U1-RNP-A bound to RNA (Varani et al., 2000). A scheme of the complete U1 RNP is shown in Figure 9.

11. Ro52

Although Ro52 and Ro60 (SS-A), shown early to be separate proteins (Chan et al., 1991), were initially suggested to be closely related, no direct interaction of the proteins could be conclusively shown. Recent studies indicated that the proteins are even localized in different cell compartments and they perform rather different functions. The 52 kDa Ro antigen was eventually identified as tripartite motif protein (TRIM) 21 ubiquitin-ligase that is over-expressed in peripheral blood mononuclear cells in SjS and SLE patients (Rhodes et al., 2002; Wada and Kamitani, 2006). Ro52 is reported to interact with several different molecules, among them calreticulin and a 78 kDa glucose-regulated protein (GRP78), also known as immunoglobulin heavy chain-binding protein (BIP) and formerly proposed as an early marker for rheumatoid arthritis (Blass et al., 2001). Taking its function into consideration, Ro52 is thought to modify the role or stability of its substrates through ubiquitination, and this modification might result in the Ro52-mediated biological events (Wada and Kamitani, 2006; Gomez-Martin et al., 2008).

12. Association between anti-Ro52 and anti-Ro60 antibodies in different autoimmune diseases

Testing for SS-A/Ro60 and Ro52 with sera from SSA/Ro related autoimmune diseases showed differing prevalences of the two autoantibodies in the different disease entities (see Figure 10). The frequencies of anti-Ro52 antibodies and anti-Ro60 were comparable in all groups except the myositis and scleroderma cohort. The prevalences of anti-Ro52 reactivitiy without anti-Ro60 reactivity varied in the different groups from 14.5 % in SLE to 37.5 % in the myositis group. In the SjS group, 51.7 % of anti-Ro52 sera had also antibodies to Ro60.

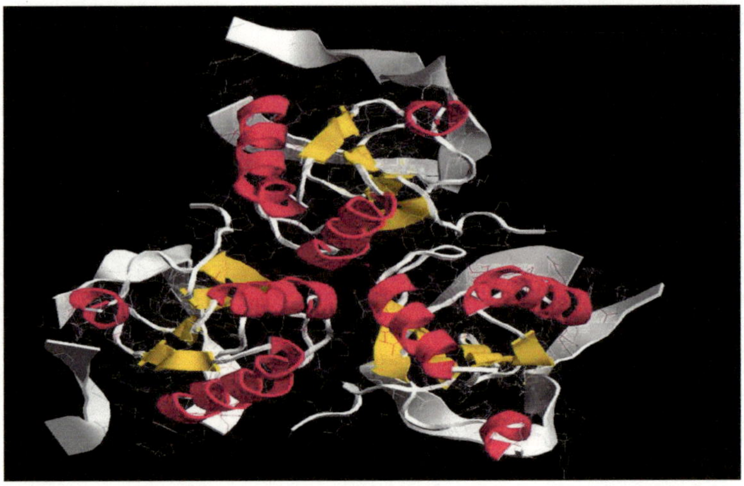

Fig. 8. U1 RNP-A bound to RNA (grey) (Varani et al., 2000).

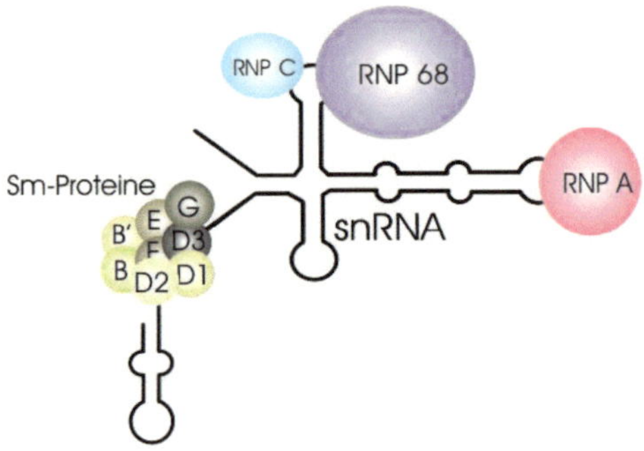

Fig. 9. Schematic view of the snRNP.

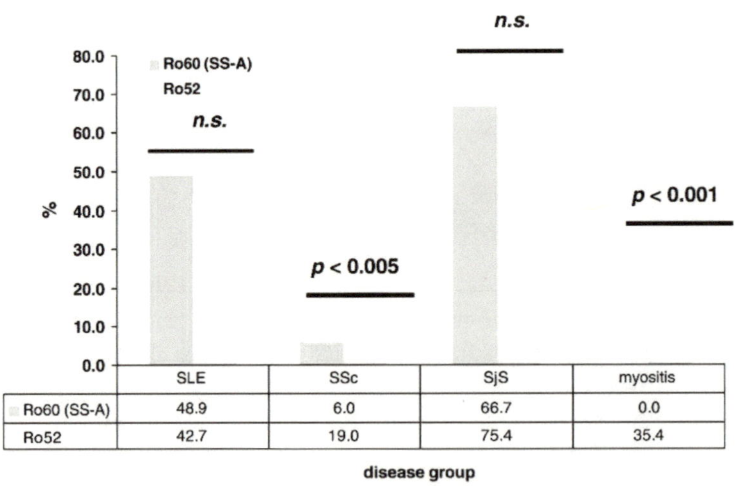

Fig. 10. Anti Ro antibody profiles in different disease groups (Schulte-Pelkum et al., 2008).

13. Coincidence of anti-Ro52 and anti-Jo-1 in patients with polymyositis

A high degree of correlation was found in a group of myositis sera tested for aab against Jo-1 and Ro52: a panel of 43 sera of myositis patients revealed reactivities against Ro52 and Jo-1 in 70 % (*p*=0.0002, Odds ratio=14.17, kappa=0.54) of Jo-1 positive sera when tested with ELISA (Dr. Fooke Laboratorien) and ALBIA. 22 (24) sera were found positive for anti-Jo-1 by ELISA and ALBIA (numbers in brackets), 16 (17) of these were also found positive for anti-Ro52 (72 % by ELISA, 70.8 % by ALBIA). These observations underline previous conclusions (Peene et al., 2002) that anti-Ro52 is indeed an independent aab in myositis. Rutjes et al. (Rutjes et al., 1997) found anti-Ro52 reactivity in 58 % of Jo-1 positive myositis sera, an observation confirmed in the subsequent years by Rozman et al. (2000), Brouwer et al. (2001) and Koenig et al. (2007) (Rozman et al., 2000; Brouwer et al., 2001; Koenig et al., 2007). In contrast, Langguth et al. (Langguth et al., 2007) indicated that isolated anti-Ro52 reactivity has limited clinical value in a non-obstetric population, a conclusion that could not be confirmed. Our study demonstrated the importance of detecting anti-Ro52 and anti-Ro60 aab separately when considering the diagnosis of patients and in particular myositis patients. This perspective was not included in the study performed by Langguth and colleagues.

It can be concluded that anti-Ro52 clearly differs in reactivity from anti-Ro60 (SS-A): Anti-Ro52 is seen in relatively high frequency in myositis and SSc. Anti-Ro52 has a prevalence of up to 35 % in myositis and in this disease group co-occurs in up to 72 % of anti-Jo-1 positive sera. In our opinion it is strongly recommend that diagnostic assays and kits should test anti-Ro52 and anti-Ro60 (SS-A) separately (Schulte-Pelkum et al., 2008; Schulte-Pelkum et al., 2009).

14. Acknowledgements

I thank Dr. M. Fooke of Dr. Fooke Laboratorien GmbH for all the encouragement and the support. Also thanks M. Petschinka (Dr. Fooke Laboratorien GmbH) for technical assistance and support with the preparation of the data. Also I would like to thank Dr. C. Hentschel for quick help with needed data, and Dr. M. Mahler for his data. Thanks also to Dr. rer. nat. habil. W. Schoessler.

15. References

Aberg, A., Yaremchuk, A., Tukalo, M., RASMUSSEN, B., and Cusack, S. (1997). Crystal structure analysis of the activation of histidine by Thermus thermophilus histidyl-tRNA synthetase. Biochemistry *36*, 3084-3094.

Allmang, C., Petfalski, E., Podtelejnikov, A., Mann, M., Tollervey, D., and Mitchell, P. (1999). The yeast exosome and human PM-Scl are related complexes of 3' --> 5' exonucleases. *Genes Dev 13*, 2148-2158.

Benveniste, O., Drouot, L., Jouen, F., Charuel, J.L., Bloch-Queyrat, C., Behin, A., Amoura, Z., Marie, I., Guiguet, M., Eymard, B., Gilbert, D., Tron, F., Herson, S., Musset, L., and Boyer, O. (2011). Anti-signal recognition particle auto-antibody levels correlate with creatine kinase activity in patients with necrotizing myopathy. Arthritis Rheum.

Betteridge, Z., Gunawardena, H., North, J., Slinn, J., and McHugh, N. (2007). Anti-synthetase syndrome: a new autoantibody to phenylalanyl transfer RNA synthetase (anti-Zo) associated with polymyositis and interstitial pneumonia. Rheumatology. (Oxford) *46*, 1005-1008.

Blass, S., Union, A., Raymackers, J., Schumann, F., Ungethum, U., Muller-Steinbach, S., de Keyser, F., Engel, J.M., and Burmester, G.R. (2001). The stress protein BiP is overexpressed and is a major B and T cell target in rheumatoid arthritis. Arthritis Rheum *44*, 761-771.

Bluthner, M., Mahler, M., Muller, D.B., Dunzl, H., and Bautz, F.A. (2000a). Identification of an alpha-helical epitope region on the PM/Scl-100 autoantigen with structural homology to a region on the heterochromatin p25beta autoantigen using immobilized overlapping synthetic peptides. J. Mol. Med. *78*, 47-54.

Bluthner, M., Mahler, M., Muller, D.B., Dunzl, H., and Bautz, F.A. (2000b). Identification of an alpha-helical epitope region on the PM/Scl-100 autoantigen with structural homology to a region on the heterochromatin p25beta autoantigen using immobilized overlapping synthetic peptides. J Mol Med *78*, 47-54.

Brouwer, R., Hengstman, G.J., Vree, E.W., Ehrfeld, H., Bozic, B., Ghirardello, A., Grondal, G., Hietarinta, M., Isenberg, D., Kalden, J.R., Lundberg, I., Moutsopoulos, H., Roux-Lombard, P., Vencovsky, J., Wikman, A., Seelig, H.P., van Engelen, B.G., and van Venrooij, W.J. (2001). Autoantibody profiles in the sera of European patients with myositis. Ann Rheum Dis *60*, 116-123.

Brouwer, R., Vree Egberts, W.T., Hengstman, G.J., Raijmakers, R., van Engelen, B.G., Seelig, H.P., Renz, M., Mierau, R., Genth, E., Pruijn, G.J., and van Venrooij, W.J. (2002). Autoantibodies directed to novel components of the PM/Scl complex, the human exosome. Arthritis Res *4*, 134-138.

Burmester, G.R., Buttgereit, F., Keitel, W., and Sieper, J. (2001). Systemkrankheiten des Bindegewebes bei anderenorts klassifizierten Krankheiten. In Interdisziplinäre klinische Rheumatologie, H.Zeidler, J.Zacher, and F.Hiepe, eds. (Berlin: Springer Verlag), pp. 960-971.

Chan, E.K., Hamel, J.C., Buyon, J.P., and Tan, E.M. (1991). Molecular definition and sequence motifs of the 52-kD component of human SS-A/Ro autoantigen. J Clin Invest *87*, 68-76.

Conrad, K., Schößler, W., and Hiepe, F. (2001a). Autoantikörper bei systemischen Autoimmunerkrankungen. (Lengerich; Berlin; Riga; Rom; Viernheim; Wien; Zagreb: Pabst Science Publishers).

Conrad, K., Schößler, W., and Hiepe, F. (2001b). Mi-2-Antikörper. In Autoantikörper bei systemischen Autoimmunerkrankungen, K.Conrad, W.Schößler, and F.Hiepe, eds. (Lengerich, Berlin, Riga, Rom, Viernheim, Wien, Zagreb: Pabst), pp. 89-90.

Conrad, K., Schößler, W., and Hiepe, F. (2001c). Polymyositis (PM) and Dermatomyositis (DM). In Autoantikörper bei systemischen Autoimmunerkrankungen, K.Conrad, W.Schößler, and F.Hiepe, eds. (Lengerich, Berlin, Riga, Rom, Viernheim, Wien, Zagreb: Pabst), pp. 203-205.

Dynan, W.S. and Yoo, S. (1998). Interaction of Ku protein and DNA-dependent protein kinase catalytic subunit with nucleic acids. Nucleic Acids Res *26*, 1551-1559.

Fiorentino, D., Chung, L., Zwerner, J., Rosen, A., and Casciola-Rosen, L. (2011). The mucocutaneous and systemic phenotype of dermatomyositis patients with antibodies to MDA5 (CADM-140): A retrospective study. J. Am. Acad. Dermatol.

Ge, Q., Nilasena, D.S., O'Brien, C.A., Frank, M.B., and Targoff, I.N. (1995). Molecular analysis of a major antigenic region of the 240-kD protein of Mi-2 autoantigen. J Clin Invest *96*, 1730-1737.

Gomez-Martin, D., Diaz-Zamudio, M., and Alcocer-Varela, J. (2008). Ubiquitination system and autoimmunity: the bridge towards the modulation of the immune response. Autoimmun. Rev. *7*, 284-290.

Gowda, K., Black, S.D., Moeller, I., Sakakibara, Y., Liu, M.C., and Zwieb, C. (1998). protein SRP54 of human signal recognition particle: cloning, expression, and comparative analysis of functional sites. Gene *207*, 197-207.

Gowda, K., Clemons, W.M., Jr., Zwieb, C., and Black, S.D. (1999). Expression, purification, and crystallography of the conserved methionine-rich domain of human signal recognition particle 54 kDa protein. protein Sci *8*, 1144-1151.

Guex, N. and Peitsch, M.C. (1997). SWISS-MODEL and the Swiss-PdbViewer: an environment for comparative protein modeling. Electrophoresis *18*, 2714-2723.

Hengstman, G.J., ter Laak, H.J., Vree Egberts, W.T., Lundberg, I.E., Moutsopoulos, H.M., Vencovsky, J., Doria, A., Mosca, M., van Venrooij, W.J., and van Engelen, B.G. (2006). Anti-signal recognition particle autoantibodies: marker of a necrotising myopathy. Ann. Rheum. Dis. *65*, 1635-1638.

Hentschel, C., Schulte-Pelkum, J., Schößler, W., Hiepe, F., and Mierau, R. (2002). A new LINE Immuno assay for the detection of myositis specific autoantibodies. Report on the 6th Dresden Symposium on Autoantibodies *4*, 649-650.

Hirakata, M., Mimori, T., Akizuki, M., Craft, J., Hardin, J.A., and Homma, M. (1992). Autoantibodies to small nuclear and cytoplasmic ribonucleoproteins in Japanese patients with inflammatory muscle disease. Arthritis Rheum *35*, 449-456.

Hirakata, M., Nakamura, S., Okano, Y., Suwa, A., Inada, S., Akizuki, M., and Hardin, J.A. (1995). Anti-alanyl tRNA synthetase (PL12) antibodies are associated with interstitial lung disease in Japanese patients. Arthritis Rheum *38*, 321.

Hirakata, M., Suwa, A., Nagai, S., Kron, M.A., Trieu, E.P., Mimori, T., Akizuki, M., and Targoff, I.N. (1999). Anti-KS: identification of autoantibodies to asparaginyl-transfer RNA synthetase associated with interstitial lung disease. J. Immunol. *162*, 2315-2320.

Hoshino, K., Muro, Y., Sugiura, K., Tomita, Y., Nakashima, R., and Mimori, T. (2010). Anti-MDA5 and anti-TIF1-gamma antibodies have clinical significance for patients with dermatomyositis. Rheumatology. (Oxford) *49*, 1726-1733.

Jafri, F., Hardin, J.A., and Dynan, W.S. (2001). A method to detect particle-specific antibodies against Ku and the DNA- dependent protein kinase catalytic subunit in autoimmune sera. J Immunol Methods *251*, 53-61.

Kaji, K., Fujimoto, M., Hasegawa, M., Kondo, M., Saito, Y., Komura, K., Matsushita, T., Orito, H., Hamaguchi, Y., Yanaba, K., Itoh, M., Asano, Y., Seishima, M., Ogawa, F., Sato, S., and Takehara, K. (2007). Identification of a novel autoantibody reactive with 155 and 140 kDa nuclear proteins in patients with dermatomyositis: an association with malignancy. Rheumatology. (Oxford) *46*, 25-28.

Kalovidouris, A.E. (1992). Immune aspects of myositis. Curr Opin Rheumatol *4*, 809-814.

Koenig, M., Fritzler, M.J., Targoff, I.N., Troyanov, Y., and Senecal, J.L. (2007). Heterogeneity of autoantibodies in 100 patients with autoimmune myositis: insights into clinical features and outcomes. Arthritis Res. Ther. *9*, R78.

Kwan, A.H., Gell, D.A., Verger, A., Crossley, M., Matthews, J.M., and Mackay, J.P. (2003). Engineering a protein scaffold from a PHD finger. Structure. (Camb.) *11*, 803-813.

Labirua, A. and Lundberg, I.E. (2010). Interstitial lung disease and idiopathic inflammatory myopathies: progress and pitfalls. Curr. Opin. Rheumatol. *22*, 633-638.

Langguth, D.M., Morris, S., Clifford, L., Wilson, R.J., Neil, J., Hogan, P.G., and Wong, R.C. (2007). Specific testing for "isolated" anti-52 kDa SSA/Ro antibodies during standard anti-extractable nuclear antigen testing is of limited clinical value. J. Clin. Pathol. *60*, 670-673.

Lejon, S., Thong, S.Y., Murthy, A., AlQarni, S., Murzina, N.V., Blobel, G.A., Laue, E.D., and Mackay, J.P. (2011b). Insights into association of the NuRD complex with FOG-1 from the crystal structure of an RbAp48.FOG-1 complex. J. Biol. Chem. *286*, 1196-1203.

Lejon, S., Thong, S.Y., Murthy, A., AlQarni, S., Murzina, N.V., Blobel, G.A., Laue, E.D., and Mackay, J.P. (2011a). Insights into association of the NuRD complex with FOG-1 from the crystal structure of an RbAp48.FOG-1 complex. J. Biol. Chem. *286*, 1196-1203.

Mahler, M., Bluthner, M., and Pollard, K.M. (2003). Advances in B-cell epitope analysis of autoantigens in connective tissue diseases. Clin. Immunol. *107*, 65-79.

Mahler, M. and Raijmakers, R. (2007a). Novel aspects of autoantibodies to the PM/Scl complex: clinical, genetic and diagnostic insights. Autoimmun. Rev. *6*, 432-437.

Mahler, M. and Raijmakers, R. (2007b). Novel aspects of autoantibodies to the PM/Scl complex: clinical, genetic and diagnostic insights. Autoimmun. Rev. *6*, 432-437.

Manchul, L.A., Jin, A., Pritchard, K.I., Tenenbaum, J., Boyd, N.F., Lee, P., Germanson, T., and Gordon, D.A. (1985). The frequency of malignant neoplasms in patients with polymyositis-dermatomyositis. A controlled study. Arch. Intern. Med. *145*, 1835-1839.

Manis, J.P., Gu, Y., Lansford, R., Sonoda, E., Ferrini, R., Davidson, L., Rajewsky, K., and Alt, F.W. (1998). Ku70 is required for late B cell development and immunoglobulin heavy chain class switching. J. Exp. Med. *187*, 2081-2089.

Maoz, C.R., Langevitz, P., Livneh, A., Blumstein, Z., Sadeh, M., Bank, I., Gur, H., and Ehrenfeld, M. (1998). High incidence of malignancies in patients with dermatomyositis and polymyositis: an 11-year analysis. Semin. Arthritis Rheum. *27*, 319-324.

Mimori, T. (1996). Structures targeted by the immune system in myositis. Curr Opin Rheumatol *8*, 521-527.

Mimori, T., Akizuki, M., Yamagata, H., Inada, S., Yoshida, S., and Homma, M. (1981). Characterization of a high molecular weight acidic nuclear protein recognized by autoantibodies in sera from patients with polymyositis- scleroderma overlap. J Clin Invest *68*, 611-620.

Nakashima, R., Imura, Y., Kobayashi, S., Yukawa, N., Yoshifuji, H., Nojima, T., Kawabata, D., Ohmura, K., Usui, T., Fujii, T., Okawa, K., and Mimori, T. (2010). The RIG-I-like receptor IFIH1/MDA5 is a dermatomyositis-specific autoantigen identified by the anti-CADM-140 antibody. Rheumatology. (Oxford) *49*, 433-440.

Nelissen, R.L., Heinrichs, V., Habets, W.J., Simons, F., Luhrmann, R., and van Venrooij, W.J. (1991). Zinc finger-like structure in U1-specific protein C is essential for specific binding to U1 snRNP. Nucleic Acids Res. *19*, 449-454.

Newkirk, M.M., van Venrooij, W.J., and Marshall, G.S. (2001). Autoimmune response to U1 small nuclear ribonucleoprotein (U1 snRNP) associated with cytomegalovirus infection. Arthritis Res. *3*, 253-258.

Nishikai, M. and Reichlin, M. (1980). Heterogeneity of precipitating antibodies in polymyositis and dermatomyositis. Characterization of the Jo-1 antibody system. Arthritis Rheum *23*, 881-888.

Parker, R. and Song, H. (2004). The enzymes and control of eukaryotic mRNA turnover. Nat. Struct. Mol. Biol *11*, 121-127.

Peene, I., Meheus, L., De, K.S., Humbel, R., Veys, E.M., and De, K.F. (2002). Anti-Ro52 reactivity is an independent and additional serum marker in connective tissue disease. Ann. Rheum. Dis. *61*, 929-933.

Peitsch, M.C., Schwede, T., and Guex, N. (2000). Automated protein modelling--the proteome in 3D. Pharmacogenomics. *1*, 257-266.

Raijmakers, R., Egberts, W.V., van Venrooij, W.J., and Pruijn, G.J. (2003). The association of the human PM/Scl-75 autoantigen with the exosome is dependent on a newly identified N terminus. J. Biol. Chem. *278*, 30698-30704.

Raijmakers, R., Renz, M., Wiemann, C., Egberts, W.V., Seelig, H.P., van Venrooij, W.J., and Pruijn, G.J. (2004). PM-Scl-75 is the main autoantigen in patients with the polymyositis/scleroderma overlap syndrome. Arthritis Rheum. *50*, 565-569.

Reeves, W.H., Nigam, S.K., and Blobel, G. (1986). Human autoantibodies reactive with the signal-recognition particle. Proc. Natl. Acad. Sci. U. S. A *83*, 9507-9511.

Rhodes, D.A., Ihrke, G., Reinicke, A.T., Malcherek, G., Towey, M., Isenberg, D.A., and Trowsdale, J. (2002). The 52 000 MW Ro/SS-A autoantigen in Sjogren's syndrome/systemic lupus erythematosus (Ro52) is an interferon-gamma inducible tripartite motif protein associated with membrane proximal structures. Immunology *106*, 246-256.

Rozman, B., Bozic, B., Kos-Golja, M., Plesivcnik-Novljan, M., and Kveder, T. (2000). Immunoserological aspects of idiopathic inflammatory muscle disease. Wien. Klin. Wochenschr. *112*, 722-727.

Rutjes, S.A., Vree Egberts, W.T., Jongen, P., Van Den, H.F., Pruijn, G.J., and van Venrooij, W.J. (1997). Anti-Ro52 antibodies frequently co-occur with anti-Jo-1 antibodies in sera from patients with idiopathic inflammatory myopathy. Clin. Exp. Immunol. *109*, 32-40.

Schulte-Pelkum, J. (2005). Entwicklung neuer Methoden zum Nachweis von Myositiden. (Berlin Erlangen.

Schulte-Pelkum, J., Fritzler, M.J., and Mahler, M. (2009). Latest update on the Ro/SS-A autoantibody system. Autoimmun. Rev. *8*, 632-637.

Schulte-Pelkum, J., Simon, T., Szmyrka-Kaczmarek, M., Fritzler, M.J., and Mahler, M. (2008). Latest Update on the Ro/SS-A Autoantibody System. 6th International Congress on Autoimmunity, Porto (Lecture).

Schwede, T., Kopp, J., Guex, N., and Peitsch, M.C. (2003). SWISS-MODEL: An automated protein homology-modeling server. Nucleic Acids Res. *31*, 3381-3385.

Seelig, H.P., Moosbrugger, I., Ehrfeld, H., Fink, T., Renz, M., and Genth, E. (1995). The major dermatomyositis-specific Mi-2 autoantigen is a presumed helicase involved in transcriptional activation. Arthritis Rheum *38*, 1389-1399.

Seelig, H.P., Renz, M., Targoff, I.N., Ge, Q., and Frank, M.B. (1996). Two forms of the major antigenic protein of the dermatomyositis- specific Mi-2 autoantigen. Arthritis Rheum *39*, 1769-1771.

Selva-O'Callaghan, A., Trallero-Araguas, E., Grau-Junyent, J.M., and Labrador-Horrillo, M. (2010). Malignancy and myositis: novel autoantibodies and new insights. Curr. Opin. Rheumatol. 22, 627-632.

Sillekens, P.T., Habets, W.J., Beijer, R.P., and van Venrooij, W.J. (1987). cDNA cloning of the human U1 snRNA-associated A protein: extensive homology between U1 and U2 snRNP-specific proteins. EMBO J. *6*, 3841-3848.

Stryer, L., Berg, J.M., and Tymoczko, J.L. (2002). The Immune System. In Biochemistry, L.Stryer, J.M.Berg, and J.L.Tymoczko, eds. (New York: W.H. Freeman & Company New York), pp. 912-979.

Targoff, I., Trieu, E., None, M., Levy-Neto, M., Prasertsuntarasai, T., and Miller, F.W. (2006a). Autoantibodies to Transcriptional Intermediary Factor 1-gamma (TIF1-g) in Dermatomyositis. ACR Meeting 1241-Presentation.
Targoff, I.N. (2000). Update on myositis-specific and myositis-associated autoantibodies. Curr Opin Rheumatol *12*, 475-481.
Targoff, I.N., Johnson, A.E., and Miller, F.W. (1990). Antibody to signal recognition particle in polymyositis. Arthritis Rheum *33*, 1361-1370.
Targoff, I.N., Mamyrova, G., Trieu, E.P., Perurena, O., Koneru, B., O'Hanlon, T.P., Miller, F.W., and Rider, L.G. (2006b). A novel autoantibody to a 155-kd protein is associated with dermatomyositis. Arthritis Rheum. *54*, 3682-3689.
Theissen, H., Etzerodt, M., Reuter, R., Schneider, C., Lottspeich, F., Argos, P., Luhrmann, R., and Philipson, L. (1986). Cloning of the human cDNA for the U1 RNA-associated 70K protein. EMBO J. *5*, 3209-3217.
Unverricht, H. (1887). Über eine eigentümliche Form von akuter Muskelentzündung mit einem der Trichinose ähnlichen Krankheitsbilde. Münchener medizinische Wochenschrift *34*, 488-492.
Van Eenennaam, H., Vogelzangs, J.H., Bisschops, L., Te Boome, L.C., Seelig, H.P., Renz, M., De Rooij, D.J., Brouwer, R., Pluk, H., Pruijn, G.J., van Venrooij, W.J., and Van Den Hoogen, F.H. (2002). Autoantibodies against small nucleolar ribonucleoprotein complexes and their clinical associations. Clin Exp Immunol *130*, 532-540.
Varani, L., Gunderson, S.I., Mattaj, I.W., Kay, L.E., Neuhaus, D., and Varani, G. (2000). The NMR structure of the 38 kDa U1A protein - PIE RNA complex reveals the basis of cooperativity in regulation of polyadenylation by human U1A protein. Nat. Struct. Biol. *7*, 329-335.
Venturini, L., You, J., Stadler, M., Galien, R., Lallemand, V., Koken, M.H., Mattei, M.G., Ganser, A., Chambon, P., Losson, R., and de The, H. (1999). TIF1gamma, a novel member of the transcriptional intermediary factor 1 family. Oncogene *18*, 1209-1217.
Wada, K. and Kamitani, T. (2006). Autoantigen Ro52 is an E3 ubiquitin ligase. Biochem Biophys. Res. Commun. *339*, 415-421.
Wagner, E.L. (1863). Fall einer seltenen Muskelkrankheit. Archiv der Heilkunde *4*, 282-283.
Walker, J.R., Corpina, R.A., and Goldberg, J. (2001). Structure of the Ku heterodimer bound to DNA and its implications for double-strand break repair. Nature *412*, 607-614.
Wang, J., Dong, X., Myung, K., Hendrickson, E.A., and Reeves, W.H. (1998). Identification of two domains of the p70 Ku protein mediating dimerization with p80 and DNA binding. J Biol Chem *273*, 842-848.
Wang, J., Dong, X., Stojanov, L., Kimpel, D., Satoh, M., and Reeves, W.H. (1997). Human autoantibodies stabilize the quaternary structure of Ku antigen. Arthritis Rheum *40*, 1344-1353.
Woodage, T., Basrai, M.A., Baxevanis, A.D., Hieter, P., and Collins, F.S. (1997). Characterization of the CHD family of proteins. Proc Natl. Acad Sci U. S. A *94*, 11472-11477.
Yamamoto, K., Miura, H., Moroi, Y., Yoshinoya, S., Goto, M., Nishioka, K., and Miyamoto, T. (1988). Isolation and characterization of a complementary DNA expressing human U1 small nuclear ribonucleoprotein C polypeptide. J. Immunol. *140*, 311-317.
Zantos, D., Zhang, Y., and Felson, D. (1994). The overall and temporal association of cancer with polymyositis and dermatomyositis. J. Rheumatol. *21*, 1855-1859.
Zhang, Y., LeRoy, G., Seelig, H.P., Lane, W.S., and Reinberg, D. (1998). The dermatomyositis-specific autoantigen Mi2 is a component of a complex containing histone deacetylase and nucleosome remodeling activities. Cell *95*, 279-289.

3

Arthrogenic Alphaviruses and Inflammatory Myopathies

Lara Herrero and Suresh Mahalingam
Institute for Glycomics
Griffith University
Australia

1. Introduction

There is increasing evidence to suggest that viruses have aetiological roles in inflammatory myopathies. It has been reported that viruses, by means of direct infection of the skeletal muscle, can cause myalgias, polymyositis, and virus-associated rhabdomyolysis. It has also been found that some viruses can cause myositis through a secondary immune-mediated phenomenon. In addition, there are emerging reports of cases of idiopathic polymyositis suspected to be associated with infectious agents, predominantly viruses.

Arthrogenic alphaviruses such as chikungunya virus (CHIKV), Ross River virus (RRV) and sindbis virus (SINV) are known to cause outbreaks of polyarthritis worldwide (Griffin, 2007). The clinical presentation of alphavirus infection includes fever, rash, arthralgia, and arthritis, however, one of the predominant features of alphaviral disease is myalgia with corresponding myositis. The recent outbreaks of CHIKV in several countries surrounding the Indian Ocean have seen millions of people affected, with case reports showing a high incidence of myalgia and skeletal muscle involvement.

The ability of these viruses to cause long-term disease sequelae persisting for months or even years after the initial infection is of particular interest. Although difficult to substantiate indefinitely, there is significant reason to suspect that this long-term impact, combined with the virus's ability to cause acute muscle damage, could make arthrogenic viruses a potential cause of idiopathic inflammatory myopathies.

The mechanisms by which alphaviruses cause musculoskeletal disease are now being unraveled with clear evidence to suggest that the viral-induced inflammatory response can lead to destruction of striated muscle fibres, providing a possible cause for the symptoms of myalgia. In recent years, the use of animal models of alphavirus-induced myositis has increased our understanding of the inflammatory myopathies caused by these viruses. Using these animal models it has been shown that in the acute phase of infection, skeletal muscle is the major site of viral replication, resulting in striated muscle fibre destruction (Lidbury *et al.*, 2000; Morrison *et al.*, 2006). In the sub-acute phase of infection, the virus triggers an extensive inflammatory immune response, resulting in the influx of inflammatory cells and production of soluble mediators, leading to extensive myositis. The use of animal models has been instrumental in elucidating the role of alphaviruses as triggers of inflammatory myopathies.

This chapter will discuss the role of alphavirus infections as triggers of myositis, including how animal models are being used to dissect the pathobiology of disease and identify potential drug candidates to ameliorate disease.

2. Alphaviruses

Alphaviruses are a group of mosquito-transmitted viruses of the *Togaviridae* family. The virus particle is approximately 60 nm in size and is comprised of a single-strand of ribonucleic acid (RNA) of approximately twelve kilobases, encased in a nucleocapsid with a lipid membrane envelope. The RNA genome is divided into two regions, the non-structural and the structural regions. The non-structural region encodes four nonstructural proteins (nsPs; nsP1 to nsP4), and the structural region encodes the capsid protein (C) and three glycoproteins (E1, E2 and E3). The glycoproteins E1 and E2 protrude from the viral lipid envelope and are the most external and immunodominant epitopes being exposed to a significant amount of immune pressure.

The *Alphavirus* genus can be classified into two subgroups depending on differences in disease aetiologies; the Old World and the New World alphaviruses. The Old World alphaviruses, including RRV, o'nyong-nyong (ONNV), Semliki Forest virus (SFV), SINV, mayaro virus (MAYV), Barmah Forest virus (BFV) and CHIKV, typically cause fever, rash, myalgia, arthralgia and arthritis in humans, with symptoms often persisting for several months to years following infection (Table 1) (Suhrbier & La Linn, 2004). The New World alphaviruses, including Venezuelan equine encephalitis virus (VEEV), Eastern equine encephalitis virus (EEEV) and Western equine encephalitis virus (WEEV), cause severe disease in humans targeting the central nervous system (CNS), often resulting in encephalitis (Johnston & Peters, 1996), and are not associated with myositis. This chapter will focus on Old World alphaviruses.

Old World alphaviruses have been associated with large outbreaks of disease worldwide. These outbreaks are often explosive in nature, affecting many thousands to millions of people such as the 1959-1962 outbreak of ONNV fever in Africa, involving an estimated two million cases (Lanciotti *et al.*, 1998; Posey *et al.*, 2005; Williams *et al.*, 1965), the 1979-1980 outbreak of RRV in the South Pacific, resulting in more than 60,000 reported cases (Harley *et al.*, 2001) and the 2005-2006 outbreak of CHIKV in India with at least 1.5 million people affected (Josseran *et al.*, 2006; Kalantri *et al.*, 2006; Yergolkar *et al.*, 2006). In addition to the larger outbreaks, alphaviruses are also known to cause smaller, sporadic outbreaks such as that of MAYV in Brazil in 1978 and 2008 (Azevedo *et al.*, 2009; Pinheiro *et al.*, 1981), outbreaks of SINV in Finland and Sweden as the causative agent of Pogosta and Ockelbo diseases respectively (Kurkela *et al.*, 2004; Skogh & Espmark, 1982) and the recent 2009 outbreaks of CHIKV in Thailand, Singapore, Malaysia and Indonesia (Hapuarachchi *et al.*, 2010; Higgs & Ziegler, 2010; Ng *et al.*, 2009a; Thavara *et al.*, 2009; Theamboonlers *et al.*, 2009). Although the predominant clinical feature in most alphaviral outbreaks is the typical arthritis/arthralgia, a second important feature of the disease is myalgia.

The course of a typical alphavirus infection first involves the bite of an infected mosquito, resulting in subcutaneous inoculation of the virus. This is then followed by the initial viral replication and systemic viraemic spread. The primary viraemia marks the acute phase of the infection. Infection progresses to secondary sites where the virus can replicate, however, by this stage the body mounts an immune response to counteract the virus. It is at this point that specific clinical signs and symptoms of disease commence, which correlate closely to the immune inflammatory response, and mark the sub-acute phase of infection. The sub-acute phase can last several weeks, and there have been numerous cases documented where disease symptoms have lasted for months to years, thereby marking the chronic stage of alphaviral infection. In all three stages of alphaviral infection; acute, sub-acute and chronic, there is clear evidence of inflammatory response in the muscle and symptoms of myalgia.

Old World alphavirus	Geographic distribution	Cases	Comments
Ross River (RRV)	Australia West Pacific	~5,000 pa in Australia	Reported in travelers and visiting US military personnel
Barmah Forest (BFV)	Australia	~1500-2000 pa in Australia	Probably underdiagnosed due to similarity with RRV
Sindbis group (SINV)	Africa, Asia, Australia	Rare *	Although differently named, probably all the same virus
Karelian fever	Russia	Rare	Outbreaks occur frequently in Europe
Ockelbo	Sweden	30 pa	
Pogosta	Finland	100–200 pa	
Mayaro (MAYV)	South America	Small sporadic epidemics, underdiagnosed due to circulating dengue	Reported in travelers in Europe and the USA
O'nyong-nyong (ONNV)	Central and East Africa	Small sporadic epidemics, >2 million 1959–1962 epidemic	
Igbo Ora	Central Africa	Rare	Serologically related to ONNV and CHIKV
Chikungunya (CHIKV)	South and East Asia, Africa, West Pacific	Recurrent epidemics, anywhere from a thousand to a million cases reported annually since it re-emergence in 2005	Large epidemics in countries around the Indian Ocean from 2005-present. Reported in travelers in Europe and the USA

*Cases believed to be under reported world-wide

These viruses are generally transmitted by mosquitos and constitute over 40 members, several of which cause polyarthritis/arthralgia/myalgia in humans. pa, per annum.

Table 1. Old World viruses of the *Alphavirus* genus.

2.1 Ross River virus (RRV)

RRV was first isolated in 1959 in Queensland, Australia and was identified as an arbovirus causing polyarthritis by the early 1960s. It circulates endemically in Australia and the South Pacific (Harley *et al.*, 2001). Like all alphaviruses, the virus is maintained in transmission cycles between its mosquito vector and vertebrate hosts. In the case of RRV the predominant vectors are the mosquitoes *Culex annulirostris* and *Aedes vigilax* and the vertebrate hosts are commonly found to be native marsupials (Harley *et al.*, 2001; Old & Deane, 2005; Oliveira *et al.*, 2006). In Australia, there are between 5,000 to 8,000 cases of RRV reported annually (Harley *et al.*, 2001), with patients displaying symptoms of arthritis, arthralgia, myalgia, fatigue, febrile illness and rash (Fraser, 1986; Harley *et al.*, 2002; Harley *et al.*, 2001).

The characteristic feature of RRV-infection in its acute stage is a febrile illness, which is frequently ignored by patients. Following the non-specific fever, comes the onset of RRV-specific symptoms, such as rash, arthritis, arthralgia and myalgia. It is at this sub-acute stage that patients generally seek medical attention, with infection confirmed by the detection of virus-specific IgM/IgG in the serum. The acute symptoms can last for weeks to months, however chronic disease associated with RRV infection in some cases has been reported to last up to a year or more (Mylonas *et al.*, 2002).

A survey conducted in southeast Queensland of 67 adult patients with RRV disease found that RRV disease was often severe at onset, with patients presenting predominantly with polyarthralgia. Around one third to one half also experienced rash, fever, myalgia, and/or fatigue. In all but 2% of cases, symptoms resolved over an average 3 to 6-month period. In the 2% of cases, symptoms appeared to last longer than 1 year (Mylonas *et al.*, 2002). These clinical features are common in RRV-infected patients.

2.1.1 Models of RRV disease

A small animal model of RRV-disease has been developed in 20-24 day old C57BL/6 mice (Lidbury *et al.*, 2008; Morrison *et al.*, 2007; Morrison *et al.*, 2006), subcutaneously infected with RRV. The infection progresses with virus titre peaking in the first 24-48 hours post-infection (p.i.), with virus detected in the serum, skeletal muscles and joints, indicative of productive infection. Disease onset is observed by 4-5 days p.i., with clinical disease signs that include ruffled fur and weight loss. By 7-12 days p.i., peak disease is reached, with severe hind limb dysfunction observed to the point of paralysis, loss of grip strength and severe weight loss; at this point viraemia is no longer detectable. The infection elicits an inflammatory response, detectable primarily within the muscle tissues, with severe myositis observed in the skeletal muscle (Figure 1). By 15-21 days p.i., the disease signs resolve, with mice regaining hind limb function and beginning to gain weight. By 30 days p.i. mice show no signs of disease, although myositis is still evident (Figure 1F). Interestingly, histology of the myofibres shows the presence of centralized nuclei indicative of muscle fibre regeneration (Morrison *et al.*, 2006).

2.2 Chikungunya virus (CHIKV)

CHIKV was first isolated during an outbreak of dengue-like fever in Tanzania in 1952 (Robinson, 1955). Due to the similarities in febrile illness, it is possible that CHIKV may have been assumed as dengue fever for hundreds of years (Carey, 1971). The word 'chikungunya' comes from the Makonde language of Tanzania, and means 'that which bends up', which describes the clinical signs of disease frequently observed in CHIKV-infected patients (Griffin, 2007). The current geographical distribution of CHIKV covers the continents of Africa and Asia including India and the islands of the Indian Ocean. The original vector of CHIKV is *Aedes aegypti* with transmission cycles existing between vector and monkeys, however *Aedes albopictus* has been implicated as the vector responsible for a number of the recent outbreaks and the resulting spread of CHIKV into new global regions.

Since its identification in 1952 (Ross, 1956), laboratory-confirmed outbreaks of CHIKV have occurred annually in south and central Africa and South East Asia (Higgs & Ziegler, 2010). Recently, the re-emergence of CHIKV in the French island of La Réunion saw a third of the population infected (more than 250,000 people) (Renault *et al.*, 2007). The virus then rapidly spread to the Indian Ocean, India and South East Asia, with estimates as high as five million reported cases since 2006 (Josseran *et al.*, 2006; Kalantri *et al.*, 2006; Yergolkar *et al.*, 2006). CHIKV cases have also been reported among travellers in Europe and the USA (Liumbruno *et al.*, 2008) with a localised outbreak occurring in Italy (Enserink, 2007). Currently the virus continues to circulate and cause sporadic outbreaks in the Asia Pacific region, the most recent being the 2009 outbreaks in South East Asia affecting more than 100,000 people (Centers-for-Disease-Control-and-Prevention, 15 August 2010; Thavara *et al.*, 2009; Theamboonlers *et al.*, 2009).

Typical symptoms of CHIKV infection are abrupt febrile illness, headache, arthralgia, myalgia and in some cases maculopapular rash. Similar to other alphaviruses the incubation period for CHIKV ranges from 3 to 7 days, and as few as 5% of the CHIKV cases are asymptomatic. The acute signs and symptoms usually resolve in less than 2 weeks, but arthralgia and myalgia may linger for weeks, months or even years (Couderc & Lecuit, 2009; Jaffar-Bandjee *et al.*, 2009). This acute phase of infection is frequently more severe in both newborns and elderly patients who often have an extremely high viral load (Jaffar-Bandjee *et al.*, 2009). As with other alphaviruses the sub-acute phase, defined by the presence of arthralgia and myalgia, appears to be largely modulated by the immune system's response to the invading pathogen. The chronic phase of CHIKV infection has been studied more extensively than that of other alphaviruses and appears to be associated with the persistence of specific IgM and chronic arthralgia/myalgia (Jaffar-Bandjee *et al.*, 2009). It is postulated that the ongoing symptoms may be linked to the virus's capacity to persist in tissues by mechanisms that currently remain ill-characterised.

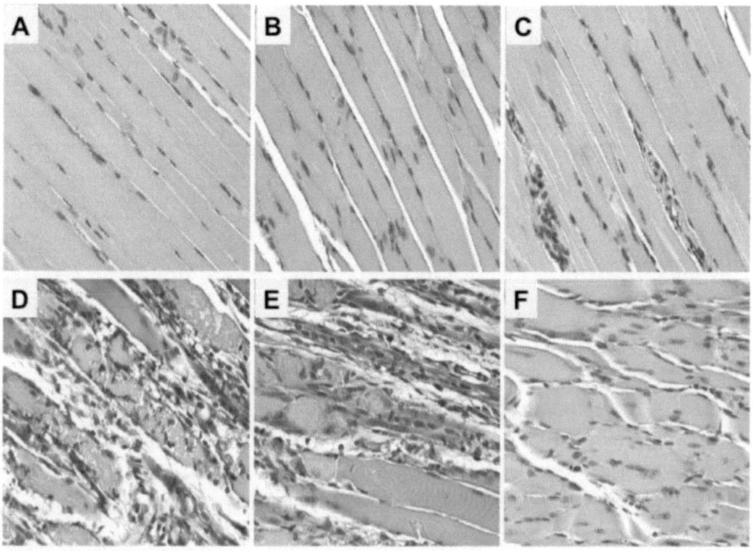

Fig. 1. RRV induces inflammation in hind limb skeletal muscle tissue of C57BL/6 mice. Mice were infected with RRV or mock-infected with diluent (PBS). At 3, 5, 7, 10, and 30 days post-infection (p.i.), mice were sacrificed, quadriceps removed, 5 µm sections generated then H&E stained. (A) Mock infection, (B) RRV 3 days p.i., (C) RRV 5 days p.i., (D) RRV 7 days p.i., (E) RRV 10 days p.i. and (F) RRV 30 days p.i. (magnification, x200). Copyright © 2006, American Society for Microbiology. All Rights Reserved. Journal of Virology, Jan. 2006, p.737–749 Vol. 80, No. 2 0022-538X/06/$08.00_0doi:10.1128/JVI.80.2. 737– 749.2006.

2.2.1 Models of CHIKV disease

Currently three different mouse models of CHIKV infection have been developed. Neonatal C57BL/6 inbred mice and CD-1 outbred mice were found to be susceptible to CHIKV infection, showing an age-dependent disease severity with a model established in 14-day-old mice (Couderc *et al.*, 2008; Morrison *et al.*, 2011; Ziegler *et al.*, 2008). These models show extensive myositis in the skeletal muscle at 7-10 days p.i. during the stage of sub-acute infection (Morrison *et al.*, 2011). Subcutaneous infection of adult C57BL/6 mice leads to a self-limiting disease characterised by arthritis, tenosynovitis and myositis. Histological studies revealed a pronounced infiltration of monocytes, macrophages and natural killer (NK) cells in muscle tissues and synovial membranes indicative of myositis and arthritis (Gardner *et al.*, 2010). Finally, adult mice partially deficient in the type I interferon (IFN) receptor (IFN-α/βR+/-) developed mild CHIKV infection which closely resembles the course of human infection, with virus recovered from muscles, joints and skin (Couderc *et al.*, 2008).

In addition to the use of small animal models, some studies have utilized non-human primates to investigate the mechanisms of CHIKV disease. A model was developed in cynomolgus macaques (*Macaca fascicularis*) to closely mimic the human disease and to test the effectiveness of immunological interventions (Labadie *et al.*, 2010). In this model, viraemia peaked at two days p.i. and subsided by 15 days p.i., with extensive mononuclear cell infiltration in the lymphoid tissues and liver of infected macaques. Long-term infection was also observed, with the virus persisting in the lymphoid organs, liver, joints and muscles. However, the major limitation with this study was the lack of pathology observed in muscle and joint tissues, which is not consistent with observations in humans.

2.3 Sindbis virus (SINV)

SINV is found world-wide and is the most widely distributed of all known arboviruses (Tesh, 1982). It was first identified in 1952, being isolated from *Culex* mosquitoes collected in the village of Sindbis near Cairo (Taylor *et al.*, 1955). The first description of clinical symptoms of SINV infection came from a single case in Uganda in 1961 and included fever, malaise, pains in the joints, muscles and tendons, and rash (Malherbe *et al.*, 1963).

In Europe, SINV is the causative agent of Ockelbo, Pogosta, and Karelian fever, all of which exhibit significant morbidity. These fevers are named according to the regions where they circulate, despite being similar in clinical presentations. The major symptoms in addition to joint and muscle inflammation are fever, fatigue, headache and rash (Laine *et al.*, 2004). The diagnosis is based on the clinical picture and serology. The musculoskeletal symptoms of SINV infection may also continue long-term with chronic SINV-associated disease symptoms being identified in a number of cases 2.5 years after the onset (Laine *et al.*, 2000).

SINV outbreaks occur in Europe in common cycles. In 1981 Sweden reported 54 cases (Ockelbo), Russia 200 cases (Karelian) and Finland 300 cases (Pogosta) of clinically and serologically diagnosed SINV infection (Brummer-Korvenkontio *et al.*, 2002; Espmark & Niklasson, 1984; L'Vov D *et al.*, 1982). Outbreaks of Pogosta disease have thus far emerged every seven years since the first outbreak was noted in 1974, including a large outbreak in 2002 (Sane *et al.*, 2010).

2.3.1 Models of SINV disease

Several mouse models of SINV infection have been developed; one of particular relevance involves the subcutaneous injection of neonatal outbred mice with SINV. In this model, primary replication of the virus occurs in the skin, fibroblasts and connective tissues, followed by systemic viraemia (Johnson, 1965). The SINV-induced inflammatory response is characterised by extensive virus replication in extraneural tissues and induction of high levels of pro-inflammatory cytokines and corticosterone, with mice frequently dying of inflammatory disease by day 5 p.i. (Klimstra *et al.*, 1999; Trgovcich *et al.*, 1996; Trgovcich *et al.*, 1997). Although these studies show the onset of myositis in skeletal muscle, the major limitation of this model is the rapid mortality.

2.4 Other alphaviruses

Barmah Forest virus (BFV) is a closely related alphavirus and shares a similar distribution to RRV. BFV infection is believed to be largely under-diagnosed due to the similarity to RRV in disease presentation and geographic distribution (McGill, 1995). However, the clinical disease presentation of BFV infection has been documented to involve arthralgia and

myalgia, suggesting that this is another alphavirus with the potential for causing an inflammatory myopathy (Jacups *et al.*, 2008).
O'nyong-nyong virus (ONNV) is an alphavirus antigenically related to CHIKV. It was first isolated in East Africa and continues to circulate endemically in Africa producing a similar disease presentation to CHIKV-infection. Between 1959 and 1962 there was a large outbreak of ONNV in East Africa involving an estimated 2 million people in which 71% of infected patients suffered from myalgia (Posey *et al.*, 2005; Williams *et al.*, 1965). In 1996-1997 ONNV re-emerged in south-central Uganda (Kiwanuka *et al.*, 1999) and is another alphavirus with the potential to cause global outbreaks of disease.
Mayaro virus (MAYV) was first isolated in 1954 and is endemic to South America where it causes sporadic cases and smaller outbreaks of disease that manifest with fever, headaches, athralgia and myalgia (Anderson *et al.*, 1957). Cases of MAYV infection and outbreaks have been documented in Trinidad, Surinam, Brazil, Bolivia, French Guinea and Peru (Tesh *et al.*, 1999). Moreover, imported cases of MAYV infection have been recently reported in two European countries demonstrating a potential for this virus to spread to non-endemic areas (Hassing *et al.*, 2010; Receveur *et al.*, 2010). A study of cases of MAYV in Peru by Tesh et al. found myalgia to be a predominant symptom with a prevalence of 77.3%. The strong level of muscle involvement in MAYV infection, coupled with the incidences of MAYV spread into other regions makes this an important virus causing myosits.
Semliki Forest virus (SFV) was first isolated in 1942 in Uganda from *Aedes abnormalis* mosquitoes in the Semliki Forest. Despite SFV being the most extensively studied member of the alphavirus genus, the virus has rarely been documented as causing disease in humans. The few reported cases of human disease have involved headache, arthralgia and myalgia, presentations that are commonly associated with other alphavirus disease manifestation. In 1987 an outbreak of SFV was recorded in the Central African Republic with severe and prolonged myalgia as a major clinical symptom (Mathiot *et al.*, 1990).

3. Tissue tropism and myositis in acute alphavirus infection

During the acute phase of a viral infection the cells and tissues that are infected can affect both the progression and clinical attributes of the disease. In CHIKV infection, skeletal muscle is the primary site of virus infection and replication, resulting in muscle fibre destruction and subsequent myositis. One of the difficulties in studying infection with CHIKV and other alphaviruses is that the incubation period and acute phase of infection, at the onset of primary viraemia, often produces non-specific symptoms that patients do not report and therefore clinicians are rarely able to document the early stages of infection. Furthermore, since alphaviruses produce non-fatal diseases, histopathological studies in humans are generally uncommon.
There have been numerous studies on alphaviral tropism *in vitro*, but these studies can only provide limited information on the mechanisms of the acute phase of infection, as they may not fully relate to the natural course of virus infection *in vivo*. The establishment of animal models of disease, in mice and macaques, has helped in progressing the understanding of alphavirus pathogenesis. In particular, cells derived from muscle tissues have been identified as sites of infection. Infected muscle cells undergo cell death, leading to muscle tissue damage and myositis, which commences at the sub-acute phase of infection.

3.1 Models of acute alphavirus infection *in vivo*

In animal models of RRV and CHIKV infection, virus initially replicates at the site of inoculation before being disseminated through the blood stream to other tissues such as skeletal muscle and joint tissues (Gardner *et al.*, 2010; Labadie *et al.*, 2010; Morrison *et al.*, 2011; Morrison *et al.*, 2006). Replication in skeletal muscle results in severe necrotic myositis with extensive myofibre destruction (Couderc & Lecuit, 2009). The damage to the skeletal muscle was clearly demonstrated using Evan's Blue dye (EBD) staining of affected tissues. EBD is commonly used to identify disrupted tissues as the tissues become permeable to EBD uptake. Following viral infection and replication, muscle tissues exhibit extensive tissue destruction, shown by prominent EBD staining (Figure 2). The occurrence of tissue pathology following viral infection and replication may correspond to the onset of myositis.

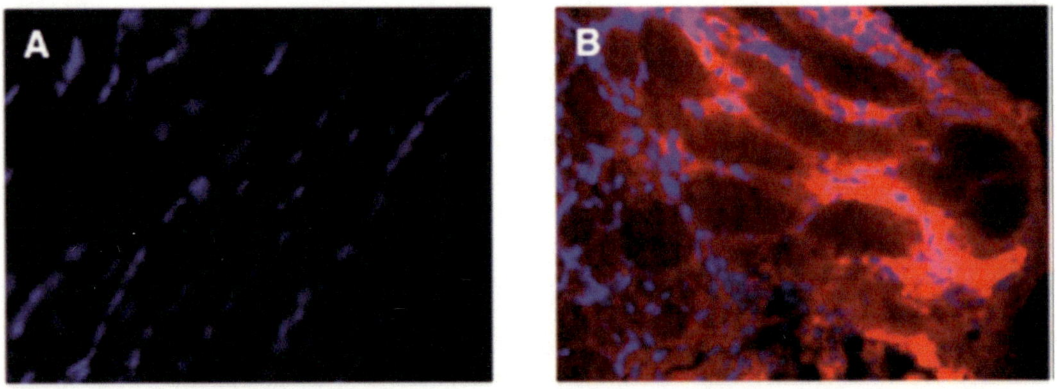

Fig. 2. RRV-infection causes skeletal tissue damage in mice. C57BL/6 mice were mock-infected (A) or infected with RRV (B). At 10 days p.i. mice were injected with 1% Evans Blue dye (EBD) and six hours later mice were sacrificed, quadriceps muscle removed and 10 µm cryosections generated. The uptake of EBD (red) and DAPI (blue; for nuclei staining) was visualised by fluorescence microscopy (magnification, x200).

Within the skeletal muscle, the cells targeted by the virus have been identified as fibroblasts and muscle satellite cells. In CHIKV-infected IFN-α/β receptor deficient mice, fibroblasts within the skeletal muscles and joint connective tissues were found to be the main target for infection (Couderc *et al.*, 2008). Analysis of CHIKV-infected human muscle, joint and skin biopsy samples confirmed these observations, with fibroblasts and muscle satellite cells identified as major targets in peripheral tissues (Couderc & Lecuit, 2009; Ozden *et al.*, 2007).

3.2 Cells susceptible to alphavirus infection *in vitro*

There are a number of *in vitro* studies demonstrating the permissibility of various cells to alphavirus infection. Although these studies have limitations, they provide insight into the cell types that may be the target of infection *in vivo*. CHIKV and RRV are known to infect cells of epithelial and fibrobast origin and some immune cells (Sourisseau *et al.*, 2007).
Myogenic progenitor cells have been shown to be permissive to CHIKV infection (Ozden *et al.*, 2007). A study by Sourisseau et al., characterised permissibility to CHIKV infection in a number of human cell types. The study demonstrated that several cells that can be found within muscle tissues such as primary fibroblasts, endothelial cells and immune cells such as monocyte-derived macrophages were susceptible to CHIKV infection (Sourisseau *et al.*,

2007). Virus infection and replication in these cells *in vitro* results in rapid shut down of host cell transcription and translation resulting in cytopathic effect (CPE) and cell death. Studies of CHIKV in epithelial (HeLa) cells *in vitro* have shown infection can lead to apoptosis which may help explain the destruction of muscle fibres seen *in vivo* (Sourisseau et al., 2007).

4. Sub-acute alphavirus infection and myositis

Severe forms of alphavirus disease result in chronic incapacitating myalgia, arthralgia and arthritis. One of the major reasons for the lack of information on the mechanisms of how these viruses cause musculoskeletal disease is due to the absence of studies in humans. Patients often only report on the symptoms they feel, and in most cases the acute phase of infection often go unreported, and the full extent of the disease not properly documented. One of the key questions is whether the symptoms of arthralgia and myalgia are a result of myositis and if so, how is the inflammatory process triggered. In recent years, the use of animal models of alphaviral-induced disease has assisted in unraveling the pathobiology of infection. By combining the clinical findings from human cases with findings from animal models, a clearer understanding of how alphaviruses cause myalgia and myositis is emerging (see Figure 3 for an overview).

4.1 Clinical observations for sub-acute alphavirus induced myopathies

There have been several studies on the clinical presentation of RRV disease, however most of these studies have focused largely on clinical reports based on patient feedback and limited biochemical and immunological analyses of patient's blood. There have been a limited number of studies on human synovial tissues. These studies have focused on the synovial fluid to determine the nature of the cellular infiltrates (Fraser, 1986; Fraser *et al.*, 1981). Unfortunately, these studies did not extend to muscle tissues. Similarly, studies on human SINV infection with Pogosta disease mainly involved analysis of human serum for antibody and viral antigen detection.

Human CHIKV infection has been clinically well documented (Chow *et al.*, 2011; Pialoux *et al.*, 2007; Powers & Logue, 2007; Simon *et al.*, 2007; Sissoko *et al.*, 2010; Taubitz *et al.*, 2007). The serology profile during the course of infection has been documented by numerous studies, showing that viraemia lasts 5-7 days (acute infection), with a subsequent IgM+/IgG- sub-acute infection progressing for a further week until IgG antibodies are detected and in some cases IgM was still detectable (Staikowsky *et al.*, 2009). Interestingly, it has been reported that levels of IgM have remained high for months and even years in many cases of alphavirus infection (Chopra *et al.*, 2008; Kurkela *et al.*, 2005; Niklasson *et al.*, 1988). In addition, it has been suggested that the presence of IgM may serve as a marker for viral persistence, whereby latent infection may be linked to the long term disease sequelae and chronic pathologies associated with alphavirus infection, including the on-going inflammatory myopathies (Jaffar-Bandjee *et al.*, 2009)

A study by Ozden et al., analysed muscle biopsies of CHIKV-infected patients providing new insight into CHIKV pathogenesis in muscle tissues (Ozden *et al.*, 2007). Patients were either IgM+ or IgG+ without detectable viraemia and were therefore classified as being in the sub-acute or recurring stage of infection. In a CHIKV patient presenting with recurrent symptoms including fever, arthralgia and myalgia, histological analysis of muscle biopsies demonstrated atrophy and necrosis (Figure 4A and 4D) and vacuolization of muscle fibres (Figure 4B) and interstitial mixed acute and chronic inflammation (Figure 4C). Viral antigens were detected in the periphery of muscle fibres in single cells (Figure 5B, 5C) or in groups of cells (Figure 5A, 5D). Viral antigen was also detected (to lower levels) in the muscle biopsy of a patient with recurrent infection (Figure 5F), indicating that muscle satellite cells may harbour persistent alphaviral infection.

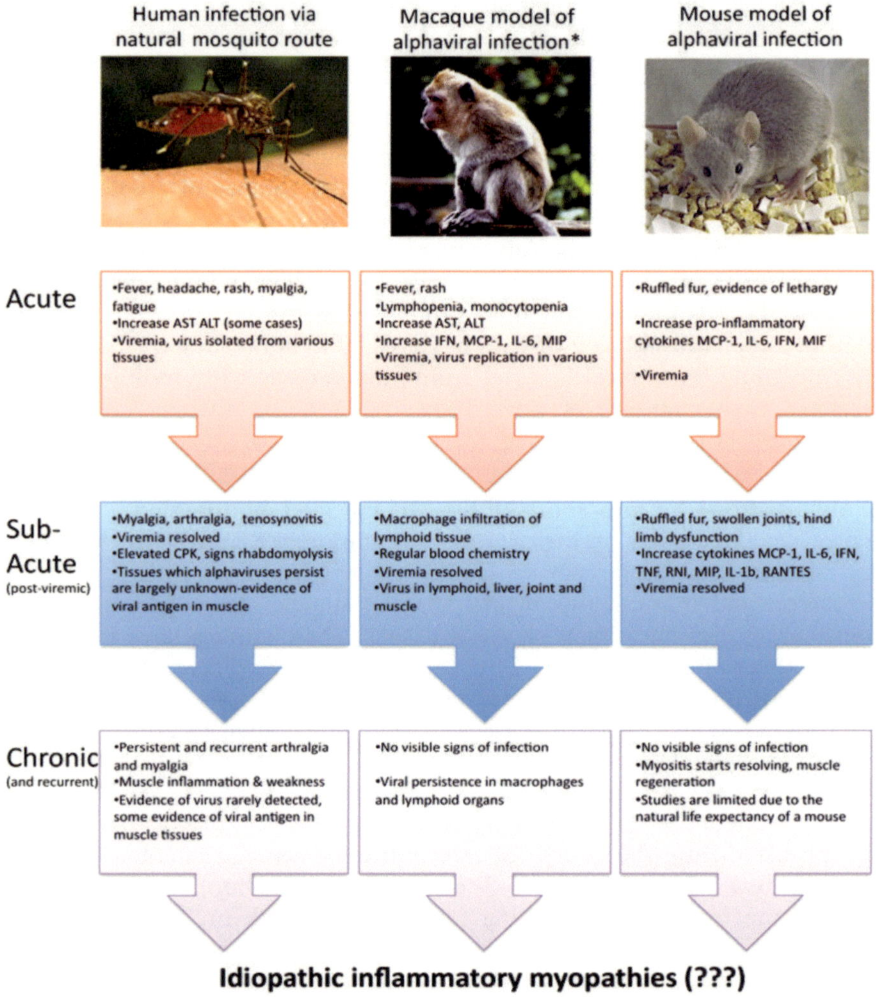

*Modeled on CHIKV infection (Labadie et al., 2010)

Fig. 3. Comparison of symptoms resulting from naturally human alphavirus infection, laboratory-infected nonhuman primate model of CHIKV, and laboratory-infected alphavirus mouse-models. Infection is broken down into three stages: acute, sub-acute, and chronic. The acute phase is defined by the presence of viraemia, the sub-acute phase is defined by the presence of IgM+ antibodies and the chronic phase is defined by IgG+ conversion. The chronic phase in humans includes persistent and recurrent myalgia and arthralgia that can last for months to years and may possibly result in symptoms synonymous with idiopathic inflammatory myopathies. Aspartate transaminase (AST) and alanine transaminase (ALT), monocyte chemoattractant protein (MCP)-1, tumour necrosis factor (TNF), interferon (IFN), Interleukin (IL), macrophage inflammatory protein (MIP), RANTES (CCL5) and reactive nitrogen intermediates (RNI).

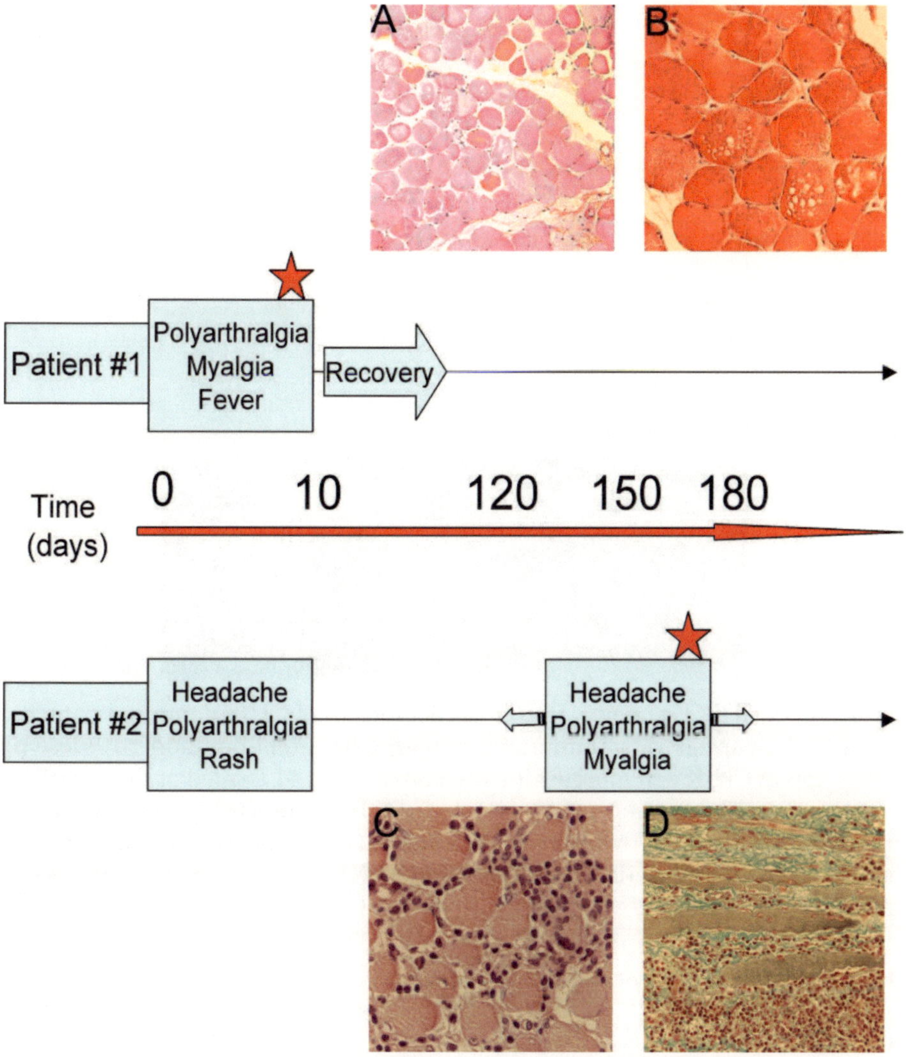

Fig. 4. Time-course and histopathological data concerning CHIKV-infected patients. Patient #1, quadriceps biopsy was obtained during the CHIKV epidemic outbreak in the Reunion Island, presented a classical clinical picture of CHIKV infection. In addition, signs of rhabdomyolysis were reported. The muscle biopsy was performed on the quadriceps muscle 10 days post disease onset (illustrated by the red star). Patient #2 complained, in January 2006, of headaches, arthralgia and a rash; around three months later, she was admitted to hospital with a classical clinical picture of CHIKV infection, including myalgia. A biopsy was performed in the quadriceps muscle during this recurrent phase of the disease (red star). (A) and (B): Sections from the muscle biopsy of patient #1 H&E stained. (A) at x60 magnification showing lack of cellular infiltrates. Atrophy and necrosis of muscle fibres could be seen, as well as central nuclei (arrow). (B): at x140 magnification showing vacuolization of muscle fibres. (C) and (D): Sections from the muscle of patient #2 showing an important mononuclear infiltration in H&E stained at x140 magnification (C) and fibrosis in Masson's trichrome stained sections at x80 magnification (D). © 2007 Ozden et al., 2007.

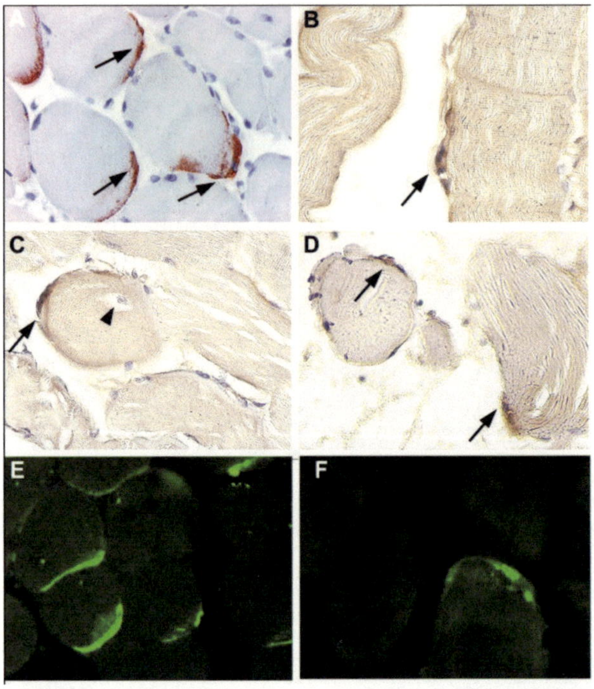

Fig. 5. Detection of CHIKV antigens from muscle biopsies of CHIKV infected patients. Detection of CHIKV antigens by immunofluorescence (IF) and immunoperoxydase (IP). (A–D): Detection of CHIKV in muscle biopsys from patient #1 located at the periphery of the myotubes, as multiple cells per microscopic field (A, D), or as single cell per field (B, C). Some immunoreactive cells (arrows) were detected at the periphery of muscle fibres with central nuclei (C, arrowhead). (E, F): Detection of CHIKV by IF in muscle biopsy sections from patient #1 (E) and #2 (F). Magnification: ×300(A,C,D,E,F); ×400(B). © 2007 Ozden et al.

4.2 Cellular factors in alphavirus induced myopathies

Histopathological analysis of patients with a range of myopathies has demonstrated inflammatory infiltrates in the muscle tissues, primarily macrophages (Hewer & Goebel, 2008) and mononuclear cells. Infiltration of these cells is characteristic of idiopathic inflammatory myopathies. However, due to the lack of suitable animal models the mechanism by which inflammatory myopathies occur and the role that macrophages and mononuclear cells play in tissue pathology is poorly understood.

In animal models of alphavirus induced disease, the inflammatory response seen in the joint, bone and skeletal muscle tissue following an acute infection is predominantly regulated by the innate immune system (Morrison *et al.*, 2007; Morrison *et al.*, 2006). The inflammatory infiltrates consist of macrophages, NK cells, CD4+ and CD8+ T cells. The key role of macrophages and monocytes in the pathogenesis of alphavirus disease was first identified using the mouse model of RRV infection (Lidbury *et al.*, 2000). The selective depletion of macrophages by treatment of mice with macrophage-toxic agents such as silica or carrageenan, was found to almost entirely abrogate disease and the clearance of macrophages from damaged tissue correlated with recovery (Lidbury *et al.*, 2000). The high degree of macrophage and monocyte infiltration into infected tissues and joints has also been confirmed in the models of CHIKV infection (Gardner *et al.*, 2010; Morrison *et al.*, 2011).

The exact role that macrophages play in mediating disease is an area of ongoing research. It has been shown that infiltrating macrophages are a key mediator of muscle tissue destruction by mechanisms which involve the production of soluble factors such as macrophage inflammatory protein (MIP)-1, IFN-γ, interleukin (IL)-1β, reactive nitogen intermediates (RNI), tumour necrosis factor (TNF)-α, and monocyte chemoattractant protein (MCP)-1 (Lidbury *et al.*, 2008). In the macaque model of CHIKV infection, an up-regulation of IFN-α/β, IFN-γ, MCPs, IL-6 and TNF-α was detected, all synonymous with a strong, macrophage-induced inflammatory response (Labadie *et al.*, 2010). IL-1β, RNI and TNF-α are factors known to trigger apoptosis (Bhaumik & Khar, 1998; Griffin & Hardwick, 1997; Roulston *et al.*, 1999) while MCP-1 and MIP-1 are involved in amplifying the inflammatory response (Carr *et al.*, 1994; Lidbury *et al.*, 2008; Ren *et al.*, 2010; Wolpe *et al.*, 1988).

Macrophages have also been implicated as a cellular reservoir for alphavirus persistence and therefore a contributing factor in the development of chronic disease symptoms. There have been numerous studies showing long-term persistence of RRV in macrophages *in vitro* (Linn *et al.*, 1996; Linn *et al.*, 1998; Way *et al.*, 2002) however how this pertains to human infection is largely unknown. Recently, the study by Labadie et al., has shown macrophages act as a cellular reservoir for the persistence of CHIKV during the late stages of infection in macaques. This is the first *in vivo* study to show that CHIKV persistence in macrophages may be responsible for the long-lasting symptoms observed in humans. A study of viral persistence in macrophages during human infection has demonstrated evidence of CHIKV antigens in perivascular synovial macrophages in a CHIKV patient 18 months after the initial infection (Hoarau *et al.*, 2010). Thus, it is reasonable to speculate that viral persistence in macrophages may trigger low levels of macrophage activation long term, which may contribute to chronic disease symptoms.

To investigate the role of both T cells and the adaptive immune system in the development of RRV disease, studies were done on RAG-1 deficient mice, which lack functional T and B lymphocytes. Morrison et al., infected RAG-1 deficient with RRV and monitored for clinical signs of disease (Morrison *et al.*, 2006). RAG-1 deficient mice developed disease signs similar to wild-type mice. Histological analysis revealed extensive myositis in the skeletal muscle with the inflammatory infiltrates identified as macrophages and NK cells, similar to observations in wild-type mice. Taken together, the results show that the adaptive immune response does not play a critical role in the development of RRV disease (Morrison *et al.*, 2006). Furthermore, the population of infiltrating CD4+ and CD8+ T cells found in the skeletal muscles of wild-type mice does not appear to play a role in the development of myositis as the absence of T and/or B cell functions does not affect disease development or outcome. Similar studies have been done using SINV infection in immunodeficient SCID or RAG-1 deficient mice. The studies found the clinical outcomes of SINV infection in immunodeficient neonatal mice to be comparable to that in immunocompetent neonatal mice (Burdeinick-Kerr *et al.*, 2009; Levine & Griffin, 1993). Results of these studies suggest that the adaptive immune response does not play a role in the development of RRV-induced myositis and is not essential in the clinical outcome of alphaviral disease.

4.3 Soluble factors in alphavirus induced myopathies

There have been limited studies on the measurement of pro-inflammatory factors in serum and synovial aspirates taken from confirmed cases of RRV infection. The levels of complement factor C3a, MCP-1, TNF-α, IFN-γ and RNI were all elevated in RRV patients

(Lidbury *et al.*, 2008; Morrison *et al.*, 2007). Furthermore, cells obtained from synovial fluid have been found to be mononuclear in nature being mainly monocytes and activated macrophages (Clarris *et al.*, 1975; Fraser *et al.*, 1981). In terms of RRV-induced myopathies, the limitations encountered in studying the pathogenesis in humans, particularly in investigating the role of soluble factors, have been achieved using a mouse model of RRV-disease.

Animal models have been used to determine the role of various cytokines and chemokines in the development of alphaviral-induced myopathies. Studies have shown that IFN-γ, TNF-α, IL-1β, IL-6, macrophage inflammatory protein (MIP)-1α, MCP-1, MCP-2, and MCP-3 are up-regulated in response to RRV infection (Lidbury *et al.*, 2008; Rulli *et al.*, 2009). The high levels of these factors in diseased tissues implicate their role in RRV-induced myositis (Lidbury *et al.*, 2008; Rulli *et al.*, 2009). Recently, a study by Rulli et al., showed that the MCPs inhibitor, bindarit, reduced RRV disease symptoms by decreasing myositis and muscle tissue destruction (Rulli *et al.*, 2009). Bindarit down-regulated the production of chemokines MCP-1, -2 and -3, resulting in the reduction of macrophage recruitment into muscle tissues. These findings suggest a potential application of bindarit in the treatment of alphaviral-induced musculoskeletal disease such as myositis (Rulli *et al.*, 2009).

Several additional soluble factors have also been shown to play a role in the myositis that develops during the sub-acute phase of alphaviral infection. Studies using the RRV mouse model have shown that the complement component 3 (C3) contributes to the destructive phase of the inflammatory disease and promotes the development of severe myositis (Morrison *et al.*, 2008). The main function of the complement system is to eliminate invading organisms. It is activated through a number of different pathways and is centered around the action of the protein C3. In the mouse model of RRV disease, C3 activation products were detected at the sites of RRV-induced inflammation and C3 was found to be critical for myositis and the tissue destruction phase of RRV-induced inflammatory myopathies (Morrison *et al.*, 2007). Furthermore, mice deficient in functional receptor for C3 (CR3; CD11b deficient mice) showed significantly reduced disease symptoms and tissue destruction following RRV infection (Morrison *et al.*, 2008), confirming the critical role of complement in the regulation of inflammatory processes at the site of alphaviral-induced myositis. These studies show complement to be a potential target for anti-viral therapies in treating alphavirus induced myositis.

Similar to studies with RRV, analysis of serum samples from CHIKV-infected patients has also shown elevated levels of cytokines and chemokines. Of particular interest is the up-regulation of IL-6, TNF-α, IL-1β, IFN-α, interferon-inducible protein-10 (IP-10) and monokine induced by IFN-γ (MIG) (Hoarau *et al.*, 2010; Ng *et al.*, 2009b). There has been an association between high levels of viraemia in acute CHIKV-infected patients and a higher production of pro-inflammatory cytokines such as IL-6 and TNF-α (Chow *et al.*, 2011). Presentation of chronic disease symptoms has also been associated with elevated levels of IL-6 and granulocyte macrophage colony-stimulating factor (GM-CSF)(Chow *et al.*, 2011). Whereas in patients who have fully recovered from disease, high levels of eotaxin and hepatocyte growth factor have been detected (Chow *et al.*, 2011).

Analysis of pro-inflammatory mediators in an adult C57BL/6 mouse model of CHIKV disease revealed an up-regulation in the expression of TNF-α, MCP-1, IFN-γ, IL-6 and IFN-α/β in the sera of infected mice (Gardner *et al.*, 2010). These results were consistent with findings using the macaque model of CHIKV disease where IFNs were shown to play an important role in CHIKV pathogenesis, with IFN-α/β and IFN-γ, along with IL-6 and MCP-1, up-regulated at 2-10 days p.i. (Labadie *et al.*, 2010).

In patients with idiopathic inflammatory myopathies, the levels of several cytokines including MCP-1 and TNF-α are elevated (Bartoli *et al.*, 2001). A large number of studies have suggested a role for IL-1β, IFN-α and TNF-α as mediators of inflammatory myopathies (Lundberg, 2000; Lundberg & Dastmalchi, 2002; Salomonsson & Lundberg, 2006). TNF has been extensively implicated in idiopathic inflammatory myopathies and is a potential therapeutic target. Enbrel® is an anti-TNF-α drug used to treat rheumatoid arthritis; has also given promising results in the treatment of myositis (Sprott *et al.*, 2004). Although TNF is similarly increased in alphavirus disease and myositis, Enbrel® treatment has been shown to both increase virus titre and alphavirus myositis (Zaid *et al.*, 2011). Therefore the use of anti-TNF therapy is not recommended in people presenting with myositis in which alphaviruses have not been ruled out as a potential causative agent.

4.4 Muscle enzymes in alphavirus induced myopathies

In addition to the roles of cytokines and chemokines in mediating alphavirus-induced myositis, muscle enzymes are also implicated in disease. Studies from the Reunion outbreak have found myalgia to be a major symptom of CHIKV infection (Paquet *et al.*, 2006). Elevated levels of creatine phosphokinase (CPK), a muscle enzyme marker for idiopathic inflammatory myopathies, and rhabdomyolysis have been reported in cases of CHIKV-infection (Lundberg, 2001). Ozden et al., analysed muscle biopsies of CHIKV-infected patients and in one case, a CHIKV-infected patient in the sub-acute phase presented with rhabdomyolysis with elevated CPK (41600 IU/mL) in addition to symptoms of myalgia and elevated myoglobin. Demonstrating a similarity between idiopathic inflammatory myopathies and alphavirus-induced myositis (Ozden *et al.*, 2007).

5. Alphaviruses and idiopathic inflammatory myopathies (IIM)

The term idiopathic inflammatory myopathies (IIM) is used to describe myopathy arising from an unknown cause which involves inflammation of the muscles. The term encompasses a group of three related muscles disorders (Polymyositis, Dermatomyositis and Body Inculsion Myositis), which can be distinguished by clinical, histopathological, and immunological features (Lundberg & Dastmalchi, 2002).

Identification of possible triggers for IIM has been the topic of numerous studies with a focus on investigating the potential role of infectious agents in the aetiology of IIM. It has long been suspected that infectious agents may have a direct role in IIM with bacteria and viruses (notably retroviruses and entroviruses) being frequently implicated (Ytterberg, 1996). As muscle inflammation is one of the primary symptoms of the acute and sub-acute stages of viral infection, it is thought that the onset of an idiopathic inflammatory myopathy could be triggered by a chronic underlying viral infection.

The ability of alphaviruses to cause persistent and chronic infections has been recently studied with the demonstration of the presence of viral antigens in the muscle and synovial tissue of infected patients (Hoarau *et al.*, 2010; Ozden *et al.*, 2007). Invading pathogens can cause muscle tissue damage in both direct (by means of infection), and indirect (involving immune mediated damage) mechanisms. The question that remains is whether, in cases of IIM where virus antigen is no-longer detected, is it possible that virus persistence at an earlier stage triggers an immune response which continues for prolonged periods? There

have been numerous studies on the potential long-term disease sequelae due to alphavirus infection, suggesting that long-term chronic illness, lasting for years, may occur (Fraser, 1986; Harley *et al.*, 2002; Laine *et al.*, 2000; Mylonas *et al.*, 2002; Niklasson & Espmark, 1986; Niklasson *et al.*, 1988). However these studies have been unable to conclusively demonstrate alphaviruses as the cause of the symptoms presented. A lack of differential diagnosis, combined with potential underdiagnosis of other conditions that may exist concurrently in patients, and the lack of experimental long-term disease models, has led to the uncertainty regarding the level of long-term alphavirus disease.
Current medical practice requires cultures and/or other direct diagnostic tests to confirm the causative agents of infectious myositis. In the absence of such diagnosis the clinical manifestations observed in a patient are termed idiopathic. It is suspected that the time between the primary infection and the related immunological clinical representation is so great that clinicians are ill-equipped to make a proper diagnosis using current medical practices. Therefore what is in reality an infectious myositis becomes inaccurately diagnosed as an idiopathic inflammatory myopathy.

6. Conclusion

The increasing frequency and severity of alphavirus epidemics highlights the importance of these viruses in the incidence of inflammatory myopathies. At present, knowledge is lacking in the clinical aspects of human myositis following alphavirus infections with speculation that virus persistence in the muscle and macrophages may explain the recurrent and chronic symptoms of myalgia. In addition the correlation between a previous exposure to an alphavirus infection and the development of idiopathic inflammatory myopathies is ill-defined, with current diagnostic tests unable to isolate alphaviruses or detect alphavirus antigen in the presenting patient. It is evident that further research is needed to fully understand the aetiology and pathobiology of alphavirus-induced inflammatory myopathies. The establishment of animal models of chronic alphavirus disease would be of immense benefit in bridging the gap in our understanding of the role of viral infections in chronic myositis. Such a model will also be of value in dissecting disease mechanisms as well as investigate new treatment modalities.

7. References

Anderson, C. R., Downs, W. G., Wattley, G. H., Ahin, N. W. & Reese, A. A. (1957). Mayaro virus: a new human disease agent. II. Isolation from blood of patients in Trinidad, B.W.I. *Am J Trop Med Hyg* 6, 1012-1016.

Azevedo, R. S., Silva, E. V., Carvalho, V. L., Rodrigues, S. G., Nunes-Neto, J. P., Monteiro, H., Peixoto, V. S., Chiang, J. O., Nunes, M. R. & Vasconcelos, P. F. (2009). Mayaro fever virus, Brazilian Amazon. *Emerg Infect Dis* 15, 1830-1832.

Bartoli, C., Civatte, M., Pellissier, J. F. & Figarella-Branger, D. (2001). CCR2A and CCR2B, the two isoforms of the monocyte chemoattractant protein-1 receptor are up-regulated and expressed by different cell subsets in idiopathic inflammatory myopathies. *Acta Neuropathol* 102, 385-392.

Bhaumik & Khar (1998). Cytokine-induced production of NO by macrophages induces apoptosis and immunological rejection of AK-5 histiocytic tumor. *Apoptosis* 3, 361-368.

Brummer-Korvenkontio, M., Vapalahti, O., Kuusisto, P., Saikku, P., Manni, T., Koskela, P., Nygren, T., Brummer-Korvenkontio, H. & Vaheri, A. (2002). Epidemiology of Sindbis virus infections in Finland 1981-96: possible factors explaining a peculiar disease pattern. *Epidemiol Infect* 129, 335-345.

Burdeinick-Kerr, R., Govindarajan, D. & Griffin, D. E. (2009). Noncytolytic clearance of sindbis virus infection from neurons by gamma interferon is dependent on Jak/STAT signaling. *J Virol* 83, 3429-3435.

Carey, D. E. (1971). Chikungunya and dengue: a case of mistaken identity? *J Hist Med Allied Sci* 26, 243-262.

Carr, Roth, Luther, Rose & Springer (1994). Monocyte chemoattractant protein1acts as a T-lymphocyte chemoattractant. *ProcNatdAcadSci* 91, 3652-3656.

Centers-for-Disease-Control-and-Prevention (15 August 2010). Chikungunya fever in Asia and the Indian Ocean. In *Outbreak Notice*.

Chopra, A., Anuradha, V., Lagoo-Joshi, V., Kunjir, V., Salvi, S. & Saluja, M. (2008). Chikungunya virus aches and pains: an emerging challenge. *Arthritis Rheum* 58, 2921-2922.

Chow, A., Her, Z., Ong, E. K., Chen, J. M., Dimatatac, F., Kwek, D. J., Barkham, T., Yang, H., Renia, L., Leo, Y. S. & Ng, L. F. (2011). Persistent arthralgia induced by Chikungunya virus infection is associated with interleukin-6 and granulocyte macrophage colony-stimulating factor. *J Infect Dis* 203, 149-157.

Clarris, B. J., Doherty, R. L., Fraser, J. R., French, E. L. & Muirden, K. D. (1975). Epidemic polyarthritis: a cytological, virological and immunochemical study. *Aust N Z J Med* 5, 450-457.

Couderc, T., Chretien, F., Schilte, C., Disson, O., Brigitte, M., Guivel-Benhassine, F., Touret, Y., Barau, G., Cayet, N., Schuffenecker, I., Despres, P., Arenzana-Seisdedos, F., Michault, A., Albert, M. L. & Lecuit, M. (2008). A mouse model for Chikungunya: young age and inefficient type-I interferon signaling are risk factors for severe disease. *PLoS Pathog* 4, e29.

Couderc, T. & Lecuit, M. (2009). Focus on Chikungunya pathophysiology in human and animal models. *Microbes Infect* 11, 1197-1205.

Enserink, M. (2007). Epidemiology. Tropical disease follows mosquitoes to Europe. *Science* 317, 1485.

Espmark, A. & Niklasson, B. (1984). Ockelbo disease in Sweden: epidemiological, clinical, and virological data from the 1982 outbreak. *Am J Trop Med Hyg* 33, 1203-1211.

Fraser, J. R. (1986). Epidemic polyarthritis and Ross River virus disease. *Clin Rheum Dis* 12, 369-388.

Fraser, J. R., Cunningham, A. L., Clarris, B. J., Aaskov, J. G. & Leach, R. (1981). Cytology of synovial effusions in epidemic polyarthritis. *Aust N Z J Med* 11, 168-173.

Gardner, J., Anraku, I., Le, T. T., Larcher, T., Major, L., Roques, P., Schroder, W. A., Higgs, S. & Suhrbier, A. (2010). Chikungunya virus arthritis in adult wild-type mice. *J Virol* 84, 8021-8032.

Griffin, D. E. (2007). Alphaviruses. In *Fields virology*, 5th edn, pp. 1023-1059. Edited by D. M. Knipe: Lippincott Williams & Wilkins.

Griffin, D. E. & Hardwick, J. M. (1997). Regulators of apoptosis on the road to persistent alphavirus infection. *Annu Rev Microbiol* 51, 565-592.

Hapuarachchi, H. C., Bandara, K. B., Sumanadasa, S. D., Hapugoda, M. D., Lai, Y. L., Lee, K. S., Tan, L. K., Lin, R. T., Ng, L. F., Bucht, G., Abeyewickreme, W. & Ng, L. C. (2010). Re-emergence of Chikungunya virus in South-east Asia: virological evidence from Sri Lanka and Singapore. *J Gen Virol* 91, 1067-1076.

Harley, D., Bossingham, D., Purdie, D. M., Pandeya, N. & Sleigh, A. C. (2002). Ross River virus disease in tropical Queensland: evolution of rheumatic manifestations in an inception cohort followed for six months. *Med J Aust* 177, 352-355.

Harley, D., Sleigh, A. & Ritchie, S. (2001). Ross River virus transmission, infection, and disease: a cross-disciplinary review. *Clin Microbiol Rev* 14, 909-932, table of contents.

Hassing, R. J., Leparc-Goffart, I., Blank, S. N., Thevarayan, S., Tolou, H., van Doornum, G. & van Genderen, P. J. (2010). Imported Mayaro virus infection in the Netherlands. *J Infect* 61, 343-345.

Hewer, E. & Goebel, H. H. (2008). Myopathology of non-infectious inflammatory myopathies - the current status. *Pathol Res Pract* 204, 609-623.

Higgs, S. & Ziegler, S. A. (2010). A nonhuman primate model of chikungunya disease. *J Clin Invest* 120, 657-660.

Hoarau, J. J., Jaffar Bandjee, M. C., Krejbich Trotot, P., Das, T., Li-Pat-Yuen, G., Dassa, B., Denizot, M., Guichard, E., Ribera, A., Henni, T., Tallet, F., Moiton, M. P., Gauzere, B. A., Bruniquet, S., Jaffar Bandjee, Z., Morbidelli, P., Martigny, G., Jolivet, M., Gay, F., Grandadam, M., Tolou, H., Vieillard, V., Debre, P., Autran, B. & Gasque, P. (2010). Persistent chronic inflammation and infection by Chikungunya arthritogenic alphavirus in spite of a robust host immune response. *J Immunol* 184, 5914-5927.

Jacups, S. P., Whelan, P. I. & Currie, B. J. (2008). Ross River virus and Barmah Forest virus infections: a review of history, ecology, and predictive models, with implications for tropical northern Australia. *Vector Borne Zoonotic Dis* 8, 283-297.

Jaffar-Bandjee, M. C., Das, T., Hoarau, J. J., Krejbich Trotot, P., Denizot, M., Ribera, A., Roques, P. & Gasque, P. (2009). Chikungunya virus takes centre stage in virally induced arthritis: possible cellular and molecular mechanisms to pathogenesis. *Microbes Infect* 11, 1206-1218.

Johnson, R. T. (1965). Virus invasion of the central nervous system: a study of sindbis virus infection in the mouse using fluorescent antibody. *Am J Pathol* 46, 929-943.

Johnston, R. E. & Peters, C. J. (1996). *Alphaviruses*. Philadelphia, Pa: Lippincott-Raven Publishers.

Josseran, L., Paquet, C., Zehgnoun, A., Caillere, N., Le Tertre, A., Solet, J. L. & Ledrans, M. (2006). Chikungunya disease outbreak, Reunion Island. *Emerg Infect Dis* 12, 1994-1995.

Kalantri, S. P., Joshi, R. & Riley, L. W. (2006). Chikungunya epidemic: an Indian perspective. *Natl Med J India* 19, 315-322.

Kiwanuka, N., Sanders, E. J., Rwaguma, E. B., Kawamata, J., Ssengooba, F. P., Najjemba, R., Were, W. A., Lamunu, M., Bagambisa, G., Burkot, T. R., Dunster, L., Lutwama, J. J., Martin, D. A., Cropp, C. B., Karabatsos, N., Lanciotti, R. S., Tsai, T. F. & Campbell, G. L. (1999). O'nyong-nyong fever in south-central Uganda, 1996-1997: clinical features and validation of a clinical case definition for surveillance purposes. *Clin Infect Dis* 29, 1243-1250.

Klimstra, W. B., Ryman, K. D., Bernard, K. A., Nguyen, K. B., Biron, C. A. & Johnston, R. E. (1999). Infection of neonatal mice with sindbis virus results in a systemic inflammatory response syndrome. *J Virol* 73, 10387-10398.

Kurkela, S., Manni, T., Myllynen, J., Vaheri, A. & Vapalahti, O. (2005). Clinical and laboratory manifestations of Sindbis virus infection: prospective study, Finland, 2002-2003. *J Infect Dis* 191, 1820-1829.

Kurkela, S., Manni, T., Vaheri, A. & Vapalahti, O. (2004). Causative agent of Pogosta disease isolated from blood and skin lesions. *Emerg Infect Dis* 10, 889-894.

L'Vov D, K., Skvortsova, T. M., Kondrashina, N. G., Vershinskii, B. V. & Lesnikov, A. L. (1982). [Etiology of Karelia fever--a new arbovirus infection]. *Vopr Virusol* 27, 690-692.

Labadie, K., Larcher, T., Joubert, C., Mannioui, A., Delache, B., Brochard, P., Guigand, L., Dubreil, L., Lebon, P., Verrier, B., de Lamballerie, X., Suhrbier, A., Cherel, Y., Le Grand, R. & Roques, P. (2010). Chikungunya disease in nonhuman primates involves long-term viral persistence in macrophages. *J Clin Invest* 120, 894-906.

Laine, M., Luukkainen, R., Jalava, J., Ilonen, J., Kuusisto, P. & Toivanen, A. (2000). Prolonged arthritis associated with sindbis-related (Pogosta) virus infection. *Rheumatology (Oxford)* 39, 1272-1274.

Laine, M., Luukkainen, R. & Toivanen, A. (2004). Sindbis viruses and other alphaviruses as cause of human arthritic disease. *J Intern Med* 256, 457-471.

Lanciotti, R. S., Ludwig, M. L., Rwaguma, E. B., Lutwama, J. J., Kram, T. M., Karabatsos, N., Cropp, B. C. & Miller, B. R. (1998). Emergence of epidemic O'nyong-nyong fever in Uganda after a 35-year absence: genetic characterization of the virus. *Virology* 252, 258-268.

Levine, B. & Griffin, D. E. (1993). Molecular analysis of neurovirulent strains of Sindbis virus that evolve during persistent infection of scid mice. *J Virol* 67, 6872-6875.

Lidbury, B. A., Rulli, N. E., Suhrbier, A., Smith, P. N., McColl, S. R., Cunningham, A. L., Tarkowski, A., van Rooijen, N., Fraser, R. J. & Mahalingam, S. (2008). Macrophage-derived proinflammatory factors contribute to the development of arthritis and myositis after infection with an arthrogenic alphavirus. *J Infect Dis* 197, 1585-1593.

Lidbury, B. A., Simeonovic, C., Maxwell, G. E., Marshall, I. D. & Hapel, A. J. (2000). Macrophage-induced muscle pathology results in morbidity and mortality for Ross River virus-infected mice. *J Infect Dis* 181, 27-34.

Linn, M. L., Aaskov, J. G. & Suhrbier, A. (1996). Antibody-dependent enhancement and persistence in macrophages of an arbovirus associated with arthritis. *J Gen Virol* 77, 407–411.

Linn, M. L., Mateo, L., Gardner, J. & Suhrbier, A. (1998). Alphavirus-specific cytotoxic T lymphocytes recognize a cross-reactive epitope from the capsid protein and can eliminate virus from persistently infected macrophages. *J Virol* 72, 5146-5153.

Liumbruno, G. M., Calteri, D., Petropulacos, K., Mattivi, A., Po, C., Macini, P., Tomasini, I., Zucchelli, P., Silvestri, A. R., Sambri, V., Pupella, S., Catalano, L., Piccinini, V., Calizzani, G. & Grazzini, G. (2008). The Chikungunya epidemic in Italy and its repercussion on the blood system. *Blood Transfus* 6, 199-210.

Lundberg, I. E. (2000). The role of cytokines, chemokines, and adhesion molecules in the pathogenesis of idiopathic inflammatory myopathies. *Curr Rheumatol Rep* 2, 216-224.

Lundberg, I. E. (2001). The physiology of inflammatory myopathies: an overview. *Acta Physiol Scand* 171, 207-213.

Lundberg, I. E. & Dastmalchi, M. (2002). Possible pathogenic mechanisms in inflammatory myopathies. *Rheum Dis Clin North Am* 28, 799-822.

Malherbe, H., Strickland-Cholmley, M. & Jackson, A. L. (1963). Sindbis virus infection in man. Report of a case with recovery of virus from skin lesions. *S Afr Med J* 37, 547-552.

Mathiot, C. C., Grimaud, G., Garry, P., Bouquety, J. C., Mada, A., Daguisy, A. M. & Georges, A. J. (1990). An outbreak of human Semliki Forest virus infections in Central African Republic. *Am J Trop Med Hyg* 42, 386-393.

McGill, P. E. (1995). Viral infections: alpha-viral arthropathy. *Baillieres Clin Rheumatol* 9, 145-150.

Morrison, T. E., Fraser, R. J., Smith, P. N., Mahalingam, S. & Heise, M. T. (2007). Complement contributes to inflammatory tissue destruction in a mouse model of Ross River virus-induced disease. *J Virol* 81, 5132-5143.

Morrison, T. E., Oko, L., Montgomery, S. A., Whitmore, A. C., Lotstein, A. R., Gunn, B. M., Elmore, S. A. & Heise, M. T. (2011). A mouse model of chikungunya virus-induced musculoskeletal inflammatory disease: evidence of arthritis, tenosynovitis, myositis, and persistence. *Am J Pathol* 178, 32-40.

Morrison, T. E., Simmons, J. D. & Heise, M. T. (2008). Complement receptor 3 promotes severe ross river virus-induced disease. *J Virol* 82, 11263-11272.

Morrison, T. E., Whitmore, A. C., Shabman, R. S., Lidbury, B. A., Mahalingam, S. & Heise, M. T. (2006). Characterization of Ross River virus tropism and virus-induced inflammation in a mouse model of viral arthritis and myositis. *J Virol* 80, 737-749.

Mylonas, A. D., Brown, A. M., Carthew, T. L., McGrath, B., Purdie, D. M., Pandeya, N., Vecchio, P. C., Collins, L. G., Gardner, I. D., de Looze, F. J., Reymond, E. J. & Suhrbier, A. (2002). Natural history of Ross River virus-induced epidemic polyarthritis. *Med J Aust* 177, 356-360.

Ng, L. C., Tan, L. K., Tan, C. H., Tan, S. S., Hapuarachchi, H. C., Pok, K. Y., Lai, Y. L., Lam-Phua, S. G., Bucht, G., Lin, R. T., Leo, Y. S., Tan, B. H., Han, H. K., Ooi, P. L., James, L. & Khoo, S. P. (2009a). Entomologic and virologic investigation of Chikungunya, Singapore. *Emerg Infect Dis* 15, 1243-1249.

Ng, L. F., Chow, A., Sun, Y. J., Kwek, D. J., Lim, P. L., Dimatatac, F., Ng, L. C., Ooi, E. E., Choo, K. H., Her, Z., Kourilsky, P. & Leo, Y. S. (2009b). IL-1beta, IL-6, and RANTES as biomarkers of Chikungunya severity. *PLoS One* 4, e4261.

Niklasson, B. & Espmark, A. (1986). Ockelbo disease: arthralgia 3-4 years after infection with a Sindbis virus related agent. *Lancet* 1, 1039-1040.

Niklasson, B., Espmark, A. & Lundstrom, J. (1988). Occurrence of arthralgia and specific IgM antibodies three to four years after Ockelbo disease. *J Infect Dis* 157, 832-835.

Old, J. M. & Deane, E. M. (2005). Antibodies to the Ross River virus in captive marsupials in urban areas of eastern New South Wales, Australia. *J Wildl Dis* 41, 611-614.

Oliveira, N. M., Broom, A. K., Mackenzie, J. S., Smith, D. W., Lindsay, M. D., Kay, B. H. & Hall, R. A. (2006). Epitope-blocking enzyme-linked immunosorbent assay for detection of antibodies to Ross River virus in vertebrate sera. *Clin Vaccine Immunol* 13, 814-817.

Ozden, S., Huerre, M., Riviere, J. P., Coffey, L. L., Afonso, P. V., Mouly, V., de Monredon, J., Roger, J. C., El Amrani, M., Yvin, J. L., Jaffar, M. C., Frenkiel, M. P., Sourisseau, M., Schwartz, O., Butler-Browne, G., Despres, P., Gessain, A. & Ceccaldi, P. E. (2007). Human muscle satellite cells as targets of Chikungunya virus infection. *PLoS One* 2, e527.

Paquet, C., Quatresous, I., Solet, J. L., Sissoko, D., Renault, P., Pierre, V., Cordel, H., Lassalle, C., Thiria, J., Zeller, H. & Schuffnecker, I. (2006). Chikungunya outbreak in Reunion: epidemiology and surveillance, 2005 to early January 2006. *Euro Surveill* 11, E060202 060203.

Pialoux, G., Gauzere, B. A., Jaureguiberry, S. & Strobel, M. (2007). Chikungunya, an epidemic arbovirosis. *Lancet Infect Dis* 7, 319-327.

Pinheiro, F. P., Freitas, R. B., Travassos da Rosa, J. F., Gabbay, Y. B., Mello, W. A. & LeDuc, J. W. (1981). An outbreak of Mayaro virus disease in Belterra, Brazil. I. Clinical and virological findings. *Am J Trop Med Hyg* 30, 674-681.

Posey, D. L., O'Rourke, T., Roehrig, J. T., Lanciotti, R. S., Weinberg, M. & Maloney, S. (2005). O'Nyong-nyong fever in West Africa. *Am J Trop Med Hyg* 73, 32.

Powers, A. M. & Logue, C. H. (2007). Changing patterns of chikungunya virus: re-emergence of a zoonotic arbovirus. *J Gen Virol* 88, 2363-2377.

Receveur, M., Ezzedine, K., Pistone, T. & Malvy, D. (2010). Chikungunya infection in a French traveller returning from the Maldives, October, 2009. *Euro Surveill* 15, 19494.

Ren, Guo, Guo, Lenz, Qian, Koenen & al, e. (2010). Polymerization of MIP-1 chemokine (CCL3 and CCL4) and clearance of MIP-1 by insulin-degrading enzyme. *The EMBO Journal* 29, 3952-3966.

Renault, P., Solet, J. L., Sissoko, D., Balleydier, E., Larrieu, S., Filleul, L., Lassalle, C., Thiria, J., Rachou, E., de Valk, H., Ilef, D., Ledrans, M., Quatresous, I., Quenel, P. & Pierre, V. (2007). A major epidemic of chikungunya virus infection on Reunion Island, France, 2005-2006. *Am J Trop Med Hyg* 77, 727-731.

Robinson, M. C. (1955). An epidemic of virus disease in Southern Province, Tanganyika Territory, in 1952-53. I. Clinical features. *Trans R Soc Trop Med Hyg* 49, 28-32.

Ross, R. W. (1956). The Newala epidemic. III. The virus: isolation, pathogenic properties and relationship to the epidemic. *J Hyg (Lond)* 54, 177-191.

Roulston, A., Marcellus, R. C. & Branton, P. E. (1999). Viruses and apoptosis. *Annu Rev Microbiol* 53, 577-628.

Rulli, N. E., Guglielmotti, A., Mangano, G., Rolph, M. S., Apicella, C., Zaid, A., Suhrbier, A. & Mahalingam, S. (2009). Amelioration of alphavirus-induced arthritis and myositis in a mouse model by treatment with bindarit, an inhibitor of monocyte chemotactic proteins. *Arthritis Rheum* 60, 2513-2523.

Salomonsson, S. & Lundberg, I. E. (2006). Cytokines in idiopathic inflammatory myopathies. *Autoimmunity* 39, 177-190.

Sane, J., Guedes, S., Kurkela, S., Lyytikainen, O. & Vapalahti, O. (2010). Epidemiological analysis of mosquito-borne Pogosta disease in Finland, 2009. *Euro Surveill* 15.

Simon, F., Parola, P., Grandadam, M., Fourcade, S., Oliver, M., Brouqui, P., Hance, P., Kraemer, P., Ali Mohamed, A., de Lamballerie, X., Charrel, R. & Tolou, H. (2007). Chikungunya infection: an emerging rheumatism among travelers returned from Indian Ocean islands. Report of 47 cases. *Medicine (Baltimore)* 86, 123-137.

Sissoko, D., Ezzedine, K., Moendandze, A., Giry, C., Renault, P. & Malvy, D. (2010). Field evaluation of clinical features during chikungunya outbreak in Mayotte, 2005-2006. *Trop Med Int Health* 15, 600-607.

Skogh, M. & Espmark, A. (1982). Ockelbo disease: epidemic arthritis-exanthema syndrome in Sweden caused by Sindbis-virus like agent. *Lancet* 1, 795-796.

Sourisseau, M., Schilte, C., Casartelli, N., Trouillet, C., Guivel-Benhassine, F., Rudnicka, D., Sol-Foulon, N., Le Roux, K., Prevost, M. C., Fsihi, H., Frenkiel, M. P., Blanchet, F., Afonso, P. V., Ceccaldi, P. E., Ozden, S., Gessain, A., Schuffenecker, I., Verhasselt, B., Zamborlini, A., Saib, A., Rey, F. A., Arenzana-Seisdedos, F., Despres, P., Michault, A., Albert, M. L. & Schwartz, O. (2007). Characterization of reemerging chikungunya virus. *PLoS Pathog* 3, e89.

Sprott, H., Glatzel, M. & Michel, B. A. (2004). Treatment of myositis with etanercept (Enbrel), a recombinant human soluble fusion protein of TNF-alpha type II receptor and IgG1. *Rheumatology (Oxford)* 43, 524-526.

Staikowsky, F., Talarmin, F., Grivard, P., Souab, A., Schuffenecker, I., Le Roux, K., Lecuit, M. & Michault, A. (2009). Prospective study of Chikungunya virus acute infection in the Island of La Reunion during the 2005-2006 outbreak. *PLoS One* 4, e7603.

Suhrbier, A. & La Linn, M. (2004). Clinical and pathologic aspects of arthritis due to Ross River virus and other alphaviruses. *Curr Opin Rheumatol* 16, 374-379.

Taubitz, W., Cramer, J. P., Kapaun, A., Pfeffer, M., Drosten, C., Dobler, G., Burchard, G. D. & Loscher, T. (2007). Chikungunya fever in travelers: clinical presentation and course. *Clin Infect Dis* 45, e1-4.

Taylor, R. M., Hurlbut, H. S., Work, T. H., Kingston, J. R. & Frothingham, T. E. (1955). Sindbis virus: a newly recognized arthropodtransmitted virus. *Am J Trop Med Hyg* 4, 844-862.

Tesh, R. B. (1982). Arthritides caused by mosquito-borne viruses. *Annu Rev Med* 33, 31-40.

Tesh, R. B., Watts, D. M., Russell, K. L., Damodaran, C., Calampa, C., Cabezas, C., Ramirez, G., Vasquez, B., Hayes, C. G., Rossi, C. A., Powers, A. M., Hice, C. L., Chandler, L. J., Cropp, B. C., Karabatsos, N., Roehrig, J. T. & Gubler, D. J. (1999). Mayaro virus disease: an emerging mosquito-borne zoonosis in tropical South America. *Clin Infect Dis* 28, 67-73.

Thavara, U., Tawatsin, A., Pengsakul, T., Bhakdeenuan, P., Chanama, S., Anantapreecha, S., Molito, C., Chompoosri, J., Thammapalo, S., Sawanpanyalert, P. & Siriyasatien, P. (2009). Outbreak of chikungunya fever in Thailand and virus detection in field population of vector mosquitoes, Aedes aegypti (L.) and Aedes albopictus Skuse (Diptera: Culicidae). *Southeast Asian J Trop Med Public Health* 40, 951-962.

Theamboonlers, A., Rianthavorn, P., Praianantathavorn, K., Wuttirattanakowit, N. & Poovorawan, Y. (2009). Clinical and molecular characterization of chikungunya virus in South Thailand. *Jpn J Infect Dis* 62, 303-305.

Trgovcich, J., Aronson, J. F. & Johnston, R. E. (1996). Fatal Sindbis virus infection of neonatal mice in the absence of encephalitis. *Virology* 224, 73-83.

Trgovcich, J., Ryman, K., Extrom, P., Eldridge, J. C., Aronson, J. F. & Johnston, R. E. (1997). Sindbis virus infection of neonatal mice results in a severe stress response. *Virology* 227, 234-238.

Way, S. J., Lidbury, B. A. & Banyer, J. L. (2002). Persistent Ross River virus infection of murine macrophages: an in vitro model for the study of viral relapse and immune modulation during long-term infection. *Virology* 301, 281-292.

Williams, M. C., Woodall, J. P., Corbet, P. S. & Gillett, J. D. (1965). O'nyong-nyong Fever:An epidemic virus disease in East Africa. 8. Virus isolations from Anopheles mosquitoes. *Trans R Soc Trop Med Hyg* 59, 300-306.

Wolpe, S. D., Davatelis, G., Sherry, B., Beutler, B., Hesse, D. G., Nguyen, H. T., Moldawer, L. L., Nathan, C. F., Lowry, S. F. & Cerami, A. (1988). Macrophages secrete a novel heparin-binding protein with inflammatory and neutrophil chemokinetic properties. *J Exp Med* 167, 570–581.

Yergolkar, P. N., Tandale, B. V., Arankalle, V. A., Sathe, P. S., Sudeep, A. B., Gandhe, S. S., Gokhle, M. D., Jacob, G. P., Hundekar, S. L. & Mishra, A. C. (2006). Chikungunya outbreaks caused by African genotype, India. *Emerg Infect Dis* 12, 1580-1583.

Ytterberg, S. R. (1996). Infectious agents associated with myopathies. *Curr Opin Rheumatol* 8, 507-513.

Zaid, A., Rulli, N. E., Rolph, M. S., Suhrbier, A. & Mahalingam, S. (2011). Disease exacerbation by etanercept in a mouse model of alphaviral arthritis and myositis. *Arthritis Rheum* 63, 488-491.

Ziegler, S. A., Lu, L., da Rosa, A. P., Xiao, S. Y. & Tesh, R. B. (2008). An animal model for studying the pathogenesis of chikungunya virus infection. *Am J Trop Med Hyg* 79, 133-139.

4

The Antisynthetase Syndrome

Jan Tore Gran and Øyvind Molberg
Department of Rheumatology, Oslo University Hospital, Rikshospitalet, Oslo, Norway

1. Introduction

The antisynthetase syndrome (ASS) was first described by Marguerie and coworkers in 1990 as a triad of polymyositis, diffuse interstitial lung disease (ILD) and serum autoantibodies to aminoacyl transfer RNA synthetases (anti-ARS) (1). Later, cohort studies have indicated that 20-25 % of patients diagnosed with polymyositis (PM) or dermatomyositis (DM) have anti-ARS antibodies (2-4). In most cases, these anti-ARS+ PM/DM patients also have ILD. The ILD is, in fact, the major determinant of morbidity and mortality in the ASS.

The most common of the anti-ARS, anti-Jo-1, was first described in 1980. Three years later, the Jo-1 antigen was identified as histidyl-tRNA synthetase (5;6). In recent case series, the anti-Jo-1 antibody accounts for 68-87% of the anti-ARS observed in ASS (7-9). The seven other anti-ARS identified (Table 1) are all rare, but their relative frequencies have not been extensively studied (7;8). With very few exceptions, each patient has only one anti-ARS antibody (10). More than half of the anti-ARS+ patients also possess anti-SSA autoantibodies (8;9;11) and then most frequently anti-Ro52 (11).

2. Disease definition

At present, there is no internationally accepted definition of ASS and no classification criteria have been established. Consequently, the clinical characteristics of published ASS cases vary substantially. Some studies have included all patients with anti-ARS, regardless of clinical manifestations, while others have selected patients according to predefined clinical features.

As it is generally agreed upon that ILD is the clinical hallmark of ASS, this clinical feature is regarded mandatory for the diagnosis of ASS by most workers. The finding of ILD in 64-100 % of patients possessing anti-Jo-1 autoantibodies underlines the close association between anti-ARS and ILD (3;9;12-17). In one study (3), anti-ARS were found in 3% of DM without ILD as opposed to 63% in DM with ILD, further emphazising the importance of pulmonary disease in ASS. Thus, ILD is an important but not a compulsory feature of ASS diagnosis.

In ASS, the extent and severity of myopathy may vary considerably (18). Usually, the myositis is less severe than in DM and PM without anti-ARS. Some cases develop clinically overt myositis, others present with hypomyopathic or even amyopathic disease. Thus, a diagnosis of ASS should be considered even in the absence of myositis.

Criteria for the ASS have been proposed recently (19). These criteria suggest that a diagnosis of ASS could be made in the presence of positive serologic testing for an anti-ARS plus one of the following; myositis, ILD, arthritis, fever, Raynaud`s phenomenon or Mechanic`s hands. We feel, however, that ILD and myositis represent the most important clinical features of ASS, hence at least one of them should be included in such classification criteria. It is thus tentatively suggested that a diagnosis of definite ASS should require anti-ARS and either ILD and/or inflammatory myopathy plus at least one other clinical criterion commonly found in this syndrome (Table 2). A diagnosis of probable ASS would be met when either ILD and/or inflammatory is present in a patient with anti-ARS.

3. Epidemiology

ASS is a rare disease, but its frequency in the general population is not known. In most studies, the estimated population prevalence of PM/DM is around 15/100 000 (refs). If 25% of the PM/DM patients have anti-ARS, then the prevalence of the anti-ARS should be least 3-4/100 000. ASS has been reported in both Caucasian, Asian and Afro-American patients, but it is known if the prevalence of the disease differs between ethnic groups.

The age at onset among adults ranges from 19 to 82 years with a mean age at onset varying from 43 to 60 yrs (2;3;9;12;20). Very few children and adolescents with ASS have been reported. A female dominance, with about twice as many females as men affected, has been found in most series (3;9;12).

4. Pathology

Muscle. The results of histological examination of muscle tissue are somewhat conflicting. In one early study (21), the authors demonstrated prominent perimysial inflammation with fragmentation and perifascicular myopathic changes whereas endomysial inflammation was uncommon. Consequently, these findings suggested a dermatomyositis pattern in ASS rather than polymyositis. In subsequent reports, the picture has become less clear as a polymyositis pattern has been more commonly observed than a dermatomyositis pattern (13;22). Some studies have, however, concluded with similar frequencies of polymyositis and dermatomyositis in ASS (8;23). In our own experience, the majority of cases exhibit changes compatible with a diagnosis of dermatomyositis. The frequent occurrence of dermatological lesions to some extent supports a closer relationship to dermatomyositis than to polymyositis. Moreover, the frequent findings of vasculopathic changes at nail fold capillaroscopy may also favor a vasculopathic genesis rather than a myopathic one. Further studies of muscle and vessel pathology in ASS are clearly warranted.

Lung. Limited pathologic case series have shown that the ILD in ASS encompasses various histologic subtypes and both non-specific interstitial pneumonia (NSIP), usual interstitial pneumonia (UIP), cryptogenic organizing pneumonia (COP) and diffuse alveolar damage (DAD) may be diagnosed (20;24;25).

5. Genetics

Most works on the genetics of ASS have been confined to candidate genes in the very polymorphic Human Leukocyte Antigen (HLA) region. All the published studies confirm that the HLA-DRB1*0301, DQA1*0501 and DQB1*0201genes are risk factors for the development of anti-Jo-1+ ASS (7).

6. Disease mechanisms

Already in the 1980's it was speculated that the *in vivo* formation of anti-histidyl tRNA synthetase antibodies was driven by viral infections, possibly through molecular mimicry between viral proteins and histidyl tRNA synthetase (HRS) (26). The basic idea was that the cross-reactive anti-HRS (anti-Jo-1) caused damage through its ability to inhibit HRS and/or through formation of immune complexes . Although never backed by experimental evidence, the viral hypothesis is still highlighted in many reviews on ASS.

More recent studies have focused more on auto-antigenic properties of the HRS molecule per se. A very interesting finding in this respect, was that soluble HRS acted as a chemokine and attracted CD4+ T cells (27). In inflamed tissues marked by cell destruction and high concentrations of free HRS this mechanism could contribute to the breaking of tolerance (27). Another observation has been that HRS expression is upregulated in regenerating muscle cells. Areas with active myositis should thus have very high expression of HRS. Together, these studies indicate that muscle inflammation *per se* may increase the levels of HRS and the likelihood of initiating immune responses to HRS, at least in genetically susceptible individuals. Whether similar mechanisms are operative in the lung is not known, but it has been suggested that HRS adopts a more immunogenic conformation in the lung than in blood cells (28). Previously, it was shown that T cells from the blood of both ASS patients and healthy individuals often recognized HRS (29). No data on T cell or B cell reactivities to HRS in inflamed muscle or lung exist, but CD4+ T cells from the bronchoalveolar lavage fluid of two anti-Jo-1+ ASS patients have been shown to contain the same T cell receptor gene family (30).

7. Clinical features

Disease onset. At onset of disease, respiratory symptoms are present in 40-60 % of patients. In one case series (3), the onset of ILD preceded the onset of myositis in 33%, while myositis and ILD developed simultaneously in 60%. Myositis preceding ILD was observed in only 7% of the patients. At onset of disease, patients may also present with constitutional symptoms such as fever (seen in 35-90% of the patients), loss of appetite and weight loss (2;3;31;32). Other features seen at onset of ASS are joint pain, arthritis, tenosynovitis, and Raynaud`s phenomenon.

Respiratory symptoms. The reported frequency of ILD in ASS varies, depending on patient selection and the sensitivity of the tests applied to detect ILD (18). Most reports indicate that the frequency of ILD in the ASS is in the range of 70-95 % (3;9;12-14;16;31), but some few case series have found lower frequencies (2;33). The frequency of ILD appears to be highest among ASS patients who are anti-PL12 positive, as ILD was diagnosed in 90-100% of PL-12 positives as compared to 50-75% in Jo-1 positives (20;34).

Most frequently, patients complain of shortness of breath and cough. The lung disease may present very acute, subacute or asymptomatic ILD with development of clinically apparent ILD later on. Consequently, the type of onset may be classified into three groups, type I acute, type II gradual and type III asymptomatic. Such a classification may be important for predicting outcome and selecting optimal treatment.

Muscle weakness is reported at onset of disease in 20-50 % of patients. Most commonly, it involves the proximal and axial muscles (31;33). Patients may also report muscular stiffness and pain. The muscular component is thus indistinguishable from that seen in PM and DM.

However, muscle involvement is less frequent and usually milder than in non-ASS patients (18). The reported accumulated incidence of myositis ranges from 40-94% (3).
The tendency to milder myositis among cases with PL-12 was further supported by the findings of a frequency of 60% PL-12 among patients without clinically evident myositis (35). ASS may also present with a hypo- or even amyopathic dermatomyositis pattern.
Skin symptoms. Dermatological features are frequently encountered in ASS, being observed in 7-70% of the various reports (3;9;12;14;32;33). Mechanic`s hands appear as fissuring and scaling of the lateral and distal aspects of the hand, and is rarely seen in conditions other than ASS. In ASS, this clinical feature is seen in 0-32% of cases (3;9;12;31-33). Histological examinations of biopsy specimens of Mechanic`s hands have displayed mononuclear cell infiltrates around the blood vessels and mucin deposition in the dermis (36). As in DM, heliotrophic rash is seen in 7-38% (3;14;31;36). Gottron`s lesions appearing on bony prominences such as finger knockles are observed in 9-69% of patients (3;31;33;36). Microvascular changes presenting as periungual erythema may also be seen (1). Although infrequently reported, V-sign and Shawl-sign may also develop in ASS.
Joint pain or swelling. Arthritis is a frequent clinical manifestation of ASS, being seen in 42-82% of reported cases (2;3;9;12;14;36). Although rare, a subluxating arthropathy involving the distal joints of the fingers (37) is a rather characteristic feature of ASS. ASS may also present as a symmetric inflammatory polyarthritis initially indistinguishable from that of rheumatoid arthritis (38). Tenosynovitis has also been reported. Joint pain without signs of inflammation also occur frequently in ASS (66-89%) (2;32).
Gastrointestinal symptoms. Involvement of the gastrointestinal canal is usually restricted to the distal parts of the oesophagus. The incidence of distal oesophageal dysmotility evidently depends on the tests used to identify the abnormality, but is diagnosed in 5-52% of the reports (9;12;31-33). Oesophageal disease is an important clinical feature of ASS as dysphagia leading to aspiration may further damage the already compromised pulmonal function. In patients with end stage interstitial lung disease, this manifestation may restrict patients`possibilitis of being accepted for lung transplantation. Routine examinations using barium enema x-ray is therefore recommended to diagnose oesophageal dysmotility which should be treated vigorously.
Vascular symptoms. Clinical signs of vasculopathy may appear. Raynaud`s phenomenon accompanies ASS in 30-50 % of cases (2;3;9;12;14;20;32). Skin necrosis and ischemic ulcera have also been observed in ASS (39). Pulmonary arterial hypertension has not been subjected to studies aimed at detecting its true incidence that is using echocardiography to screen all cases. It is, however, infrequently observed in DM and PM, and in one study (43) PAH was diagnosed by echocardiography in 16 of 198 consecutive cases (0,8%). It was thus concluded that mild to severe PAH is a rare complication of IIM (43). In ASS, cases with fatal (40) and acute (41-43) PAH have been observed. In our patient cohort of 67 cases of ASS, PAH diagnosed by right heart catherization was observed in nine cases and represented a frequent cause of death in this syndrome.
Other clinical features seen rather commonly in ASS include, sicca symptoms (8-54%) (2;9;31;32), sclerodactyli (12) and subcutaneous calcinosis (44). Glomerulonephritis may be seen (45).
Clinical features stratified by anti-aaRS. In general, the similarities of the clinical features among patients possessing different ASS are rather impressive. Some differences have, however, been suggested. Due to low numbers of non-Jo-1 positive ASS patients reported, it is prudent that these differences are considered preliminary and interpreted cautiously.

Among PL-12 positive ASS, the histological features of ILD is predominantly of the NSIP pattern (20), while myositis is mostly mild (34). In one study (20), CK levels increased to up to twice the normal level in only two individuals. Interestingly, two of these cases were diagnosed with PAH.

Patients with anti-PL7 autoantibodies may also show different clinical features when compared to Jo-1 positives. Anti-PL-7 autoantibodies have been associated with milder muscle weakness (46) and almost all patients reported have had ILD (46;47). Seven patients with anti-OJ autoantibodies were described by Sato et al (48) of whom all had ILD, and four presented muscle weakness and polyarthritis. None had Raynaud`s phenomenon or sclerodactyli. In a study of eight patients with anti-KS autoantibodies, 88% had ILD 25% (49).

Other clinical associations. Anti-SSA antibodies, anti-Ro52 in particular, occur in more than 50% of ASS (8;11) and have been associated with more severe lung fibrosis (13). In one study (50) patients without anti SSA autoantibodies more often lacked fibrosis on the initial CT scans compared to patients possessing these autoantibodies. In another study (33), patients with such autoantibodies seemed to be predisposed to the development of a more severe ILD as assessed by both HRCT and lung function tests.

8. Disease associations

Cancer. The increased risk of cancer in DM is well documented. In one study of 103 patients with DM, 15 patients had concomitant malignancy (51) and the risk of cancer was highest among those without myositis-specific autoantibodies. Thus, ASS was suspected to provide some protection against the development of cancer. However, subsequent case reports of concurrent ASS and cancer appeared (52;53), clearly showing that ASS does not provide total protection against development of malignant disease. Whether or not the risk of cancer is less in ASS compared to other IIM remains to be studied. However, in a recent study from Japan , 4.8 % of patients with DM and concomitant cancer possessed anti-Jo-1 antibody as opposed to 15.9 % in DM patients without malignant disease (54). Although these findings may indicate some protective effect of anti-ARS against development of malignancy, further studies are warranted to corroborate such an association.

Other immune-mediated disorders. Approximately 5-8 % of anti-ARS cases manifest as overlap syndromes with another connective tissue disease such as systemic lupus erythematosus, systemic sclerosis and Sjøgren`s syndrome (55).

9. Evaluation and diagnosis

Assessment of the respiratory system. The diagnosis of ASS associated ILD is based on HRCT of lungs. Ground glass opacities, subpleural fibrosis and bronchiectasies, all due to compromise of the alveolar-capillary interface, may be observed early in the disease course. In some cases, the progression of ILD is severe, culminating in end stage pulmonal disease (honeycombing) after a rather short disease duration. In other cases, more limited abnormalities on HRCT are seen with little impact on lung function.

Lung function tests typically reveals a restrictive pattern with FVC or total lung capacity less than 80% of the predicted value for age and height and a decrease in the diffusing capacity for carbon monoxide. As lung function tests are readily reproducible and minimally invasive, such tests are recommended both for uncovering occult ILD and for monitoring disease severity and disease progression. Lung biopsy offers unclear prognostic value (19), and is not recommended as a routine procedure in the evaluation of ASS.

Assessment of the musculoskeletal system. Evaluation of muscular involvement reveals in the majority of cases significant elevations of creatin kinase (CK). Compared to PM, the elevations of CK are often modest, in the majority of cases not exceeding 5000 IU/ml (2;3;9). In a few cases, however, the myositis is severe, exhibiting CK levels of several thousands and causing severe muscular weakness. MRI will in cases of clinically overt disease show oedema initially, and by time development of fibrosis, fatty deposits and atrophy. In hypomyopathic patients, MRI and CK levels may be normal in spite of muscular weakness. In other cases of hypomyopathic ASS, there are no muscle complaints while CK levels may be elevated or MRI may show signs of inflammation. Amyopathic ASS denotes a condition in which neither clinical symptoms nor laboratory abnormalities are present.

10. Assessment of other organ systems

Further evaluation of patients with ASS should include barium oesophageal x-ray which in more than 25 % of cases will reveal distal oesophageal dysmotility. Diagnosis and proper treatment of oesophageal dysmotility is important to avoid further damage to the lungs by aspiration. Another important disease complication is represented by pulmonary hypertension, either pre- or post capillary. Echocardiography should therefore be considered in the work-up of ASS. If PAH is suggested by echocardiography, the diagnosis should be verified by right heart catherization. Capillaroscopy may show reduced capillary density (56), and in two studies nailfold capillary changes were detected in 31 and 89%, respectively (3;9). Whether or not the occurrence of such vasculopathic changes differ between those with a histologic pattern of dematomyositis as oppsoded to polymyositis remains to be studied.

11. Evaluation of disease activity and disease severity

Biomarkers for disease activity and disease severity have been incompletely studied in ASS. Whether or not traditional markers for acute phase responses such as SR and CRP correlate with the actual activity and progression of disease remains to be seen. In the initial phases of disease, an acute phase response may be evident. One study suggested that levels of anti-Jo-1 autoantibodies correlated with disease activity (12), but these findings await confirmation. Thus, further research of ASS biomarkers for disease activity and disease severity should be strongly encouraged.

12. Treatment

Treatment of ASS is a challenge as no controlled trials have been performed and recommendations are based on single case reports and small patient series.

Standard treatment regimes include corticosteroids in addition to immunosuppressives. The role of corticosteroids in ASS associated ILD and their potential impact on disease course and patient survival is, however, unclear. Corticosteroids have little prospective evidence supporting their use (19), but their well documented intense anti-inflammatory efficacy suggests that they may be an essential part of initial therapeutic regimen. Moreover, the efficacy of corticosteroids in suppressing myositis is well documented. Thus, most clinicians regard corticosteroids as a basic part of the therapeutic regimen of ASS. In acute or subacute pulmonary disease, high doses of oral glucocorticosteroids are usually administered (1 mg/kg/day). At some centers, intravenous methylprednisolon in doses of 500-1000 mg/day for 2-3 consecutive days are used as initial treatment. It should be noted, however, that there are no studies that clearly show the superiority of intravenous to oral corticosteroid treatment. In gradually developing ILD (type II) moderate doses of corticosteroids (0.5 mg/day initially) are most often preferred.

There is unfortunately no general consensus to what immunosuppressives that should be preferred in addition to corticosteroids in ASS. Although placebo-controlled trials are lacking, favorable experiences with cyclophosphamide in other connective tissue diseases have led many clinicians to prefer this drug as an adjunct to steroids. The choice of immunosuppressive treatment, however, clearly depends on the severity and extent of disease. In moderate to mild cases, a combination of oral glucocorticosteroids and either cyclophosphamide, azathioprine or methotrexate may be recommended. However, in our experience this regimen is insufficient in cases with acute and rapidly progressing ILD. Although based on retrospective case series, we recommend a combination of oral corticosteroids, cyclophosphamide and the anti-CD-20 monoclonal antibody rituximab as induction therapy in type I ASS (57). The efficacy of rituximab has also been reported in several case reports (58;59).

Others have experienced favorable effect of calcineurin inhibitors such as cyclosporin A (60) and tacrolimus (23). Another therapeutic option is mycophenolate mofetil and for myositis methotrexate may be valuable as an adjunct to corticosteroids. Clearly, multicenter randomised controlled studies of the efficacy of immunosuppressive therapy in ASS is highly warranted.

In end stage pulmonary disease, lung transplantation appears the only therapeutic option, but is rarely accepted due to oesophageal dysmotility. The dermatological manifestations may be favorable treated by hydroxychloroquine.

13. Disease outcome

The final outcome of ASS largely depends on the type and progression of ILD. Myositis have usually limited impact on outcome. The majority of patients run a chronic disease course (24) and will require immunosuppressive therapy for several years. Unfortunately, no follow-up study including a large number of patients have been performed to display the impact of ASS on functional outcome and quality of life. In one study of 12 patients followed for 5.5 years, muscle function improved in all and pulmonary function normalized in 1/3 (32).

In a study of 32 patients (61), patients with acute onset and respiratory insufficiency were compared to those with a gradual onset of ILD. The percentage of patients in whom the ILD improved at three months was significantly higher among those with acute onset. However, most patients with ILD progression after 12 months were among those with acute onset. Other studies have also shown an association between acute and subacute onset and poor prognosis (62).

Whether or not the pattern of HRCT findings is indicative of final outcome is a matter of debate. Ground glass opacities, initially thought to represent reversible inflammation have been associated with a better response to therapy (63), hence a more favorable outcome. However, ground glass opacities may also represent fine reticular fibrosis, and some studies have suggested a poor prognosis in patients demonstrating such changes (64). Finally, mortality appears to have little relationship to biopsy subtype (19).

Mortality and causes of death in ASS have been rarely subjected to investigation. After an average of 5.5 years, only one of 12 patients succumed ((32) and mortality was estimated to 8%. Others have found a cumulative mortality of 14% (9). At present, the overal annual mortality of ASS cannot be exactly assessed, but it can be concluded that ASS is associated with excess mortality.
In general, the mortality in IIM has improved during the last decades, from a 5-year survival of 65% in the 1960ies compared to 75-96% in the last decade (65). If modern therapy and more aggressive therapy have had the same impact on ASS remains to be seen.

14. Future perspectives

ASS represent a rather newly defined disease entity whose etiopathogenesis remains incompletely understood. The disease course is usually chronic and ASS is most likely associated with decreased survival. Due to its low incidence large scale prospective investigations are few. Knowledge about the clinical aspects of ASS has accumulated, while outcome, prognostic markers, biomarkers for disease activity, treatment, mortality and risk of cancer have been insufficiently investigated.

Anti-Jo-1	histidyl
Anti-PL-12	alanyl
Anti-PL-7	threonyl
Anti-EJ	glycyl
Anti-OJ	isoleucyl
Anti-KS	asparaginyl
Anti-Zo	phenylalanyl
Anti-Ha	tyrosyl

Table 1. Antisynthetase autoantibodies.

Antisynthetase autoantibody demonstrated on two separate occasions	Plus at least one of the following
Plus	Arthritis/arthralgia
Either Interstitial lung disease	Raynaud`s phenomenon
And/or Inflammatory muscle disease	Gottron`s paples or sign
	Mechanic`s hands
	D

Table 2. Suggested classification criteria for ASS.

15. Reference

[1] Marguerie C, Bunn CC, Beynon HL, Bernstein RM, Hughes JM, So AK et al. Polymyositis, pulmonary fibrosis and autoantibodies to aminoacyl-tRNA synthetase enzymes. Q J Med 1990; 77(282):1019-38.
[2] Hengstman GJ, Brouwer R, Egberts WT, Seelig HP, Jongen PJ, van Venrooij WJ et al. Clinical and serological characteristics of 125 Dutch myositis patients. Myositis specific autoantibodies aid in the differential diagnosis of the idiopathic inflammatory myopathies. J Neurol 2002; 249(1):69-75.

[3] Matsushita T, Hasegawa M, Fujimoto M, Hamaguchi Y, Komura K, Hirano T et al. Clinical evaluation of anti-aminoacyl tRNA synthetase antibodies in Japanese patients with dermatomyositis. J Rheumatol 2007; 34(5):1012-8.

[4] O'Hanlon TP, Carrick DM, Targoff IN, Arnett FC, Reveille JD, Carrington M et al. Immunogenetic risk and protective factors for the idiopathic inflammatory myopathies: distinct HLA-A, -B, -Cw, -DRB1, and -DQA1 allelic profiles distinguish European American patients with different myositis autoantibodies. Medicine (Baltimore) 2006; 85(2):111-27.

[5] Mathews MB, Bernstein RM. Myositis autoantibody inhibits histidyl-tRNA synthetase: a model for autoimmunity. Nature 1983; 304(5922):177-9.

[6] Nishikai M, Reichlin M. Heterogeneity of precipitating antibodies in polymyositis and dermatomyositis. Characterization of the Jo-1 antibody system. Arthritis Rheum 1980; 23(8):881-8.

[7] Chinoy H, Salway F, Fertig N, Shephard N, Tait BD, Thomson W et al. In adult onset myositis, the presence of interstitial lung disease and myositis specific/associated antibodies are governed by HLA class II haplotype, rather than by myositis subtype. Arthritis Res Ther 2006; 8(1):R13.

[8] Koenig M, Fritzler MJ, Targoff IN, Troyanov Y, Senecal JL. Heterogeneity of autoantibodies in 100 patients with autoimmune myositis: insights into clinical features and outcomes. Arthritis Res Ther 2007; 9(4):R78.

[9] Selva-O'Callaghan A, Labrador-Horrillo M, Solans-Laque R, Simeon-Aznar CP, Martinez-Gomez X, Vilardell-Tarres M. Myositis-specific and myositis-associated antibodies in a series of eighty-eight Mediterranean patients with idiopathic inflammatory myopathy. Arthritis Rheum 2006; 55(5):791-8.

[10] Mimori T, Imura Y, Nakashima R, Yoshifuji H. Autoantibodies in idiopathic inflammatory myopathy: an update on clinical and pathophysiological significance. Curr Opin Rheumatol 2007; 19(6):523-9.

[11] Rutjes SA, Vree Egberts WT, Jongen P, Van Den Hoogen F, Pruijn GJ, van Venrooij WJ. Anti-Ro52 antibodies frequently co-occur with anti-Jo-1 antibodies in sera from patients with idiopathic inflammatory myopathy. Clin Exp Immunol 1997; 109(1):32-40.

[12] Stone KB, Oddis CV, Fertig N, Katsumata Y, Lucas M, Vogt M et al. Anti-Jo-1 antibody levels correlate with disease activity in idiopathic inflammatory myopathy. Arthritis Rheum 2007; 56(9):3125-31.

[13] Vancsa A, Csipo I, Nemeth J, Devenyi K, Gergely L, Danko K. Characteristics of interstitial lung disease in SS-A positive/Jo-1 positive inflammatory myopathy patients. Rheumatol Int 2009; 29(9):989-94.

[14] Mielnik P, Wiesik-Szewczyk E, Olesinska M, Chwalinska-Sadowska H, Zabek J. Clinical features and prognosis of patients with idiopathic inflammatory myopathies and anti-Jo-1 antibodies. Autoimmunity 2006; 39(3):243-7.

[15] Yoshifuji H, Fujii T, Kobayashi S, Imura Y, Fujita Y, Kawabata D et al. Anti-aminoacyl-tRNA synthetase antibodies in clinical course prediction of interstitial lung disease complicated with idiopathic inflammatory myopathies. Autoimmunity 2006; 39(3):233-41.

[16] Richards TJ, Eggebeen A, Gibson K, Yousem S, Fuhrman C, Gochuico BR et al. Characterization and peripheral blood biomarker assessment of anti-Jo-1 antibody-positive interstitial lung disease. Arthritis Rheum 2009; 60(7):2183-92.

[17] Kang EH, Nakashima R, Mimori T, Kim J, Lee YJ, Lee EB et al. Myositis autoantibodies in Korean patients with inflammatory myositis: anti-140-kDa polypeptide antibody is primarily associated with rapidly progressive interstitial lung disease independent of clinically amyopathic dermatomyositis. BMC Musculoskelet Disord 2010; 11:223.
[18] Labirua A, Lundberg IE. Interstitial lung disease and idiopathic inflammatory myopathies: progress and pitfalls. Curr Opin Rheumatol 2010; 22(6):633-8.
[19] Connors GR, Christopher-Stine L, Oddis CV, Danoff SK. Interstitial lung disease associated with the idiopathic inflammatory myopathies: what progress has been made in the past 35 years? Chest 2010; 138(6):1464-74.
[20] Hervier B, Wallaert B, Hachulla E, Adoue D, Lauque D, Audrain M et al. Clinical manifestations of anti-synthetase syndrome positive for anti-alanyl-tRNA synthetase (anti-PL12) antibodies: a retrospective study of 17 cases. Rheumatology (Oxford) 2010; 49(5):972-6.
[21] Mozaffar T, Pestronk A. Myopathy with anti-Jo-1 antibodies: pathology in perimysium and neighbouring muscle fibres. J Neurol Neurosurg Psychiatry 2000; 68(4):472-8.
[22] Fathi M, Vikgren J, Boijsen M, Tylen U, Jorfeldt L, Tornling G et al. Interstitial lung disease in polymyositis and dermatomyositis: longitudinal evaluation by pulmonary function and radiology. Arthritis Rheum 2008; 59(5):677-85.
[23] Wilkes MR, Sereika SM, Fertig N, Lucas MR, Oddis CV. Treatment of antisynthetase-associated interstitial lung disease with tacrolimus. Arthritis Rheum 2005; 52(8):2439-46.
[24] Koreeda Y, Higashimoto I, Yamamoto M, Takahashi M, Kaji K, Fujimoto M et al. Clinical and pathological findings of interstitial lung disease patients with anti-aminoacyl-tRNA synthetase autoantibodies. Intern Med 2010; 49(5):361-9.
[25] Yousem SA, Gibson K, Kaminski N, Oddis CV, Ascherman DP. The pulmonary histopathologic manifestations of the anti-Jo-1 tRNA synthetase syndrome. Mod Pathol 2010; 23(6):874-80.
[26] Mathews MB, Bernstein RM. Myositis autoantibody inhibits histidyl-tRNA synthetase: a model for autoimmunity. Nature 1983; 304(5922):177-9.
[27] Suber TL, Casciola-Rosen L, Rosen A. Mechanisms of disease: autoantigens as clues to the pathogenesis of myositis. Nat Clin Pract Rheumatol 2008; 4(4):201-9.
[28] Levine SM, Raben N, Xie D, Askin FB, Tuder R, Mullins M et al. Novel conformation of histidyl-transfer RNA synthetase in the lung: the target tissue in Jo-1 autoantibody-associated myositis. Arthritis Rheum 2007; 56(8):2729-39.
[29] Ascherman DP, Oriss TB, Oddis CV, Wright TM. Critical requirement for professional APCs in eliciting T cell responses to novel fragments of histidyl-tRNA synthetase (Jo-1) in Jo-1 antibody-positive polymyositis. J Immunol 2002; 169(12):7127-34.
[30] Englund P, Wahlstrom J, Fathi M, Rasmussen E, Grunewald J, Tornling G et al. Restricted T cell receptor BV gene usage in the lungs and muscles of patients with idiopathic inflammatory myopathies. Arthritis Rheum 2007; 56(1):372-83.
[31] Hausmanowa-Petrusewicz I, Kowalska-Oledzka E, Miller FW, Jarzabek-Chorzelska M, Targoff IN, Blaszczyk-Kostanecka M et al. Clinical, serologic, and immunogenetic features in Polish patients with idiopathic inflammatory myopathies. Arthritis Rheum 1997; 40(7):1257-66.
[32] Spath M, Schroder M, Schlotter-Weigel B, Walter MC, Hautmann H, Leinsinger G et al. The long-term outcome of anti-Jo-1-positive inflammatory myopathies. J Neurol 2004; 251(7):859-64.

[33] La CR, Lo Mo NA, Locaputo A, Dolzani F, Trotta F. In patients with antisynthetase syndrome the occurrence of anti-Ro/SSA antibodies causes a more severe interstitial lung disease. Autoimmunity 2006; 39(3):249-53.
[34] Kalluri M, Sahn SA, Oddis CV, Gharib SL, Christopher-Stine L, Danoff SK et al. Clinical profile of anti-PL-12 autoantibody. Cohort study and review of the literature. Chest 2009; 135(6):1550-6.
[35] Friedman AW, Targoff IN, Arnett FC. Interstitial lung disease with autoantibodies against aminoacyl-tRNA synthetases in the absence of clinically apparent myositis. Semin Arthritis Rheum 1996; 26(1):459-67.
[36] Mii S, Kobayashi R, Nakano T, Harada H, Okada M, Matsui Y et al. A histopathologic study of mechanic's hands associated with dermatomyositis: a report of five cases. Int J Dermatol 2009; 48(11):1177-82.
[37] Meyer O, Charlanne H, Cherin P, Allanore Y, Coquerelle P, Grardel B et al. Subluxing arthropathy: an unusual manifestation of the antisynthetase syndrome. Ann Rheum Dis 2009; 68(1):152-3.
[38] Mumm GE, McKown KM, Bell CL. Antisynthetase syndrome presenting as rheumatoid-like polyarthritis. J Clin Rheumatol 2010; 16(7):307-12.
[39] Disdier P, Bolla G, Harle JR, Pache X, Weiller-Merli C, Marco MS et al. [Digital necrosis disclosing antisynthetase syndrome]. Ann Dermatol Venereol 1994; 121(6-7):493-5.
[40] Chatterjee S, Farver C. Severe pulmonary hypertension in Anti-Jo-1 syndrome. Arthritis Care Res (Hoboken) 2010; 62(3):425-9.
[41] Taniguchi Y, Horino T, Kato T, Terada Y. Acute pulmonary arterial hypertension associated with anti-synthetase syndrome. Scand J Rheumatol 2010; 39(2):179-80.
[42] Cavagna L, Prisco E, Montecucco C, Caporali R. Pulmonary arterial hypertension in antisynthetase syndrome: Comment on the article by Chatterjee and Farver. Arthritis Care Res (Hoboken) 2011; 63(4):633-4.
[43] Minai OA. Pulmonary hypertension in polymyositis-dermatomyositis: clinical and hemodynamic characteristics and response to vasoactive therapy. Lupus 2009; 18(11):1006-10.
[44] Queiro-Silva R, Banegil I, de Dios-Jimenez de Aberasturi JR, Belzunegui-Otano J, Gonzalez-Beneitez C, Figueroa-Pedrosa M. Periarticular calcinosis associated with anti-Jo-1 antibodies sine myositis. Expanding the clinical spectrum of the antisynthetase syndrome. J Rheumatol 2001; 28(6):1401-4.
[45] Frost NA, Morand EF, Hall CL, Maddison PJ, Bhalla AK. Idiopathic polymyositis complicated by arthritis and mesangial proliferative glomerulonephritis: case report and review of the literature. Br J Rheumatol 1993; 32(10):929-31.
[46] Yamasaki Y, Yamada H, Nozaki T, Akaogi J, Nichols C, Lyons R et al. Unusually high frequency of autoantibodies to PL-7 associated with milder muscle disease in Japanese patients with polymyositis/dermatomyositis. Arthritis Rheum 2006; 54(6):2004-9.
[47] Sato S, Hirakata M, Kuwana M, Nakamura K, Suwa A, Inada S et al. Clinical characteristics of Japanese patients with anti-PL-7 (anti-threonyl-tRNA synthetase) autoantibodies. Clin Exp Rheumatol 2005; 23(5):609-15.
[48] Sato S, Kuwana M, Hirakata M. Clinical characteristics of Japanese patients with anti-OJ (anti-isoleucyl-tRNA synthetase) autoantibodies. Rheumatology (Oxford) 2007; 46(5):842-5.

[49] Hirakata M, Suwa A, Takada T, Sato S, Nagai S, Genth E et al. Clinical and immunogenetic features of patients with autoantibodies to asparaginyl-transfer RNA synthetase. Arthritis Rheum 2007; 56(4):1295-303.

[50] Mileti LM, Strek ME, Niewold TB, Curran JJ, Sweiss NJ. Clinical characteristics of patients with anti-Jo-1 antibodies: a single center experience. J Clin Rheumatol 2009; 15(5):254-5.

[51] Chinoy H, Fertig N, Oddis CV, Ollier WE, Cooper RG. The diagnostic utility of myositis autoantibody testing for predicting the risk of cancer-associated myositis. Ann Rheum Dis 2007; 66(10):1345-9.

[52] Legault D, McDermott J, Crous-Tsanaclis AM, Boire G. Cancer-associated myositis in the presence of anti-Jo1 autoantibodies and the antisynthetase syndrome. J Rheumatol 2008; 35(1):169-71.

[53] Rozelle A, Trieu S, Chung L. Malignancy in the setting of the anti-synthetase syndrome. J Clin Rheumatol 2008; 14(5):285-8.

[54] Azuma K, Yamada H, Ohkubo M, Yamasaki Y, Yamasaki M, Mizushima M et al. Incidence and predictive factors for malignancies in 136 Japanese patients with dermatomyositis, polymyositis and clinically amyopathic dermatomyositis. Mod Rheumatol 2011; 21(2):178-83.

[55] Park CK, Kim TJ, Cho YN, Kim IS, Lee HJ, Lee KE et al. Development of antisynthetase syndrome in a patient with rheumatoid arthritis. Rheumatol Int 2011; 31(4):529-32.

[56] Mercer LK, Moore TL, Chinoy H, Murray AK, Vail A, Cooper RG et al. Quantitative nailfold video capillaroscopy in patients with idiopathic inflammatory myopathy. Rheumatology (Oxford) 2010; 49(9):1699-705.

[57] Sem M, Molberg O, Lund MB, Gran JT. Rituximab treatment of the anti-synthetase syndrome: a retrospective case series. Rheumatology (Oxford) 2009; 48(8):968-71.

[58] Ball EM, Savage EM, Pendleton A. Refractory anti-synthetase syndrome treated with rituximab. Rheumatology (Oxford) 2010; 49(5):1013.

[59] Frikha F, Rigolet A, Behin A, Fautrel B, Herson S, Benveniste O. Efficacy of rituximab in refractory and relapsing myositis with anti-JO1 antibodies: a report of two cases. Rheumatology (Oxford) 2009; 48(9):1166-8.

[60] Kotani T, Makino S, Takeuchi T, Kagitani M, Shoda T, Hata A et al. Early intervention with corticosteroids and cyclosporin A and 2-hour postdose blood concentration monitoring improves the prognosis of acute/subacute interstitial pneumonia in dermatomyositis. J Rheumatol 2008; 35(2):254-9.

[61] Tillie-Leblond I, Wislez M, Valeyre D, Crestani B, Rabbat A, Israel-Biet D et al. Interstitial lung disease and anti-Jo-1 antibodies: difference between acute and gradual onset. Thorax 2008; 63(1):53-9.

[62] Kang EH, Lee EB, Shin KC, Im CH, Chung DH, Han SK et al. Interstitial lung disease in patients with polymyositis, dermatomyositis and amyopathic dermatomyositis. Rheumatology (Oxford) 2005; 44(10):1282-6.

[63] Mino M, Noma S, Taguchi Y, Tomii K, Kohri Y, Oida K. Pulmonary involvement in polymyositis and dermatomyositis: sequential evaluation with CT. AJR Am J Roentgenol 1997; 169(1):83-7.

[64] Won HJ, Soon KD, Keun LC, Yoo B, Bum SJ, Kitaichi M et al. Two distinct clinical types of interstitial lung disease associated with polymyositis-dermatomyositis. Respir Med 2007; 101(8):1761-9.

[65] Lundberg IE, Forbess CJ. Mortality in idiopathic inflammatory myopathies. Clin Exp Rheumatol 2008; 26(5 Suppl 51):S109-S114.

5

Aminoacyl-tRNA Synthetases in Idiopathic Inflammatory Myopathies: An Update on Immunopathogenic Significance, Clinical and Therapeutic Implications

Codrina Mihaela Ancuta[1,2], Eugen Ancuta[3] and Rodica Marieta Chirieac[1]
[1]Department of Rheumatology;
[2]Gr.T.Popa Center for Biomedical Research – European Center for Translational Research; "Gr.T.Popa" University of Medicine and Pharmacy;
[3]Research Department, "Cuza-Voda" Hospital Iasi
Romania

1. Introduction

Polymyositis and dermatomyositis, the most important disease subsets in idiopathic inflammatory myopathies (IIMs), are heterogeneous conditions classically defined by a wide clinical spectrum including proximal skeletal muscle weakness, skin lesions and systemic organ involvement, particularly interstitial lung disease, in conjunction with biochemical and histopathological background of varying degrees of muscle inflammation (Gunawardena et al., 2008; Gunawardena et al., 2009; Mimori et al., 2007).

Although the exact etiology is still controversial, there is increasing evidence of aberrant autoimmunity in both entities, closely linked to different patterns of myositis-specific (MSAs) and myositis-associated autoantibodies (MAAs) (Gunawardena et al., 2009; Mimori et al., 2007).

Currently recognized as disease biomarkers, myositis-specific autoantibodies have been identified as key players in IIMs, promoting several pathogenic pathways as they target cytoplasmic and nuclear proteins involved in basic cellular processes (protein synthesis, nuclear transcription and translocation), but also being directly connected to phenotype disease profiles (Betteridge et al., 2007; Gunawardena et al., 2008; Gunawardena et al., 2009; Mimori et al., 2007).

While several subsets of myositis-specific autoantibodies targeting both classic (aminoacyl-tRNA synthetases, ARSs, signal recognition particle, SRP, and Mi-2) and newly identified (MJ, PMS1, CADM140, p-155/p-140, SAE) autoantigens have been fully described in polymyositis and dermatomyositis (Gunawardena et al., 2009; Hengstman et al., 2004; Suber et al., 2008), the most widespread group of myositis-specific autoantibodies is represented by anti-aminoacyl-tRNA synthetase autoantibodies (Gunawardena et al., 2008; Gunawardena et al., 2009).

Advancing knowledge in the field of synthetases, either antigenic or non-antigenic subtypes, has been reflected in critical association between genotype, serotype, clinical phenotype and

therapeutic potential in IIMs (Gunawardena et al., 2008; Gunawardena et al., 2009; Mammen, 2010).
In this review we emphasize current concepts regarding the pathogenic role, clinical significance and potential therapeutic implications of aminoacyl-tRNA synthetases and their specific autoantibodies in idiopathic inflammatory myopathies.

2. Aminoacyl-tRNA synthetases and their specific autoantibodies

New findings on classical and novel aminoacyl-tRNA synthetases and their corresponding autoantibodies are analyzed in this section.

2.1 Aminoacyl-tRNA synthetases (ARSs)

The aminoacyl-transfer (t) RNA synthetases (ARSs), one of the major targets for autoimmune response in IIMs, represent a distinct group of cytoplasmic enzymes that catalyze the binding of specific aminoacids to their cognate transfer RNAs (tRNAs) in an energy-dependent manner (Hirakata, 2005; Mimori et al., 2007; Wikipedia, 2011).
The ARSs are functionally-related, ubiquitously expressed enzymes involved in protein synthesis (Betteridge et al., 2007; Gunawardena et al., 2009, Shirakawa et al. 2005). A unique, immunologically and enzymatically distinct aminoacyl-tRNA is characteristically assigned to each of the currently known 20 aminoacids (Hirakata, 2005; Mammen, 2010), transferring the appropriate aminoacid to an elongated polypeptide chain (Mammen, 2010).
Eight autoantigenic synthetases have been identified so far. Six out of eight are recognized as classical ARSs and are represented by Jo-1 (histidyl-tRNA synthetase: HisRS), PL-7 (threonyl-tRNA synthetase: ThrRS), PL-12 (alanyl-tRNA synthetase: AlaRS), EJ (glycyl-tRNA synthetase: GlyRS), OJ (isoleucyl-tRNA synthetase: IsoRS) and KS (asparaginyl-tRNA synthetase: AsnRS) (Hirakata, 2005; 7, Mimori et al, 2007; Shirakawa et al., 2005).
Additionally, two novel subsets of synthetases have been recently described as being autoantigenic, including Zo (phenylalanyl-tRNA synthetase: PheRS) and YRS or Ha (α and β chains of tyrosyl-tRNA synthetase: TyrRS), respectively (Betteridge et al., 2007; Mimori et al., 2007).
Specific autoantibodies targeting the aforementioned synthetases have been commonly encountered in connective tissue disorders, particularly in 25 to 35% of patients with polymyositis and dermatomyositis (Hirakata, 2005; Mimori et al., 2007; Park et al., 2008).
Based on distinct enzymatic properties, sequence motifs, molecular structure and the site of initial aminoacylation, ARSs can be divided in two main classes (Betteridge et al., 2007; Hirakata, 2005; Woese et al., 2000; Wikipedia, 2011). Class I ARSs comprises a multi-enzymatic complex with anti-synthetasic specificity for nine different amino acids, whereas Class II ARSs are typically found free and uncomplexed in the cellular cytoplasm. Since OJ or isoleucyl-tRNA synthase is part of such multi-enzyme complex, specific anti-OJ antibodies can react also against multiple synthetases; however, the specific anti-OJ pattern is not shaped (Betteridge et al., 2007; Hirakata, 2005; Woese et al., 2000). On the other hand, five classical synthetases, both Jo-1 and non-Jo1 subtypes (PL-7, PL-12, EJ and KS), are further classified as Class II members.
It is widely accepted that not all synthetases are autoantigenic in patients diagnosed with either polymyositis or dermatomyositis (Hirakata, 2005). Besides, ARSs are not randomly targeted as several autoantibodies like anti-Jo-1 are more prevalent than the others

(Hirakata, 2005; Mimori et al., 2007), perhaps directly related to their accessibility and expression on the cell surface (Hirakata, 2005).

2.2 Anti-aminoacyl-tRNA synthetases auto-antibodies

Overall, eight different autoantibodies reacting with autoantigenic ARSs have been recognized, specifically described as anti-Jo-1 and anti-non Jo-1 antibodies. The anti-non-Jo-1 subtypes refer to us as anti-PL-7, anti-PL-12, anti-OJ, anti-EJ, anti-KS, anti-Zo and anti-YRS or anti-Ha antibodies (Hirakata, 2005; Mimori et al., 2007; Solomon et al., 2011).

Several characteristics of these anti-ARSs autoantibodies have been emphasized (Betteridge et al., 2009; Hirakata, 2005; Solomon et al., 2011; Targoff, 2008):

- they focus on functionally related protein enzymes (synthetases) implicated in normal vital cellular cycle, specifically targeting muscle and lung tissue;
- they are highly selective, each autoantibody being directed to only one synthetase;
- they are mutually exclusive in a given patient, with a few exception only a single anti-synthetase being typically found;
- they are generally associated with particular phenotypes, a characteristic clinical syndrome being known as "anti-synthetase syndrome", although distinct profiles are defined for each autoantibody; and
- they are associated with particular genotypes.

Even thought to represent only disease biomarkers, it seems that anti-synthetase autoantibodies are active players in the immunopathogenesis of polymyositis and dermatomyositis. However, if the anti-ARSs autoantibodies are simply epiphenomena or directly linked to disease mechanisms remain an open question. Several fascinating paradigms have been effectively anticipated to explain why and how certain intracellular proteins, widely originating in all cellular types, are selectively and specifically targeted in IIMs (Betteridge et al., 2009).

Anti-ARS autoantibodies are associated with anti-synthetase syndrome (ASS), classically defined by several characteristic clinical features including myositis, interstitial lung disease (ILD), arthritis, fever, Raynaud's phenomenon and "mechanic's hands", in addition to other typical skin lesions such as Gottron's papules and heliotrope rash (Betteridge et al., 2007; Betteridge et al., 2009; Gunawardena et al., 2009; Hirakata, 2005). Moreover, distinct associations between certain anti-synthetases profile and corresponding clinical pattern have actually been up-dated.

Specific anti-synthetase autoantibodies detected in polymyositis and dermatomyositis and their target are listed in Table 1.

Anti-synthetase antibody	Target autoantigen (aminoacyl-tRNA synthetase)	Frequency in IIMs (%)
Anti-Jo-1	Histidyl-tRNA synthetase	15 - 20
Anti-non-Jo-1		
• **anti-PL-7**	Threonyl- tRNA synthetase	5 – 10
• **anti-PL-12**	Alanyl- tRNA synthetase	< 5
• **anti-OJ**	Glycyl - tRNA synthetase	5 – 10
• **anti-EJ**	Isoleucyl - tRNA synthetase	< 5
• **anti-KS**	Asparaginyl- tRNA synthetase	< 5
• **anti-Zo**	Phenylalanyl-tRNA synthetase α and β chains	< 1
• **anti-YRS (anti-Ha)**	tyrosyl- tRNA synthetase	< 1

Table 1. Anti-synthetase autoantibidies in IIMs: targets and frequencies.

3. Immunopathogenic significance of aminoacyl-tRNAs in myositis

Recent evidences have highlighted the role of autoantigenic aminoacyl-tRNA synthetases and their specific autoantibodies in the initiation and progression of myositis. Although the exact sequence of events still remains under debate, several pathways are actually proposed including (i) enhanced expression of aminoacyl synthetases in different target tissues, particularly in muscle and lung, (ii) potential role of proteolytic cleavage fragments of aminoacyl-tRNA synthetases generated during inflammation and apoptosis in lesional tissues (muscle and lung), and (iii) autoantigen signaling through chemokine receptors with subsequent amplification of the inflammatory and autoimmune response (Hirakata, 2005).
A detailed insight into the ethiopathogenic mechanisms of myostis, along with genetic susceptibility and adjuvant environmental triggers will be further discussed in this section.

3.1 Enhanced aminoacyl-tRNA synthetase expression in lesional tissues

Increased synthesis of specific antibodies subsets targeting restricted series of autoantiogens in myositis has been extensively debated. Recent findings have suggested that the modification of biochemical structure of different proteins with consecutive augmented antigenicity is essential in guiding their selection as targets (Howard et al, 2003).
Moreover, posttranslational modification of proteins as well as proteolytic cleavage of autoantigens by the direct intervention of either caspases or granzyme B leading to proteolytic fragments with enhanced autoantigenicity might contribute to the initiation and propagation of autoimmunity (Casciola-Rosen et al., 1999; Darrah & Rosen, 2010; Gunawardena et al., 2009; Howard et al, 2003).
It can be hypothesized that up-regulation of certain autoantigens in specific target tissues as muscle and lung play a key role in myositis induction, as the main source of antigens (Betteridge et al., 2009; Mimori et al., 2007). Additionally, based on augmented expression of autoantigens in the lung and skeletal muscle, it has been emphasized the potential significance of distinct microenvironments in determining the specific autoimmune response in IIMs with or without lung involvement (Betteridge et al., 2009; Levine et al., 2007).
Current reports have indicated increased expression of autoantigens, both myositis-specific and myositis- associated subgroups, in muscle fibers from patients with IIMs, particularly in damaged and regenerating cells (Casciola-Rosen et al., 2005). While most autoantigens are frequently expressed in a tissue-restricted manner, aminoacyl-tRNA synthetases are targeted only in autoimmune myositis and, therefore, markedly expressed in injured muscle (Betteridge et al., 2009; Gunawardena et al., 2008; Gunawardena et al., 2009; Mimori et al., 2007).
Enhanced ARSs expression was mainly described for histidyl-tRNAsynthetase (Jo-1), supporting the hypothesis that the presence of challenger autoantigens during reparative myogenesis promotes aberrant autoimmune response (Betteridge et al., 2009; Gunawardena et al., 2008; Gunawardena et al., 2009; Mimori et al., 2007).
Concomitant up-regulation of major histocompatibility complex (MHC) class I has been already reported in the affected muscle cells, while either very low or normal levels of

myositis-specific and associated antigens are detected in normal skeletal muscle (Betteridge et al., 2009; Mimori et al., 2007).

3.2 Proteolytic granzyme B cleavage of aminoacyl-tRNA synthetase and intervention in interstitial lung disease

It is well known that the autoantigenic fragments resulted by the specific intervention of granzyme B serine protease on aminoacyl-tRNA synthetase substrates are actually essential for myositis induction and development during IIMs (Betteridge et al., 2009; Casciola-Rosen et al., 1999; Darrah & Rosen, 2010; Levine et al., 2003; Levine et al, 2007).

Besides, it has been demonstrated that the susceptibility of these antigenic synthetases to cleavage by granzyme B is highly predictive of autoantigen status in myositis (Casciola-Rosen et al., 1999). Not only histidyl-tRNA, but also two other synthetases, isoleucyl-tRNA and alanyl-tRNA synthetases, are cleaved by granzyme B leading to the release of autoantigenic epitopes (Betteridge et al., 2009; Casciola-Rosen et al., 1999; Levine et al, 2007).

Current reports support also the hypothesis that the expression of different autoantigens is not uniformly defined across all tissues and may be modified in disease-specific milieu such as inflamed muscle and lung in patients with polymyositis and dermatomyositis (Levine et al, 2007).

Interestingly, two isoforms of autoantigenic His-RS with different susceptibility to cleavage by proteolytic enzymes, and, subsequent, distinct immunogenic properties have been recently identified (Katsumata et al, 2007; Levine et al, 2007; Mammen, 2010); the granzyme B cleavage site has been detected only in the novel described conformation. Furthermore, although the overall expression of His-RS/Jo-1 in specific target tissues (muscle, lung) is the same, the novel isoform is highly expressed in the epithelium of the lung and may be one factor that generates auto-immunity at this level (Labirua & Lundberg, 2010; Lundberg & Grundtman, 2008; Mammen, 2010). Cleavage with granzyme B result in the generation of cryptic Jo-1 fragments with increased antigenicity and subsequent immune response (Shirakawa et al., 2005).

As a consequence, the aforementioned paradigm that distinct microenvironments may influence disease expression was highlighted with the identification of high expression of this new Jo-1 conformation resulted by proteolytic cleavage in the lung (Casciola-Rosen et al., 1999; Darrah & Rosen, 2010; Labirua & Lundberg, 2010; Levine et al, 2007; Lundberg & Grundtman, 2008).

Furthermore, it has been proposed that the initiating target tissue for the autoimmune response in the anti-Jo-1 syndrome is the lung with secondary attack of muscle (Gunawerdana et al., 2009). In addition, a modification of aminoacyl-tRNA synthetases in the lung could lead to production of autoantibodies (antisynthetase antibodies), a second, event being required for the immune reaction to direct against muscle or other organs (Gunawardena et al., 2008). How the anti-Jo-1 immune response originating in the lung might be redirected to skeletal muscle cells still remain an open question (Mammen, 2010).

3.3 Pro-inflammatory and chemo-attractant properties of autoantigenic aminoacyl-tRNA synthetases

Aminoacyl-tRNA synthetases and their proteolytic fragments as a result of inflammatory and apoptotic processes seem to hold chemo-attractant properties, inducing specific autoimmune response in IIMs (Hirakata, 2005).

Recent works have demonstrated that enhanced expression of autoantigenic ARSs as well as specific cytokines and chemokines pattern are broadly involved in the initial recruitment

and amplification of muscle-specific inflammatory response, since ARSs exhibit significant pro-inflammatory and specifically chemo-attractant potential (Betteridge et al. 2007; Betteridge et al. 2009; Howard, 2006).
Furthermore, the chemo-attractant properties of ARSs might contribute to their selection as targets in myositis, not only in muscle but also in lung tissue (Howard et al., 2002). This may therefore suggest a role for tRNA synthetases in the pathogenesis of myositis and interstitial lung disease itself (Betteridge et al., 2007, Betteridge et al., 2009; Howard, 2006).
Advanced studies on the ability of aminoacyl-tRNA synthetases to induce leukocyte migration have revealed distinct profiles according to the ARSs subset (Howard et al, 2003).
Therefore, histidyl-, asparaginyl- and tyrosyl-tRNA syntetases feature chemo-attractant properties and promote CD4+ and CD8+ lymphocytes, interleukin (IL)-2-activated monocytes and immature dendritic cells migration through the intervention of CCR5 and CCR3 receptors. Indeed, while His-RS specifically functions as a nonchemokine chemo-attractant for cells expressing CCR5 (Howard et al, 2003; Mammen, 2010), Asn-RS is known to generate the migration of CCR3-bearing cells (Howard et al, 2003; Kron et al., 2005).
Additionally, both aminoacyl-tRNA synthetases hold the potential to attract immature dendritic cells, participating in the initiation of an adaptive immune response with subsequent autoantibody synthesis and perpetuation of autoimmune-mediated muscle damage (Howard et al, 2003; Mammen, 2010). In fact, most autoantigens are chemotactic for immature dendritic cells, enhancing their ability to connect the innate and the adaptive immune systems (Howard, 2006).
Further, both His-tRNA and Asn-tRNA synthetases induce the activation and subsequent migration of newly cells expressing their chemokine receptor. In turn, these leukocytes perpetuate the vicious circle by releasing a wide range of other chemokines and activating other immune cells leading to magnification of inflammatory process during IIMs (Howard, 2006).
Conversely, neutrophils, mature dendritic cells and unstimulated monocytes are not influenced by the presence of ARSs (Gunawardena et al., 2009; Howard et al, 2006).
On the other hand, non-antigenic aspartyl- and lysyl-tRNA synthetases do not exert proinflammatory chemo-attractant properties, as such ARSs do not activate chemokine receptors (Gunawardena et al., 2009; Howard et al, 2003; Howard et al, 2006).
Finally, there is now increase evidence that the local abundance of pro-inflammatory autoantigenic ARSs (perhaps liberated from damaged and regenerating muscle cells) may not only provide the reason for autoantibody synthesis, but also may expand the inflammatory process and immune-mediated muscle damage (Howard et al, 2003; Kron et al., 2005; Mammen, 2010).

3.4 Anti-Jo-1 autoantibodies

It was already emphasized that not only antigenic synthetases, but also their specific autoantibodies might contribute to IIMs pathogenesis (Gunawerdana et al., 2008). This model has been validated for anti-Jo-1 autoantibodies, particularly for the association between anti-SSA/Ro-52 (and not anti-SSA/Ro-62) and anti-Jo-1, recognized as endogeneous type 1 IFN-inducer (Betteridge et al., 2009; Gunawerdana et al., 2008; Labirua & Lundberg, 2010).
The co-existence of anti-SSA/Ro with anti-Jo-1 has been reported in up to 60% of anti-Jo-1 positivity cases and seems to be essentially involved in promoting IFN synthesis (Betteridge et al., 2009; Eloranta et al., 2007; Gunawerdana et al., 2008). Moreover, up-regulation of type-1 IFN-induced genes has been depicted in IIMs (Betteridge et al., 2009; Walsh et al., 2007).

On the other hand, it is well known that IFN type 1 plays a role in the pathogenesis of myositis, being fundamentally related to disease propagation (Betteridge et al., 2009).

3.5 Cancer, myositis and anti-aminoacyl-tRNA synthetases

Since the relationship between myositis, particularly adult dermatomyositis, and cancers is well establish, there is increasing evidence for the role of the members of aminoacyl-tRNA synthetases family as autoantigenic targets in malignancies (Betteridge et al., 2009; Chinoy et al., 2007; Mimori et al., 2007); while most studies concentrate on the contribution of hystidil-tRNA, tyrosyl-tRNA, isoleucyl-tRNA, phenylalanyl-tRNA and glycil-tRNA synthetases in malignancy-associated myositis, recent data focus on preferential expression of the alpha-chain of phenylalanyl-tRNA synthetase not only in interstiatial lung disease and solid lung tumours, but also in acute myeloid leukaemia (Betteridge et al., 2009). In addition, Jo-1 is highly expressed in lung and breast adenocarcinoma (Betteridge et al., 2009; Mimori et al., 2007).

Furthermore, it has been suggested that there may be a relative increased expression of the proteolytic enzymes such as granzyme B in carcinoma cells, with subsequent increase in autoimmune fragments and cryptic epitopes, and aberrant autoimmune response in skeletal muscle (Betteridge et al., 2009; Mimori et al., 2007). Additionally research is mandatory to support the cross-reactivity to tumor-related antigens in muscle (Betteridge et al., 2009; Mimori et al., 2007).

3.6 Environmental factors

It is widely accepted that myositis occurs in genetically susceptible recipients and that external antigens could trigger an aberrant immune response in target tissues such as lungs or skeletal muscle (Gunawardena et al., 2009; Mimori et al., 2007). Besides, the paradigm of myositis with or without interstitial lung disease has been extensively highlighted based on the link between immunogenetic profiles, autoimmune targets and clinical phenotype (Betteridge et al., 2009; Labirua & Lundberg, 2010; Targoff, 2008).

Additional evidence is directed towards the key role of infection in the development of muscular damage, particularly the interaction between myogenic RNA viruses with tRNA-like structures and ARSs, with consecutive abnormal autoimmunity face to cryptic epitopes (Betteridge et al., 2009; Gunawardena et al., 2009; Mimori et al., 2007).

Molecular mimicry between myositic autoantigenic ARS substrates and viral proteins with increasing antigenicity represents an attractive hypothesis that may modulate the immune response and the development of autoimmune myositis (Mimori et al., 2007).

Also, current data support the role of several geoclimatic variables and seasonal patterns in the development of specific serologic myositis subsets; thus, in patients with anti-ARS autoantibodies, particularly anti-Jo-1 positive cases, the onset of myositios seems to peak in spring (Gunawardena et al., 2009; Sarkar et al., 2005).

4. Clinical significance of aminoacyl-tRNA synthetases and management of anti-synthetase syndrome

Considerable progress focusing on the striking association between serotype and clinical phenotype has been made in myositis.

Whereas highly selective, mutually exclusive and associated with particular genotypes with few exceptions, anti-synthetase autoantibodies are strongest associated with the anti-synthetase syndrome, a disease subset characterized by a broad clinical spectrum including varying degrees of (i) interstitial lung disease (ILD), (ii) myositis, (iii) non-erosive (poly)arthritis, (iv) fever, (v) Raynaud's phenomenon and (vi) "mechanic's hand" meaning hyperkeratosis with fissuring and hyperpigmentation along the radial and palmar aspects of the fingers (Betteridge et al., 2007; Hirakata, 2005; Mimori et al., 2007; Solomon et al., 2011).

More detailed clinical features, investigations and specific management of patients with anti-ARS antibodies have been described in several recent reports (Betteridge et al., 2009; Hirakata, 2005; Koenig, 2007; Solomon et al., 2011).

Current findings on autoantibodies in anti-synthetase syndrome have already provided important information about clinical phenotypes, course and prognosis related to anti-ARSs status (Lundberg & Grundtman, 2008; Labirua & Lundberg, 2010).

Therefore, data about antibody profile may predict the clinical course of interstitial lung disease in patients with polymyositis and dermatomyositis (Yoshifuji et al., 2006; Labirua & Lundberg, 2010; Mimori et al., 2007); anti-ARSs positive patients had significantly higher frequency of lung involvement than negative cases (70-95% versus 40%) (Mimori et al., 2007). 70% or more of the anti-ARSs positive cases have ILD and only 40-50% muscle pathology, milder than in anti-ARSs negative patients and even subclinical (Labirua & Lundberg, 2010; Lundberg & Grundtman, 2008). Moreover, in the majority of anti-ARSs positive disease, ILD was diagnosed at the same time or before the onset of myositis (Mimori et al., 2007). There is increasing evidence that ILD is commonly associated with anti-non-Jo-1 positivity, particularly with the presence of anti-PL-7 and anti-PL-12 antibodies (Labirua & Lundberg, 2010; Targoff, 2008).

Anti-ARSs positivity in patients with ILD and myositis showed more favorable clinical outcomes with better response to first-line corticosteroids, but developed significant higher recurrence rate versus anti-ARSs negative cases (Labirua & Lundberg, 2010; Mimori et al., 2007). Conversely, it seems that the 2-year prognosis of pulmonary function was not different based on anti-ARSs status (Mimori et al., 2007).

The detection of anti-ARS antibodies is an important predictor for late-onset skeletal muscle pathology in patients with ILD and the clinical course of ILD in myositis (Mimori et al., 2007).

Although patients with anti-synthetase syndrome typically develop common clinical signs and symptoms, there is increasing evidence that autoantibody profile is associated with particular clinical subgroups (Labirua & Lundberg, 2010; Mimori et al., 2007; Sato et al., 2007; Targoff, 2008). However, the exact mechanisms responsible for this clinical diversity are still unknown.

Detailed insights into clinical picture of distinct anti-synthetase syndrome are further presented and summarized in table 2.

4.1 Anti-Jo-1 positive anti-synthetase syndrome

Anti-Jo-1 (anti-HisRS) autoantibody. Anti-Jo-1 was the first discovered and characterized autoantibody from the eight currently described anti-synthetases and, in the mean time, the most common anti-ARSs antibody (Betteridge et al., 2009; Solomon et al., 2011). Most anti-Jo-1 positive patients have been diagnosed with polymyositis (20-30%), while only 5 to 10% of cases have dermatomyositis; overall, nearly 75% of all anti-ARS cases present with anti-Jo-1 positivity (Labirua & Lundberg, 2010; Mileti et al., 2009) and anti-Jo-1 is found in 15 to 20 % of all myositis patients (Mimori et al., 2007).

Anti-ARSs antibody	Anti-synthetase syndrome cinical spectrum	Clinical subsets
Anti-Jo-1	**Myositis**	Arthritis (75%); Raynaud (50%); mechanic's hand (20%)
Anti-PL-7	**Lung involvement** interstitial pneumonia	Interstitial lung disease (up to 100%); infrequent myositis (40%); polymyositis/ scleroderma overlap syndrome
Anti-PL-12	**Skin involvement** mechanic's hands Gottron's papules	Interstitial lung disease (70-100%); pulmonary hypertension; myositis (0-50% to 60-100%); amyopatic ASS (60%); Raynaud (40-100%); rare mechanic's hand
Anti-OJ	**Joint involvement** non erosive (poly)arthritis	Interstitial lung disease (95%); rare myositis or Raynaudphenomenon
Anti-KS	**Fever**	Interstitial lung disease
Anti-Zo	**Raynaud phenomenon**	Severe non-specific interstitial pneumonia, proximal myopathy, Raynaud and arthralgia
Anti-YRS/Ha		Skin rash, muscle weakness, interstitial lung disease and arthritis

Table 2. Anti-aminoacyl-tRNA synthetase antibodies, anti-synthetase syndrome and particular clinical phenotipes.

Certain genotypic, immunological, histopathological and clinical characteristics have been demonstrated among anti-Jo-1 positive patients, with particular relevance for their prognosis (Solomon et al., 2011; Zampieri et al., 2005).

Recent studies on the association between anti-Jo-1 levels and myositis activity have shown the presence of a direct correlation, even if modest, with creatine kinase levels, myositis, articular and pulmonary disease status (Gunawardena et al., 2009; Stone et al., 2007). Furthermore, it seems that anti-Jo-1 positivity is the strongest predictor of ILD in polymyositis and dermatomyositis, over 70% of those patients featuring lung disease (Solomon et al., 2011). The true incidence of myositis in anti-Jo-1 anti-synthetase syndrome is difficult to evaluate, since either biochemical or clinical significant disease might be reported (Mileti et al., 2009; Solomon et al., 2011).

A particular subset of anti-Jo-1 positive anti-synthetase syndrome has been described in patients with the association between anti-Jo-1 and anti-SSA/Ro-52; the clinical phenotype of such patients showed severe extensive lung pathology (interstiytial lung fibrosis), with higher activity and damage scores and adverse outcomes, even with aggressive immunosupresive therapy (Labirua & Lundberg, 2010)

4.2 Anti-Jo-1 negative anti-synthetase syndromes

Anti-PL-7 (anti-ThrRS) autoantibody. Clinical characteristics of anti-PL-7 positive anti-synthetase syndrome have also been described. Compared to anti-Jo-1 positive ASS, patients with anti-PL-7 positivity appear to have a higher incidence of pulmonary disease (up to 100%) associated with a lower incidence of myositis (about 40%) (Labirua & Lundberg, 2010; Mimori et al., 2007; Solomon et al., 2011). Lower serum muscle enzymes (creatinine kinase) and milder muscle pathology in Japanese cases, as well as polymyositis–scleroderma overlap syndrome with idiopathic interstitial pneumonitis, arthritis and sclerodactyly have been also reported in patients with anti-PL7 autoantibodies (Gunawardena et al., 2009; Mimori et al., 2007; Sato et al., 2007).

Anti-PL-12 (anti-AlaRS) autoantibodys. It should be noted that the clinical spectrum of anti-PL-12 positive anti-synthetase syndrome varies from interstitial lung disease (70-100%) to myositis (earlier reports 60-100%, but recent ones with a smaller proportion of 0-50%) and Raynaud's phenomenon (40-100%), but rare mechanic's hand (Hirakata, 2005; Kalluri et al., 2009; Labirua & Lundberg, 2010; Solomon et al., 2011; Tzioufas, 2001).

Moreover, compared to anti-Jo-1 positive anti-synthetase syndrome, patients with anti-PL-12 positivity account for higher incidence of lung and lower incidence of muscle pathology (Gunawardena et al., 2009; Hervier et al., 2010). In the mean time, anti-PL-12 antibodies were also revealed in up to 60% of cases presenting with amyopatic anti-synthetase syndrome and non-specific interstitial pneumonia (Gunawardena et al., 2009; Hirakata, 2005; Solomon et al., 2011).

Reports of higher pulmonary hypertension with hystologically proven intimal proliferation in the pulmonary arteries, and esophageal involvement have been registered in a limited number of cases (Hirakata, 2005; Labirua & Lundberg, 2010; Solomon et al., 2011). Finally, prognosis seems to depend on severity of ILD and the response to immunosuppressive therapy is variable (Solomon et al., 2011).

Anti-OJ (anti-IsoRS) autoantibody. Anti-OJ antibodies are found in up to 2% of polymyositis and dermatomyositis patients (Sato et al., 2007; Solomon et al., 2011). It is classically accepted the association between interstitial pneumonia and non-Jo-1 anti-ARS antibodies including anti-OJ, the reported prevalence being as high as 95%; furthermore, it seems that patients with lung disease in the absence of clinically apparent myositis are closely related to anti-OJ subset (Betteridge et al., 2009, Gunawardena et al., 2009; Mimori et al., 2007).

Additionally, one study conducted in Japanese patients has recently concluded that the presence of anti-OJ antibodies may distinguish a subtype of anti-ARS syndrome that is more closely associated with ILD than myositis or Raynaud's phenomenon (Mimori et al., 2007; Sato et al., 2007). Moreover, anti-OJ was found to be useful for the diagnosis of patients with ILD with or without myositis (Sato et al., 2007).

Anti-KS (anti-AsnRS) autoantibody. Clinical and immunogenetic characteristics have recently focused on interstitial pneumonia that may predominate in ASS with non-Jo-1 anti-ARS antibodies including anti-KS (Gunawardena et al., 2009; Mimori et al., 2007), but also on stronger association with ILD than myositis (Hirakata et al., 2007; Sato et al., 2007).

Anti-Zo (anti-PheRS) autoantibody. The newly identified anti-Zo antibodies directed against autoantigenic alpha and beta chains of PheRS have been recently detected in only one patient with typical features of ASS, namely severe non-specific interstitial pneumonia, proximal myopathy, Raynaud's phenomenon and arthralgia (Betteridge et al., 2009, Mimori et al., 2007; Solomon et al., 2011), by using proteomic analysis of immunopprecipitation and immunoblotting.

Anti-YRS or anti-Ha (anti-TyrRS) autoantibody. Another novel antibody targeting TyrRS has been identified in one case of typical clinical pattern of ASS, particularly the association between skin rash, muscle weakness, interstitial lung disease and arthritis (Hashish et al., 2005; Mimori et al., 2007).

4.3 Therapeutic consideration

Latest findings have clearly demonstrated the association between aminoacyl-tRNA synthetases and their corresponding specific autoantibodies profiles in patients with IIMs with clinical and therapeutic implications. Moreover, the prevalence, course and severity of interstitial lung disease are significantly influenced by the autoantibody pattern. Accordingly, it seems that crucial decision on possible therapeutic options and subsequent disease outcomes and prognosis are fundamentally guided by the presence of different antibodies subsets (Baer, 2006; Labirua & Lundberg, 2010).

Classically, high doses of steroids, as first-line therapy, in association with second-line immunosuppresors including azathioprine, cyclophosphamide, cyclosporine, mycophenolate mofetil or tacrolimus could be effective in such patients (Baer, 2006; Hervier et al., 2009; Labirua & Lundberg, 2010). Aggressive therapy such as intravenous immunoglobulins or newer biological are controversial, as there are no data to define firmly long-term disease outcomes in such conditions. Furthermore, advancing knowledge about the potential benefits of rituximab, an anti-CD20 monoclonal antibody, in life threatening antisynthetase syndrome provide conflicting data (Ball et al., 2010; Labirua & Lundberg, 2010; Sem et al., 2009; Vandenbroucke et al., 2009).

An attractive therapeutic approach fundamentally based on antagonists of the targeted chemokine receptors has already been proposed, but not yet validated; the design of such intervention was suggested by the paradigm of chemokine receptor mediated cell migration triggered by autoantigens like aminoacyl-tRNA synthetases (Howard, 2006).

5. Conclusion

There is now emerging evidence supporting the fundamental role of specific aminoacyl-tRNA synthetases and their corresponding autoantibodies in the initiation, propagation and expression of myositis spectrum.

Furthermore, detailed insights into the pathways of myostis emphasizes the critical contribution of up-regulated synthetase expression in target tissues, particularly in muscle and lung, proteolytic cleavage fragments generated during inflammation and apoptosis in specific microenvironments and autoantigen signaling through chemokine receptors with subsequent amplification of the inflammatory and autoimmune response.

The paradigm of distinct anti-aminoacyl-tRNA synthetase autoantibody pattern shaping the clinical features and course of the generic anti-synthetase syndrome to specific phenotypes is actually wide accepted.

Considerable progress focusing on the striking association between serotype and clinical phenotype may be the fundamental for further development of more specific therapeutic options.

6. References

Baer, A.N. (2006). Advances in the therapy of idiopathic inflammatory myopathies, *Curr Opin Rheumatol*, Vol. 18, No.3, pp. 236-241, ISSN 1040-8711

Ball, E.M.; Savage, E.M. & Pendleton, A. (2010). Refractory anti-synthetase syndrome treated with rituximab. *Rheumatology (Oxford),* Vol.49, No.5, pp. 1013; online ISSN 1462-0332, print ISSN 1462-0324

Betteridge, Z.; Gunawardena, H, North, J., Slinn, J. & McHugh, N. (2007). Anti-synthetase syndrome: a new autoantibody to phenylalanyl transfer RNA synthetase (anti-Zo) associated with polymyositis and interstitial pneumonia. *Rheumatology (Oxford),* Vol.46, pp. 1005–1008, online ISSN 1462-0332, print ISSN 1462-0324

Betteridge, Z.E.; Gunawardena, H. & McHugh, aN.J. (2009). Pathogenic mechanisms of disease in myositis: autoantigens as clues. *Curr Opin Rheumatol,* Vol.21, pp. 604–609

Casciola-Rosen, L.; Andrade, F., Ulanet, D., Wong, B.W. & Rosen, A. (1999). Cleavage by granzyme B is strongly predictive of autoantigen status: implication for initiation of autoimmunity. *J Exp Med,* Vol.190, No.6, pp. 815-825, Online ISSN: 1540-9538; Print ISSN: 0022-1007

Casciola-Rosen, L.; Nagaraju, K. & Plotz, P. (2005). Enhanced autoantigen expression in regenerating muscle cells in idiopathic inflammatory myopathy. *J Exp Med,* Vol.201, pp. 591-601; Online ISSN: 1540-9538; Print ISSN: 0022-1007

Chinoy, H.; Fertig, N., Oddis, C.V. (2007). The diagnostic utility of myositis autoantibody testing for predicting the risk of cancer-associated myositis. *Ann Rheum Dis,* Vol.66, pp.1345-1349, ISSN (printed) 0003-4967

Darrah, E. & Rosen, A. (2010). Granzyme B cleavage of autoantigens in autoimmunity. *Cell Death and Differentiation,* Vol.17, pp. 624-632, ISSN : 1350-9047

Eloranta, M.L.; Barbarosso Helmers, S., Ulfgren, A.K. (2007). A possible mechanism for endogenous activation of the type 1 interferon system in myositis patients with anti-Jo-1 or anti-Ro 52/ anti-Ro 60 autoantibodies. *Arthritis Rheum,* Vol.56, pp. 3112-3124, ISSN:1044-2626

Gunawardena, H.; Betteridge, Z.E. & McHugh, N.J. (2008). Newly identified autoantibodies: relationship to idiopathic inflammatory myopathy subsets and pathogenesis, *Curr Opin Rheumatol,* Vol.20, pp. 675–680, ISSN 1040-8711

Gunawardena, H.; Betteridge, Z.E. & McHugh, N.J. (2009). Myositis-specific autoantibodies: their clinical and pathogenic significance in disease expression. *Rheumatology (Oxford),* Vol.48, pp.607–612, online ISSN 1462-0332, print ISSN 1462-0324

Hashish, L.; Trieu, E.P., Sadanandan, P. & Targoff, I.N. (2005).Identification of autoantibodies to tyrosyl-tRNA synthetase in dermatomyositis with features consistent with anti-syhthetase syndrome (abstract). *Arthritis Rheum,* Vol.52, suppl.9, pp.312, ISSN:1044-2626

Hengstman, G.J.; van Enghelen, B.G. & van Venrooij, W.J. (2004). Myositis specific autoantibodies: changing insights in pathophysiology and clinical associations. *Curr Opin Rheumatol.* Vol. 16, pp. 692-699, ISSN 1040-8711

Hervier, B. ; Masseau, A., Mussini, J.M., Audrain, M. & Hamidou, M.A. (2009). Long-term efficacy of myciophenolate mofetil in a case of refractory antisynthetase syndrome. *Joint Bone Spine,* Vol.76, No.5, pp. 575-576, ISSN:1778-7254

Hervier, B.; Wallaert, B., Hachulla, E., Adoue, D., Lauque, D. & Audrain, M. (2010). Clinical manifestations of anti-synthetase syndrome positive for anti-alanyl-tRNA synthetase syndrome (anti-PL12) antibodies: a retrospective study of 17 cases, *Rheumatology (Oxford),* Vol.49, No.5, pp. 972-976, online ISSN 1462-0332, print ISSN 1462-0324

Hirakata, M. (2005). Autoantinodies to aminoacyl-tRNA synthetases. *Internal Medicine,* Vol.4, no.6, pp. 527-528, ONLINE, ISSN, : 1349-7235. PRINT, ISSN, : 0918-2918.

Hirakata, M.; Suwa, A., Takada, T. (2007). Clinical and immunogenetic features of patients with autoantibodies to asparagynil-transferRNA synthetase. *Arthritis Rheum,* Vol.56, pp. 1295-1303, ISSN:1044-2626

Howard, O.M. Z.; Hui, F.D., Raben, N., Nagaraju, K., Rosen, A., Casciola-Rosen, L., Hartelein, M., Kron, M., Yang, D., Yiadom, K., Dwivedi, S. Plotz, P.H. & Oppenheim, J.J. (2003). Histidyl-tRNA synthetase and asparaginyl-tRNA synthetase, autoantigens in myositis, activate chemokine receptors on T lymphocytes and immature dendritic cells. *J Exp Med,* Vol. 196, No. 6, pp. 781-791 ISSN 0022-1007

Howard,O.M.Z. (2006). Autoantigen signalling through chemokine receptors, *Curr Opin Rheumatol,* Vol.18, pp. 642–646, ISSN 1040-8711

Yoshifuji, H.; Fujii, T., Kobayashi, S., Imura, Y., Fujita, Y. & Kawabata, D. (2006). Anti-aminoacyl-tRNA synthetase antibodies in clinical course prediction if interstitial lung disease complicated with idiopathic inflammatory myopathies. *Autoimmunity,* Vol.39, No.3, pp. 233-241, ISSN 0891-6934

Kalluri, M.; Sahn, S.A., Oddis, K.V., Gharib, S.L., Christopher-Stine, L. & Danoff, S.K. (2009). Clinical profile of anti-PL12 autoantiabody. Cohort study and review of the literature, *Chest,* Vol.135, No.6, pp. 1550-1556, ISSN (Print): 0012-3692. ISSN (Online): 1931-3543

Katsumata, Y., Ridgway, W.M. & Oriss, T. (2007). Species specific immune response generated by HisRS immunization are associated with muscle and lung inflammation. *J Autoimmun,* Vol.29, pp.174-186, ISSN: 0896-8411

Koenig, M.; Fritzler, M.J., Targoff, I.N. (2007). Heterogeneity of autoantibodies in 100 patients with autoimmune myosiytis: insights into clinical features and outcomes, *Arthritis Res Ther,* Vol. 9, R.878, ISSN:1478-6362

Kron, M.A.; Petridis, M., Haertleib, M., Libranda-Ramirez, B. & Scaffidi, L.E. (2005). Do tissue levels of autoantigenic aminoacyl-tRNA synthetase predict clinical disease? *Medical Hypotheses,* Vol. 65, No.6,pp. 1124-1127, ISSN: 0306-9877

Labirua, A. & Lundberg, I.E. (2010). Interstitial lung disease and idiopathic inflammatory myopathies: progress and pitfalls, *Curr Opin Rheumatol,*Vol. 22, pp. 633–638, ISSN 1040-8711

Levine, S.; Rosen, A. & Casciola-Rosen, L.A. (2003). Anti-aminoacyl tRNA synthetase immune responses: insights into the pathogenesis of the idiopathic inflammatory myopathies. *Cur Opin Rheumatol,* Vol.15, No.6, pp. 708-713, ISSN 1040-8711

Levine, S.M.; Raben, N., Xie, D., Askin, F.B., Tuder, R., Mullins, M., Rosen, A. & Casciola-Rosen, A. (2007). Novel conformation of histidyl-transfer RNA synthetase in the lung. The target tissue in Jo-1 autoantibody-associated myositis. *Arthritis & Rheum,* Vol.56, No.8, pp. 2729-2739, ISSN:1044-2626

Lundberg, I.E. & Grundtman, C. (2008). Developments in the scientific and clinical understanding of inflammatory myopathies. *Arthritis Res Ther,* Vol. 10, pp.220, ISSN:1478-6362

Mammen, A.L. (2010). Anti-Jo-1 and other anti-tRNA synthetases autoantibodies. *Ann N Y Acad Sci,* Vol. 1184, pp. 134-153, ISSN 0077-8923

Mileti, L.M.; Strek, M.E., Niewold, T.B., Curran, J.J. & Sweiss, N.J. (2009). Clinical characteristics of patients with anti-Jo-1 antibodies: a single center experience. *J Clin Rheumatol,* Vol.15, pp. 254-255, ISSN: 1076-1608. Online ISSN: 1536-7355

Mimori, T.; Imura, Y., Nakashima, R. & Yoshifuji, H. (2007). Autoantibodies in idiopathic inflammatory myopathy: an update on clinical and pathophysiological significance, *Curr Opin Rheumatol,* Vol.19, pp. 523–529, ISSN 1040-8711

Park, S.G.; Schimmel, P. & Kim, S. (2008). Aminoacyl t RNA synthetases and their connection to disease. *Proc Natl Acad Sci USA*, Vol. 105, pp. 11043-11049

Sarkar, K.; Weinberg, C.R. & Oddis, C.V. (2005). Seasonal influence on the onset of idiopathic inflammatory myopathies in serologically defined groups. *Arthritis Rheum*, Vol.52, pp. 2433-2438, ISSN:1044-2626

Sato, S.; Kuwana, M. & Hirakata, M. (2007). Clinical characteristics of Japanese patients with anti-OJ (anti-isoleucyl-tRNA synthetase) autoantibodies. *Rheumatology (Oxford)*, Vol.46, pp. 842-845, online ISSN 1462-0332, print ISSN 1462-0324

Sem, M.; Molberg, O., Lund, M.B. & Gran, J.T. (2009). Rituximab treatment on the anti-synthetase treatment. *Rheumatology (Oxford)*, Vol.48, No.8, pp. 968-971, online ISSN 1462-0332, print ISSN 1462-0324

Shirakawa, T.; Nakamura, A., Kohama, K., Hirakata, M. & Ogihara, S. (2005). Class-specific binding of two aminoacyl-tRNA synthetases to annexin, a Ca^{2+} and phospholipid-binding protein. *Cell Structure and Function*, Vol.29, pp. 159-164, ONLINE, ISSN 1347-3700. PRINT, ISSN 0386-7196

Solomon, J; Swigris, J.J. & Brown, K.K. (2011). Myositis-related interstitial lung disease and antisynthetase syndrome. *J Bras Pneumol*, Vol. 37, No. 1, pp. 100-109, ISSN 1806-3713 print version. ISSN 1806-3756 online version

Stone, K.B.; Oddis, C.V., Fertig, N., Katsumata, Y., Lucas, M. & Vogt, M. (2007). Anti-Jo-1 antibody levels correlate with disease activity in idiopathic inflammatory myopathy. *Arthritis Rheum*, Vol.56, No.9, pp. 3125-3131, ISSN 1044-2626

Suber, T.L.; Casciola-Rosen, L. & Rosen, A. (2008). Mechanisms of disease: autoantigens as clues to the pathogenesis of myositis. *Nat Clin Pract Rheumatol*, Vol.4, pp. 201-209, ISSN (printed): 1745-8382

Targoff, I.N. (2008). Autoantibodies and their significance in myositis. *Curr Rheumatol Rep*, Vol. 10, pp.330-340, ISSN (printed): 1523-3774. ISSN (electronic): 1534-6307

Tzioufas, A.G. (2001). Antisynthetase syndrome. *Orphanet encyclopedia*, November 2001

Vanderbroucke, E.; Gruitters, J.K., Altenburg, J., Boersma, W.G., Borg, E.J. & van den Bosch, J.M. (2009). Rituximab in life threatening antisynthetase syndrome, *Rheumatol Int*, Vol.29, No.12, pp. 1499-1502, ISSN: 0172-8172

Zampieri, S.; Ghirardello, A., Iaccarino, L., Tarricone, E., Gambari, P.F. & Doria, A. (2005). Anti-Jo-1 antibodies. *Autoimmunity*, Vol.38, No.1, pp. 73-78 Zampieri, S.; Ghirardello, A., Iaccarino, L., Tarricone, E., Gambari, P.F. & Doria, A. (2005). Anti-Jo-1 antibodies. *Autoimmunity*, Vol.38, No.1, pp. 73-78, ISSN 0891-6934

Walsh, R.J.; Kong, S.W. & Yao, Y. (2007). Type -1 interferon-inducible gene expression inn blood is present and reflects disease activity in dermatomyositis and polymyositis. *Arthritis Rheum*, Vol.56, pp3784-3792, ISSN 1044-2626

Wikipedia, the free encyclopedia (2011). Aminoacyl tRNA synthetase, *Wikipedia, the free encyclopedia*, http://en.wikipedia.org/wiki/Aminoacyl_tRNA_synthetase

Woese, C.R.; Olsen, G.J., Ibba, M. & Soll, D. (2000). Aminoacyl-tRNA synthetases, the genetic code and the evolutionary process. *Microbiology and Molecular Biology Reviews*, pp.202-236, ISSN (printed): 1092-2172

6

Interstitial Lung Disease Associated with Clinically Amyopathic Dermatomyositis

Toshinori Takada[1], Eiichi Suzuki[2] and Ichiei Narita[1]
[1]Division of Respiratory Medicine, Graduate School of Medical and Dental Sciences, Niigata University
[2]Department of General Medicine, Niigata University Medical and Dental Hospital
Japan

1. Introduction

Polymyositis and dermatomyositis (PM-DM) are forms of idiopathic inflammatory myositis (Bohan & Peter, 1975, Dalakas & Hohlfeld, 2003). The diagnosis of DM is definite if the myopathy is accompanied by the characteristic rash and histopathology. If patients with DM has the typical rashes but little (hypomyopathic DM) or no (amyopathic DM) evidence of myositis for 6 months or longer, the condition is termed "clinically amyopathic DM" (Euwer & Sontheimer, 1991, Gerami et al., 2006). Although muscle strength is apparently normal, many patients with clinically amyopathic dermatomyositis have some evidence of muscle inflammation upon testing. Some clinically amyopathic dermatomyositis patients also have been observed to develop overt proximal muscle weakness years after onset of their DM skin disease. Among patients with DM or PM, interstitial lung disease is a major cause of morbidity and mortality (Fathi et al., 2008, Love et al., 1991, Marie et al., 2002). In particular, patients with clinically amyopathic dermatomyositis sometimes develop rapidly progressive interstitial lung disease that remains unresponsive to intensive immunosuppresive therapy (Mukae et al., 2009).

2. Polymyositis and dermatomyositis

2.1 Diagnostic criteria

Three sets of classification criteria have been developed for DM-PM. The original criteria formulated in 1975 by Bohan and Peter included the following features: symmetric proximal muscle weakness, characteristic electromyographic changes, elevation of serum levels of muscle-associated enzymes, evidence of chronic inflammation in muscle biopsy, and characteristic rashes of DM (Bohan & Peter, 1975). However, when these criteria were formulated, testing for myositis-specific autoantibodies was not available. In addition, inclusion body myositis was not recognized until the 1980s (Griggs et al., 1995). Thus, patients classified as DM or PM according to these criteria may have some other disorder. To address this problem, two alternative criteria have been suggested since 2004 (Hoogendijk et al., 2004, Troyanov et al., 2005). One criterion classifies patients according to a "clinicoserologic" approach relying on extensive testing for autoantibodies. Excluding inclusion body myositis, four categories of inflammatory myopathy were recognized: pure

PM, pure DM, overlap myositis, and cancer-associated myositis (Troyanov et al., 2005). The second criterion has nine categories based on clinical, histopathologic, and laboratory findings with autoantibody tests, which include amyopathic DM also called dermatomyositis sine myositis (Hoogendijk et al., 2004).

2.2 Clinically amyopathic dermatomyositis

Clinically amyopathic dermatomyositis is an umbrella designation used to refer to DM with no myositis (amyopathic DM) or DM with little myositis (hypomyopathic DM), i.e. clinically amyopathic DM = amyopathic DM + hypomyopathic DM. Patients with amyopathic DM have hallmark inflammatory skin changes of DM but no clinical evidence of proximal muscle weakness and no serum muscle enzyme abnormalities for 6 months or longer. If more extensive muscle testing is carried out, the results should be within normal limits. While, hypomyopathic DM is a condition of cutaneous DM and no clinical evidence of muscle weakness. Although muscle strength is apparently normal, patients with hypomyopathic DM have some evidence of muscle inflammation on laboratory (eg, muscle enzyme elevations), electrophysiologic, and/or radiologic evaluation. Hypomyopathic DM could also be classified into 2 groups according to degree of skeletal muscle involvement: no subjective muscle weakness but abnormalities detected by objective tests and subjective muscle weakness but no objective evidence of myopathy (el-Azhary & Pakzad, 2002). Some patients with clinically amyopathic dermatomyositis eventually develop overt proximal muscle weakness years after onset of their skin disease; however, muscle involvement may not be seen as long as six years after disease onset (Euwer & Sontheimer, 1991, Gerami et al., 2006, Stonecipher et al., 1993).

3. Interstitial lung disease associated with polymyositis and dermatomyositis

3.1 Clinical manifestations

Pulmonary involvement in PM-DM includes respiratory muscle weakness, aspiration pneumonia, infection, drug-induced pneumonia, and interstitial lung disease (Miller, 2004). interstitial lung disease occurs approximately 40 percent of patients with PM-DM. It is increasingly recognized as a serious complication and a major cause of death in this disease (Douglas et al., 2001, Fathi et al., 2008, Marie et al., 2002). High-resolution computerized tomography in combination with pulmonary function tests provides sensitive tools to detect early signs of intestitial lung disease (Selva-O'Callaghan et al., 2005). The clinical presentation of interstitial lung disease includes progressive dyspnea on exertion, nonproductive cough, and basilar rales, and a rapidly progressive syndrome (Hamman-Rich) may also occur. A rapidly progressive intestitial lung disease characterized by diffuse alveolar damage (DAD) often causes fatal respiratory failure. According to the 2002 ATS/ERS consensus classification of IIPs (2002), several histologic patterns of intestitial lung disease are associated with PM-DM; nonspecific interstitial pneumonia (NSIP) is most often found and DAD, organizing pneumonia (OP), and usual interstitial pneumonia (UIP) are also present (Douglas et al., 2001, Kang et al., 2005, Marie et al., 2002, Tansey et al., 2004, Tazelaar et al., 1990).

3.2 Treatment of interstitial lung disease associated with polymyositis and dermatomyositis

Controlled trials on the effect of different treatments for intestitial lung disease in PM-DM have not been published. Thus, the optimal treatment program for the disease has not been established. Available information on the efficacy of treatment is based on retrospective case collections or open trials.

3.2.1 Glucocorticoids

Prednisolone is considered the first-line drug for PM-DM patients with intestitial lung disease (Douglas et al., 2001, Grau et al., 1996, Hirakata & Nagai, 2000, Marie et al., 1998, Nawata et al., 1999, Oddis, 2000). It usually is started with 1 mg/kg/day or more for 4-6 weeks. Another option is to start treatment with intravenous methylprednisolone (1g/day for 3 days, if necessary repeated after 1-2 weeks) and to continue treatment with oral prednisolone. Prednisolone in the 1mg/kg/day range seems effective in suppressing the PM-DM within a few weeks in most patients, but the lung disease usually is slower to respond to therapy than is the myositis and may require treatment over several months. High doses of prednisolone may lead to serious steroid side-effects, therefore, prednisolone is gradually tapered with careful monitoring of creatine kinase, chest radiographs, and pulmonary function.

3.2.2 Immunosuppressive drugs

Although most patients respond to some degree, corticosteroid treatment as a single agent is often not sufficient to obtain improvement of intestitial lung disease. Furthermore, the high doses required over a long period are often associated with severe side-effects and the addition of an immunosuppressive drugs becomes necessary as steroid sparing agents. Selection of immunosuppressive drugs remains empirical and depends on personal experience and the relative efficacy/safety ratio (Dalakas, 1994, Oddis, 2002). Favorable outcome with immunosuppressive therapy in patients who failed to respond to steroids alone has been reported previously (Nawata et al., 1999, Shinohara et al., 1997). However, a second immunosuppressive agent is added without waiting for a response to glucocorticoid therapy or a failure of tapering (Takada et al., 2007), in particular for patients with clinically amyopathic dermatomyositis because of the high frequency of progressive interstitial lung disease.

Azathioprine (Douglas et al., 2001), or mycophenolate mofetil are often used and the comparative efficacy of these drugs is not known. Cyclophosphamide is an alternative if the patient has impending respiratory failure due to rapidly progressive interstitial lung disease with high dose glucocorticoids. Calcineurin inhibitors, cyclosporine and tacrolimus have been used in patients with inflammatory myopathy complicated by intestitial lung disease. In particular, cyclosporine has been reported to be effective to corticosteroid-resistant intestitial lung disease in PM-DM or clinically amyopathic dermatomyositis (Kameda et al., 2005, Miyake et al., 2002).

3.3 Prognostic factors associated with poor outcome of interstitial lung disease in polymyositis and dermatomyositis

Various parameters related to intestitial lung disease poor outcome in PM-DM were identified as follows: DM subtype, Hamman-Rich type presentation, initial FVC less than 60%, neutrophil alveolitis, histologic UIP, and features of clinically amyopathic dermatomyositis (Fujisawa et al., 2005, Kang et al., 2005, Marie et al., 2002). Schnabel et al. identified progressive disease, featuring ground-glass opacities on high resolution CT, and an inflammatory bronchoalveolar lavage (bronchoalveolar lavage) cell profile as indicators for intensive immunosuppressive therapy (Schnabel et al., 2003). Poor prognosis of patients with UIP was confirmed in studies with lung histology (Marie et al., 2002, Tazelaar et al., 1990). NSIP observed in PM-DM patients means the better survival compared with patients with idiopathic pulmonary fibrosis (Douglas et al., 2001) and mortality is similar to that seen in idiopathic NSIP (Tansey et al., 2004). In intestitial lung disease with clinically amyopathic dermatomyositis, although the most common finding is NSIP (Suda et al., 2006), the intestitial lung disease often takes an aggressive course even when the radiological and histological features are consistent with NSIP (Miyazaki et al., 2005). Tiju et al. reported that digital infarcts with microangiopathy may be a useful indicator for early intervention in intestitial lung disease associated with DM (Tjiu et al., 2004).

4. Interstitial lung disease associated with clinically amyopathic dermatomyositis

Patients with clinically amyopathic dermatomyositis sometimes develop rapidly progressive intestitial lung disease. It has been reported predominantly in Asia, including Japan, Hong Kong, and Taiwan (Lee et al., 2002, Mukae et al., 2009) and is often resistant to intensive therapy including high dose corticosteroids and immunosuppressive agents, resulting in fatal respiratory failure.

4.1 A case with rapidly progressive interstitial lung disease in clinically amyopathic dermatomyositis

A 46-year-old Japanese woman was admitted to a hospital because of eruption on arms to shoulders, erythema and swelling of hand joint, and dry cough for four weeks. The patient was diagnosed as dermatomyositis because of characteristic skin lesions. Chest radiograph and computed tomography on admission showed slight interstitial lung disease (Fig1A, D). Her respiratory function deteriorated in two weeks with progression of infiltrative shadow in chest radiograph and consolidation in particular around bronchovascular bundle in computed tomography (Fig1B, E). The patient was given methylprednisolone 1000mg intravenously daily for three days (pulse treatment) and transferred to our hospital.

Blood gas analysis revealed PaO_2 54.4 torr while she was breathing 3l/min oxygen by nasal plugs. Pulse treatment was followed by daily oral prednisolone 60 mg. Respiratory dysfunction became worse and finally fatal in two weeks after transfer in spite of repeated pulse treatment two more times (Fig1C). A second immunosuppressive agent was not added during hospitalization.

4.2 A case with interstitial lung disease in clinically amyopathic dermatomyositis successfully treated by corticosteroid and cyclosporin

A 31-year-old Japanese man developed bilateral hand erythema followed by fever (temperatures of more than 38°C) and hand and foot stiffness. The patient was admitted to a hospital suspected as dermatomyositis because of characteristic skin lesions. A chest radiograph and computed tomography on admission revealed reticular opacities in lower lobes (Fig2A, E). Interstitial lung disease progressed with remittent fever in three weeks. The patient was given methylprednisolone 1000mg intravenously daily for three days (pulse treatment) and transferred to our hospital.

On examination, the temperature was 38.1°C, the blood pressure 118/78 torr, the pulse 80 beats per minute, and the oxygen saturation 98% while he was breathing ambient air. The physical examination showed Gottron signs on fingers and fine crackles in bilateral back but

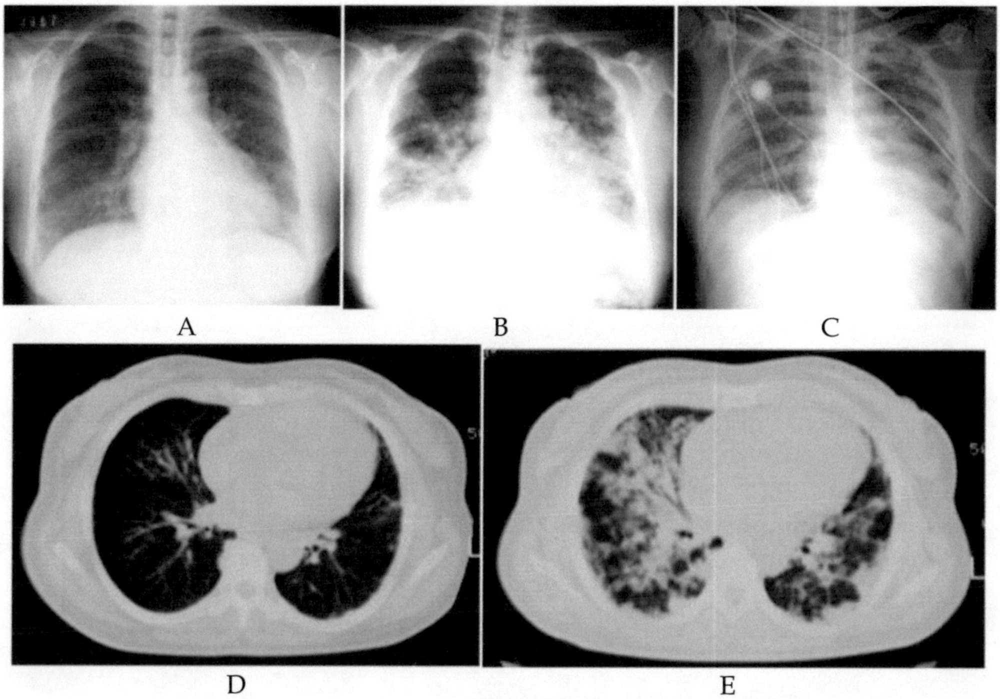

Fig. 1. Chest radiographs and computed tomography of a case with rapidly progressive interstitial lung disease associated with clinically amyopathic dermatomyositis. Very slight interstitial lung disease (A, D) deteriorated to be fatal in three months despite high dose corticosteroid treatment (B, C, E).

no muscle weakness. Interstitial lung disease deteriorated on his chest radiograph and computed tomography (Fig2B, F). The patient was diagnosed as clinically amyopathic dermatomyositis because of slight elevation of creatinin kinase (551 IU/L), mild myopathic change in electromyography, and skin diseases. Pulse treatment was repeated two more times with daily oral predonisone 60 mg and cyclosporine of maximum dose 5 mg/kg/day. Although pneumomediastinum developed during tapering of prednisolone (Fig2C, G), interstitial lung disease gradually ameliorated with only linear opacities left in the lower lobes (Fig2D, H).

4.3 A case with interstitial lung disease in clinically amyopathic dermatomyositis resistant to corticosteroid and cyclosporin

A 56-year-old Japanese woman developed finger erythema. The erythema extended to her eyelids and then body in three weeks. Being suspected as dermatomyositis, she was referred and admitted to the hospital. On examination, the temperature was 37.0°C, the blood pressure 100/70 torr, the pulse 89 beats per minute, and the oxygen saturation 94% while she was breathing ambient air. The physical examination showed heliotrope erythema on eyelids, Gottron signs on fingers, and slight fine crackles in right back but no muscle weakness. A chest radiograph and computed tomography on admission revealed consolidation with reticular opacities in lower lobes (Fig3A, D). The patient was diagnosed as clinically amyopathic dermatomyositis because of slight elevation of creatine kinase (149 IU/L), mild myopathic change in electromyography, and skin diseases.

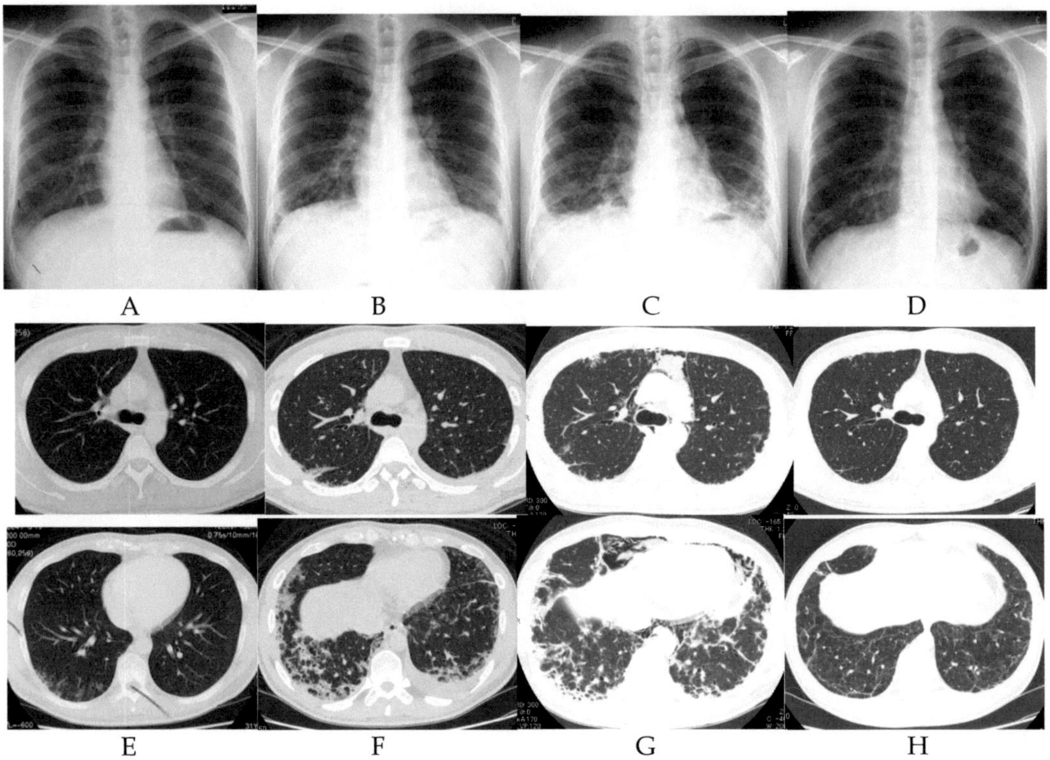

Fig. 2. Chest radiographs and computed tomography of a case with interstitial lung disease associated with clinically amyopathic dermatomyositis successfully treated by corticosteroid and cyclosporin. Interstitial lung disease progressed (A, B, E, F) with pneumomediastinum complicated (C, G), however, was finally improved (D, H).

The patient was given methylprednisolone 1000mg intravenously daily for three days (pulse treatment) followed by daily oral prednisolone 60 mg. Although respiratory functions with regard to $AaDO_2$ and consolidation in lower lobes improved by prednisolone 60 mg for a month, reticular and ground-glass opacities appeared and progressed in upper lobes with worsening of $AaDO_2$ when prednisolone was tapered to 50 mg/day (Fig3B, E). Cyclosporine of maximum dose 5 mg/kg/day and two more time pulse treatment were added with daily oral prednisolone 50 mg for another month. Interstitial lung disease gradually deteriorated in spite of the immunosuppressive therapy (Fig3C, F) and respiratory failure finally progressed to fatal in a week.

5. Characteristics of patients with interstitial lung disease in polymyositis-dermatomyositis resistant to prednisolone and cyclosporine

Cyclosporine is sometimes effective to Japanese patients with corticosteroid-resistant intestitial lung disease in PM-DM or clinically amyopathic dermatomyositis (Kameda et al., 2005, Miyake et al., 2002). However, the efficacy of cyclosporine remains limited and some patients still develop fatal respiratory failure. To clarify characteristics of fatal intestitial lung disease in PM-DM including clinically amyopathic dermatomyositis, we reviewed clinical records of PM-DM patients with intestitial lung disease.

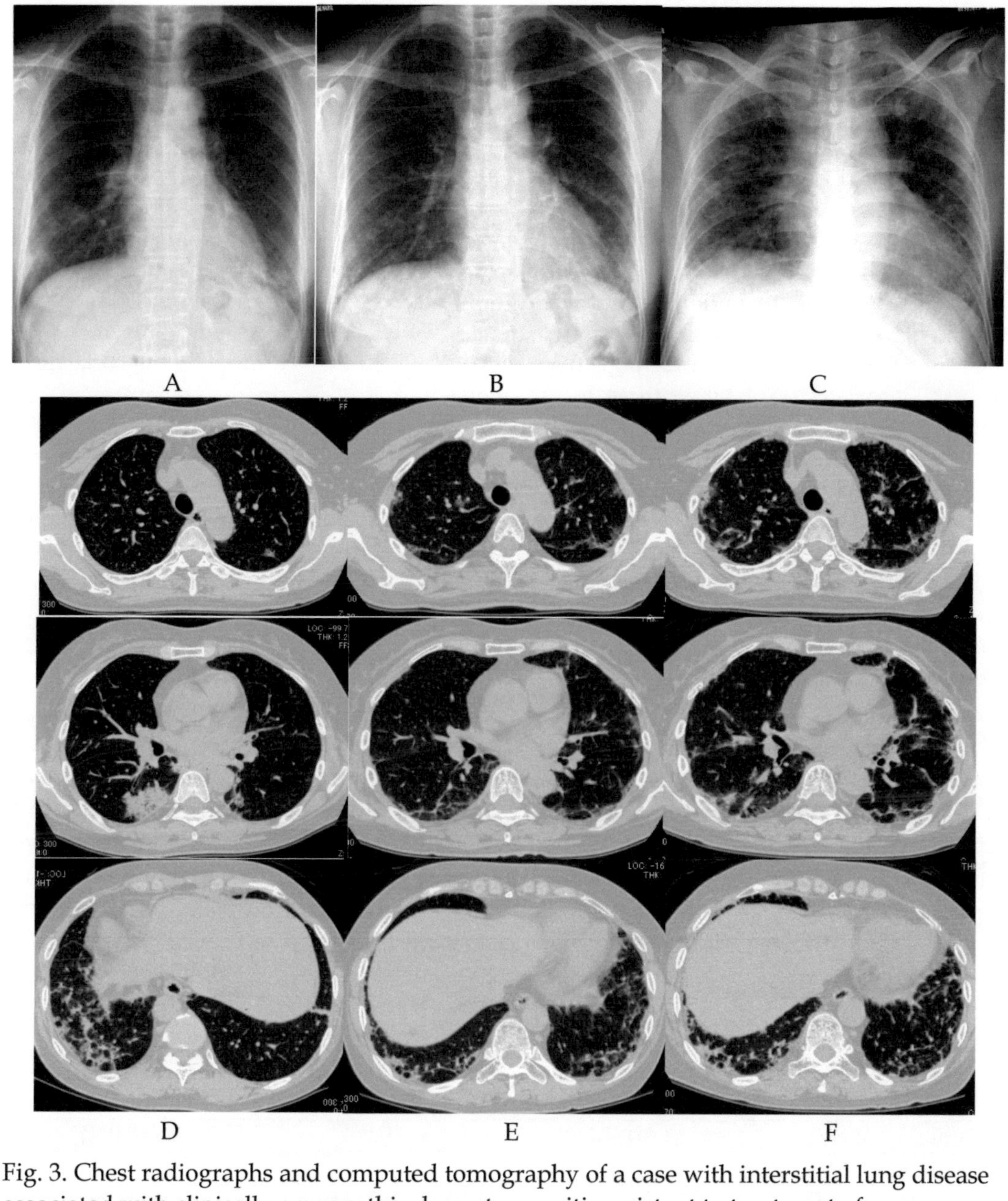

Fig. 3. Chest radiographs and computed tomography of a case with interstitial lung disease associated with clinically amyopathic dermatomyositis resistant to treatment of corticosteroid and cyclosporin. Consolidation in lower lobes was improved by corticosteroid (A, B, D, E), but reticular and ground-glass opacities appeared and progressed in upper lobes to be fatal in spite of addition of cyclosporin (C, F).

5.1 Study design

Consecutive 26 PM-DM patients with intestitial lung disease underwent initial treatment in Niigata University Medical and Dental Hospital from January 1997 to June 2006. Diagnosis of PM-DM was made according to the criteria of Bohan and Peter (Bohan & Peter, 1975). intestitial lung disease was diagnosed based on the presence of clinical symptoms, respiratory functions, and high-resolution computed tomography of the chest. Diagnosis of clinically amyopathic dermatomyositis was confirmed based on modified Euwer's criteria (Euwer & Sontheimer, 1993) as follows: 1) characteristic dermatological manifestations of classic DM, including a heliotrope rash and Gottron's papules; 2) no muscle weakness; and 3) no increases in serum muscle enzymes during the observation period. All patients received oral prednisolone 1.0mg/kg/day for initial therapy. Corticosteroid pulse therapy (methyl prednisolone, 1000mg, 3days) was added when the worsening of respiratory function was observed under the treatment of 1.0mg/kg/day prednisolone. Effect of the treatment for intestitial lung disease was evaluated two weeks later by symptoms, blood gas analysis, chest X ray, and chest high resolution CT findings. We thought intestitial lung disease steroid-resistant when three of the above four findings were not improved and added cyclosporine to prednisolone keeping a trough level of 100 to 150ng/ml. Since 2002, cyclosporine dose has been increased to achieve a trough level of 300 ng/ml for up to 4 weeks to expect the maximal immunosuppressive effect without adverse effects. Five of 26 were excluded from this study because they had received cyclosporine before the evaluation of intestitial lung disease to have a sparing effect for high dose prednisolone. Finally 21 patients with intestitial lung disease associated with PM-DM were enrolled in this study. Medical records were reviewed to obtain clinical data including history, treatment, and laboratory findings.

5.2 Demographic data of patients

Characteristics of 21 patients are shown in Table 1. Thirteen patients (61.9%) was effectively treated by corticosteroids alone. Cyclosporine was added to the other eight patients because of deterioration of intestitial lung disease even under steroid therapy. Out of these 8 steroid-resistant cases, 4 patients (19.0%) improved by addition of cyclosporine, and the other 4 patients (19.0%) showed no response to cyclosporine resulting in fatal respiratory failure. Finally, 17 patients survived and four died of respiratory failure due to progression of intestitial lung disease. All of the dead patients were diagnosed as clinically amyopathic dermatomyositis.

		Steroid-resistant cases	
	Steroid-effective cases	Cyclosporine-effective	Cyclosporine-resistant
Number of cases	13 (61.9%)	4 (19.0%)	4 (19.0%)
Sex (M/F)	2/11	3/1	2/2
Age (mean±SD)	54.5±14.3	52.0±17.7	58.8±5.1
Diagnosis			
PM	0	1	0
DM	9	2	0
CADM	4	1	4

Abbreviations: PM, polymyositis; DM, dermatomyositis; CADM, clinically amyopathic dermatomyositis

Table 1. Demographic characteristics of PM-DM with intestitial lung disease patients.

5.3 Summary of treatment

Treatment in details is shown in Table 2. All the patients initially had 1mg/kg/day prednisolone. Steroid pulse therapy (methyl prednisolone 1000mg/day, three days) was given to 11 patients. Cyclosporine was added to 7 of 11 patients. Initial trough level of cyclosporine was usually maintained at 250 to 300 ng/ml to obtain maximal immunosuppressive effect.

		Steroid-resistant cases	
	Steroid-effective cases (n=13)	Cyclosporine-effective (n=4)	Cyclosporine-resistant (n=4)
Initial dose of PS (mg/day, mean±SD)	46.2±11.2	60.0±0.0	57.5±5.0
Additional treatment			
m PSL pulse	4	0	0
cyclosporine	0	1	0
mPSL pulse, cyclosporine	0	3	4
cyclosporine trough level			
100~150ng/ml	NA	1	0
250~300ng/ml	NA	3	4

Abbreviations: PSL, prednisolone

Table 2. Treatment of PM-DM with interstitial lung disease patients.

		Steroid-resistant cases	
	Steroid-effective cases (n=13)	Cyclosporine-effective (n=4)	Cyclosporine-resistant (n=4)
WBC (/µl)	6292.3±1790.3	4 (19.0%)	4 (19.0%)
CRP (mg/dl)	0.8±1.7	4.3±4.9*	1.7±1.8
CK (IU/L)	1013.4±1272.5	2192.8±3084.4	158.5±54.2
LDH (IU/L)	679.2±362.9	733.0±795.3	499.5±81.5
AST (IU/L)	53.1±35.2	106.3±105.9	188.7±202.3
ALT (IU/L)	38.4±28.5	65.0±48.0	157.8±203.8
TP (g/dl)	6.8±0.6	6.5±0.4	6.7±0.4
Alb (g/dl)	3.6±0.6	3.0±0.3	1 (25.0)
ANA positive (%)	9 (69.2)	3 (75.0)	1 (25.0)
Jo-1 positive (%)	2 (15.4)	2 (50.0)	1 (25.0)
KL-6 (U/ml)	1127.8±454.1	769.3±570.9	797.0±180.5
BGA (torr, room air)			
PaO_2	81.8±8.8	82.7±14.1	63.4±8.6*
$PaCO_2$	41.5±3.8	36.2±4.1	37.1±1.2
$AaDO_2$ (torr)	16.4±9.0	22.1±18.6	40.3±8.0*

*P<0.01 against steroid effective group.

Table 3. Comparison of laboratory data on admission.

5.4 Laboratory findings

Laboratory findings on admission are presented in Table 3. Serum CRP level of cyclosporine-effective group was higher than that of steroid-effective group. There were no significant differences in the levels of peripheral leukocyte count, serum CK, LDH, AST, ALT, total protein, albumin, and KL-6 among thee groups. PaO_2 on admission was significantly decreased with an increase of $AaDO_2$. in cyclosporine-resistant group.
We often experience deterioration of intestitial lung disease associated with PM-DM when we perform laboratory, radiological, and neurological tests to make diagnosis of the disease. To evaluate progression of the disease during test period, we then compared changes in peripheral leukocyte count, serum CRP, CK, LDH, albumin, and $AaDO_2$ from admission to administration of prednisolone. In cyclosporine-effective group, the level of serum CRP, CK, LDH, and $AaDO_2$ significantly elevated during test period, while significant decrease of serum albumin and rapid progression of respiratory dysfunction indicated as $AaDO_2$ were observed in cyclosporine-resistant group compared with steroid-effective group (Table 4).

	Steroid-effective cases (n=13)	Steroid-resistant cases	
		Cyclosporine-effective (n=3)	Cyclosporine-resistant (n=3)
Δ WBC	-582.3±818.4	1335.0±3014.4	-516.7±692.1
Δ CRP	0.4±0.9	5.2±3.0*	0.7±0.8
Δ CK	-67.5±466.8	2076.3±2008.9*	-3.0±71.0
Δ LDH	-25.8±136.2	398.7±355.4*	-70.3±85.0§
Δ Alb	-0.2±0.4	-0.5±0.1	-1.0±0.3*§
Δ $AaDO_2$	-1.4±6.8	22.0±5.0*	53.7±34.4*

Δ =(value on admission)-(value on initial treatment)
*P<0.05 against steroid-effective group, §P<0.05 against cyclosporine-effective group.

Table 4. Changes of laboratory values from admission to initial treatment.

5.5 Bronchoalveolar lavage analysis

Bronchoalveolar lavage findings before treatment are available in 18 patients. Although there were no differences in total cell counts and frequency of alveolar macrophages, lymphocytes, and eosinophils in bronchoalveolar lavage fluid, frequency of neutrophils in cyclosporine-effective group was significantly higher than that in other two groups. In cyclosporine-resistant group, CD4/CD8 ratio was significantly higher compared with other groups (Table 5).

	Steroid-effective cases (n=12)	Steroid-resistant cases	
		Cyclosporine-effective (n=4)	Cyclosporine-resistant (n=4)
TCC ($\times 10^5$/ml)	3.2±1.4	5.5±2.8	5.6±2.4
AM (%)	51.2±20.6	49.5±31.2	61.1±23.5
Lym (%)	41.0±22.5	38.2±31.1	35.2±21.8
Neut (%)	4.2±5.1	11.2±6.1**§	1.6±2.6
Eo (%)	3.6±6.0	1.4±0.9	0.6±0.5
CD4/CD8 ratio	0.44±0.53	0.70±0.6	1.9±0.9*

*P<0.01 against steroid-effective group, **P<0.05 against steroid-effective group, §P<0.05 against cyclosporine-resistant group.

Table 5. Comparison of bronchoalveolar lavage findings.

5.6 Characteristics of patients with interstitial lung disease in polymyositis-dermatomyositis resistant to prednisolone and cyclosporine

Cyclosporin binds to cyclophilin, then the complex inhibits calcineurin phosphatase and T-cell activation (Clipstone & Crabtree, 1992). Because activated T lymphocytes, in particular $CD8^+$ T cells, may play essential roles in intestitial lung disease associated with PM-DM (Enomoto et al., 2003, Kourakata et al., 1999, Kurasawa et al., 2002), immunosuppressive therapy targeting $CD8^+$ cells should be reasonable. However, CD4/8 ratio in bronchoalveolar lavage fluid was significantly increased in cyclosporine-resistant cases compared to alive ones. Suda et al. also described that the ratio of CD4/8 lymphocytes was higher in acute/subacute intestitial lung disease than chronic intestitial lung disease in clinically amyopathic dermatomyositis, but the difference was not statistically significant (Suda et al., 2006). Increased CD4/8 ratio in bronchoalveolar lavage fluid suggests that $CD8^+$ T cells may not be major pulmonary inflammatory cells causing lung injury in PM-DM.

In this study, all of the cyclosporine-resistant cases were diagnosed as clinically amyopathic dermatomyositis and died of respiratory failure. While, five of nine patients with intestitial lung disease in clinically amyopathic dermatomyositis survived without progression of respiratory failure. Cottin et al. also described a benign form of intestitial lung disease in clinically amyopathic dermatomyositis (Cottin et al., 2003). Clinically amyopathic dermatomyositis with fatal interstitial lung disease may be a distinct clinical entity with unique clinical features.

5.7 Salvage therapy to interstitial lung disease in polymyositis-dermatomyositis

For patients with progressive intestitial lung disease in spite of the combination of glucocorticoids and a second agent, a third immunosuppressive agent may be added. High dose glucocorticoids, monthly intravenous cyclophosphamide, and cyclosporine may be used in combination for patients with intestitial lung disease in clinically amyopathic dermatomyositis, even when the intestitial lung disease is still mild. Primary intensive approach by starting immunosuppressive agents simultaneously with corticosteroids was associated with better survival than step-up approach by adding them sequentially in initial treatment for active intestitial lung disease in PM-DM (Takada et al., 2007).

In spite of the combination therapies with glucocorticoids and immunosuppressive agents, respiratory dysfunction of PM-DM patients with intestitial lung disease sometimes progresses. Although options for salvage therapy including rituximab, intravenous immune globulin, and lung transplantation are reported (Labirua & Lundberg, 2010, Shoji et al., 2010, Suzuki et al., 2009), the effects of these therapies are still unknown or limited. Recently, a case with rapidly progressive interstitial pneumonia associated with clinically amyopathic dermatomyositis successfully treated with polymyxin B-immobilized fiber column (PMX) hemoperfusion was reported (Kakugawa et al., 2008). PMX might improve oxygenation in patients with acute lung injury/ acute respiratory distress syndrome or with acute exacerbation of idiopathic pulmonary fibrosis (Kushi et al., 2005, Seo et al., 2006). This could be another option for intestitial lung disease in clinically amyopathic dermatomyositis resistant to immunosuppressive treatment.

6. Myositis-associated autoantibodies

About 30 percent of patients with DM or PM have myositis-associated autoantibodies with clinical findings of the relatively acute disease onset, constitutional symptoms, Raynaud's phenomenon, mechanic's hands, arthritis, and interstitial lung disease. Three major categories of myositis-specific autoantibodies are reported: anti-aminoacyl-tRNA synthetase antibodies, anti-SRP antibodies, and anti-Mi-2 antibodies. The presence of individual myositis antibodies may play a role in determining the disease manifestations.

6.1 Anti-aminoacyl-tRNA synthetase antibodies

A group of myositis-associated autoantibodies is strongly linked to the development of intestitial lung disease (Grau et al., 1996, Targoff, 2008). These antibodies are directed against aminoacyl-tRNA synthetase (aaRS). The most common, anti-aaRS specific for histidine (anti-Jo-1), is found in approximately 29% of patients with DM and is found even more frequently in cases with intestitial lung disease (Botha & Carney, 1999, Climent-Albaladejo et al., 2002). Others have been labeled anti-PL-7 (for threonine), anti-PL-12 (alanine), anti-EJ (glycine), anti-KS (asparagine), anti-OJ (isoleucine), and anti-Zo (phenylalanine) (Betteridge et al., 2007). Each of these antibodies has been associated with antisynthetase syndrome marked by a high frequency of intestitial lung disease compared with PM-DM without such antibodies (Targoff, 2008). Selva-O'Callaghan et al. reported that anti-aaRS negative patients with acute interstitial lung disease and pneumomediastinum had an unfavorable prognosis (Selva-O'Callaghan et al., 2005).

6.2 Anti-SRP and anti-Mi-2 antibodies

The signal recognition particle (SRP) is involved in the translocation of newly synthesized proteins into the endoplasmic reticulum. Anti-SRP antibodies are present in 4 to 6 percent of patients with acquired inflammatory and/or necrotizing myopathies (Hengstman et al., 2006). They are associated with aggressive disease with heart and lung involvement and resistance to high-dose glucocorticoids and adjunct immunosuppressive agents (Arlet et al., 2006). Anti-Mi-2 antibodies are directed against a helicase involved in transcriptional activation. They are present in 10– 30% of patients with DM (Ghirardello et al., 2005) and associated with severer cutaneous manifestations but a better response to steroid therapy (Hengstman et al., 2006).

6.3 Anti-CADM-140 antibody

A novel autoantibody associated with PM-DM was identified by screening with immunoprecipitation in 298 serum samples from patients with various connective tissue diseases or idiopathic pulmonary fibrosis. Eight out of 298 sera recognized a polypeptide of approximately 140 kd by immunoprecipitation and immunoblotting. Interestingly, all 8 patients with the antibodies had clinically amyopathic dermatomyositis and rapidly progressive interstitial lung disease with significantly higher frequency (Sato et al., 2005). Furthermore, the antibody, termed "anti-CADM-140 antibody" recognizes an antigen identified to be an RNA helicase encoded by melanoma differentiation-associated gene 5 (MDA-5) (Sato et al., 2009). RNA helicase encoded by MDA-5 is a critical molecule involved in the innate immune defense against viruses and viral infection. Although a role of anti-CADM-140 antibody in developing rapidly progressive interstitial lung disease in clinically amyopathic dermatomyositis is still unknown, this may provide a clue about the pathogenesis of the disease and lead to novel effective treatment for the disease.

6.4 A case with clinically amyopathic dermatomyositis with anti-CADM-140 antibody positive

A 45-year-old Japanese woman had complained of itchy erythema, finger joint pain, Raynaud phenomenon, and facial rush for 6 months. She was admitted to the hospital being suspected as dermatomyositis because of skin lesions, but not diagnosed definitely. Chest radiograph and computed tomography showed very slight interstitial lung disease (Fig4A, B). Although daily oral prednisolone 20mg relieved her symptoms, her skin lesions and joint pain recurred during prednisolone tapering in 10 months.

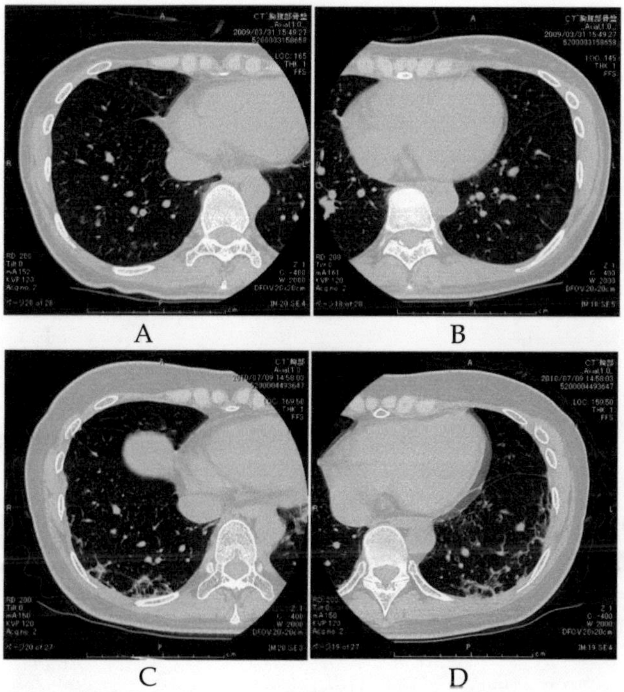

Fig. 4. Chest computed tomography of a case with interstitial lung disease associated with clinically amyopathic dermatomyositis with anti-CADM-140 antibody positive. Chest computed tomography on the first admission (A, B) and the second admission about one year later (C, D) indicated progression of interstitial lung disease in spite of daily oral prednisolone 20mg.

The patient was admitted to the hospital again. On examination, the temperature was 37.1°C, the blood pressure 101/74 torr, the pulse 89 beats per minute, and the oxygen saturation 98% while she was breathing ambient air. The physical examination showed Gottron signs on fingers, hand skin sclerosis, and Raynaud phenomenon, but no fine crackles auscultated or muscle weakness. Chest computed tomography revealed marked reticular and ground-glass opacities in lower lobes (Fig4C, D). The patient was suspected as clinically amyopathic dermatomyositis because of characteristic skin diseases. Surgical lung biopsy was performed to pathologically evaluate lung diseases. Specimens from right S2 segment contained fibrotic lesions distributed at subpleural and perivenous area and wide fibrosis extending from subpleural area with alveolar collapse (Fig5A, original magnification, x 5). Mild to moderate lymphocyte infiltration with lymph follicles in the

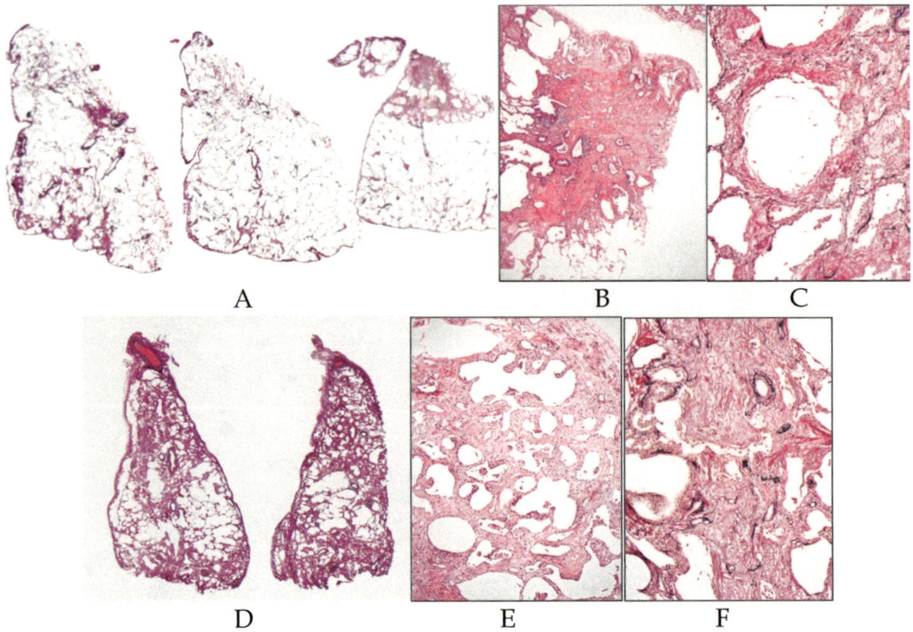

Fig. 5. Light microscopic findings of the lung specimen from a case with anti-CADM-140 antibody. Patchy fibrosing lesions were seen in the upper lobe specimens (A, B, C), while fibrotic nonspecific interstitial pneumonia (fNSIP) pattern was recognized in the specimens from lower lobe (D, E, F).

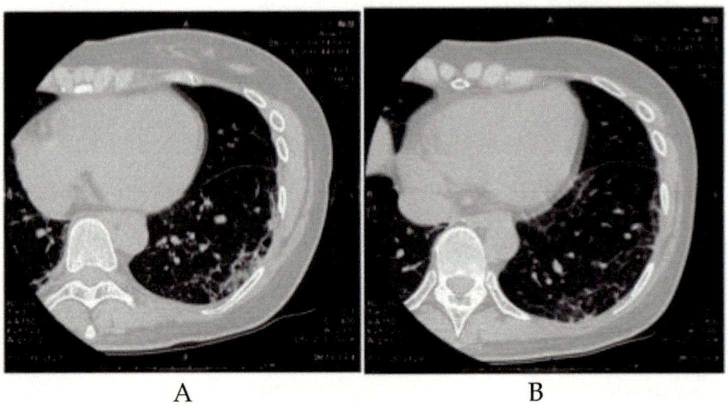

Fig. 6. Chest computed tomography of a case with interstitial lung disease associated with clinically amyopathic dermatomyositis with anti-CADM-140 antibody. Chest computed tomography on admission (A) and in treatment (B) were shown. Interstitial lung disease improved by daily intravenous methylprednisolone 500mg three days followed by daily oral prednisolone and cyclosporine for 14 days.

fibrotic lesions and ring fibrosis connecting alveolar orifices at the rim of collapsing fibrosis were seen (Fig5B, C, original magnification, x 20). Specimens from right S10 segment revealed homogenously distributed fibrotic lesions (Fig5D, original magnification, x 5). Alveolar walls were thickened by fibrosis with simplified alveolar construction and

polypoid tissue protruding into alveolar spaces was also seen (Fig5E, F, original magnification, x 20).
The patient was given methylprednisolone 500mg intravenously daily for three days followed by daily oral prednisolone 40 mg and cyclosporine of 100 to 150 mg /day. Anti-CADM-140 antibody was proven to be positive during the treatment of prednisolone and cyclosporine. Interstitial lung disease gradually ameliorated by prednisolone (Fig6A, B).

7. Conclusion

Clinically amyopathic dermatomyositis is a condition which includes the characteristic rash but little or no evidence of myositis. Patients with PM-DM, in particular clinically amyopathic dermatomyositis sometimes develop rapidly progressive intestitial lung disease. The disease is often resistant to intensive therapy including high dose corticosteroids and immunosuppressive agents, resulting in fatal respiratory failure. Although cyclophosphamide, cyclosporin, and tacrolimus were reported to be effective in treatment of refractory intestitial lung disease in PM-DM, the effect of these drugs were still limited. Our retrospective study suggested that features of glucocorticoid/cyclosporin-resistant intestitial lung disease associated with PM-DM might be 1) a subtype of clinically amyopathic dermatomyositis, 2) hypoxemia on admission and further progression of respiratory dysfunction, 3) progression of hypoalbuminemia before treatment, and 4) elevated CD4/8 ratio in bronchoalveolar lavage fluid.
A variety of serum autoantibodies are specifically detected in patients with PM-DM, including antibodies reactive with aminoacyl-transfer RNA synthetase. These autoantibodies are associated with distinct clinical subsets of PM-DM. Recently a novel PM-DM associated autoantibody, termed "anti-CADM-140 antibody" is reported. This antibody is strongly associated with clinically amyopathic dermatomyositis, in particular rapidly progressive intestitial lung disease complicated. This may provide a clue about the pathogenesis of the disease and lead to novel effective treatment for the disease.

8. Acknowledgment

The authors thank Dr. Ran Nakashima and Dr. Tsuneyo Mimori for measuring anti-CADM-140 antibody. The authors also offer special thanks to Dr. Junichi Narita for useful discussion.

9. References

(2002) American Thoracic Society/European Respiratory Society International Multidisciplinary Consensus Classification of the Idiopathic Interstitial Pneumonias. This joint statement of the American Thoracic Society (ATS), and the European Respiratory Society (ERS) was adopted by the ATS board of directors, June 2001 and by the ERS Executive Committee, June 2001. *Am J Respir Crit Care Med*. Vol. 165, No. 2: pp. 277-304

Arlet, J.B., Dimitri, D., Pagnoux, C., Boyer, O., Maisonobe, T., Authier, F.J., Bloch-Queyrat, C., Goulvestre, C., Heshmati, F., Atassi, M., Guillevin, L., Herson, S., Benveniste, O., & Mouthon, L., (2006) Marked efficacy of a therapeutic strategy associating prednisone and plasma exchange followed by rituximab in two patients with refractory myopathy associated with antibodies to the signal recognition particle (SRP). *Neuromuscul Disord*. Vol. 16, No. 5: pp. 334-336

Betteridge, Z., Gunawardena, H., North, J., Slinn, J., & McHugh, N., (2007) Anti-synthetase syndrome: a new autoantibody to phenylalanyl transfer RNA synthetase (anti-Zo) associated with polymyositis and interstitial pneumonia. *Rheumatology (Oxford)*. Vol. 46, No. 6: pp. 1005-1008

Bohan, A. & Peter, J.B., (1975) Polymyositis and dermatomyositis (first of two parts). *N Engl J Med*. Vol. 292, No. 7: pp. 344-347.

Botha, J.A. & Carney, I.K., (1999) A 59-year-old female with increasing dyspnoea, an unusual rash and myalgia. Diagnosis: dermatomyositis with associated interstitial lung disease. *Respiration*. Vol. 66, No. 4: pp. 377-379

Climent-Albaladejo, A., Saiz-Cuenca, E., Rosique-Roman, J., Caballero-Rodriguez, J., & Galvez-Munoz, J., (2002) Dermatomyositis sine myositis and antisynthetase syndrome. *Joint Bone Spine*. Vol. 69, No. 1: pp. 72-75

Clipstone, N.A. & Crabtree, G.R., (1992) Identification of calcineurin as a key signalling enzyme in T-lymphocyte activation. *Nature*. Vol. 357, No. 6380: pp. 695-697

Cottin, V., Thivolet-Bejui, F., Reynaud-Gaubert, M., Cadranel, J., Delaval, P., Ternamian, P.J., & Cordier, J.F., (2003) Interstitial lung disease in amyopathic dermatomyositis, dermatomyositis and polymyositis. *Eur Respir J*. Vol. 22, No. 2: pp. 245-250

Dalakas, M.C., (1994) How to diagnose and treat the inflammatory myopathies. *Semin Neurol*. Vol. 14, No. 2: pp. 137-145

Dalakas, M.C. & Hohlfeld, R., (2003) Polymyositis and dermatomyositis. *Lancet*. Vol. 362, No. 9388: pp. 971-982

Douglas, W.W., Tazelaar, H.D., Hartman, T.E., Hartman, R.P., Decker, P.A., Schroeder, D.R., & Ryu, J.H., (2001) Polymyositis-dermatomyositis-associated interstitial lung disease. *Am J Respir Crit Care Med*. Vol. 164, No. 7: pp. 1182-1185.

el-Azhary, R.A. & Pakzad, S.Y., (2002) Amyopathic dermatomyositis: retrospective review of 37 cases. *J Am Acad Dermatol*. Vol. 46, No. 4: pp. 560-565

Enomoto, K., Takada, T., Suzuki, E., Ishida, T., Moriyama, H., Ooi, H., Hasegawa, T., Tsukada, H., Nakano, M., & Gejyo, F., (2003) Bronchoalveolar lavage fluid cells in mixed connective tissue disease. *Respirology*. Vol. 8, No. 2: pp. 149-156

Euwer, R.L. & Sontheimer, R.D., (1991) Amyopathic dermatomyositis (dermatomyositis sine myositis). Presentation of six new cases and review of the literature. *J Am Acad Dermatol*. Vol. 24, No. 6 Pt 1: pp. 959-966

Euwer, R.L. & Sontheimer, R.D., (1993) Amyopathic dermatomyositis: a review. *J Invest Dermatol*. Vol. 100, No. 1: pp. 124S-127S

Fathi, M., Vikgren, J., Boijsen, M., Tylen, U., Jorfeldt, L., Tornling, G., & Lundberg, I.E., (2008) Interstitial lung disease in polymyositis and dermatomyositis: longitudinal evaluation by pulmonary function and radiology. *Arthritis Rheum*. Vol. 59, No. 5: pp. 677-685

Fujisawa, T., Suda, T., Nakamura, Y., Enomoto, N., Ide, K., Toyoshima, M., Uchiyama, H., Tamura, R., Ida, M., Yagi, T., Yasuda, K., Genma, H., Hayakawa, H., Chida, K., & Nakamura, H., (2005) Differences in clinical features and prognosis of interstitial lung diseases between polymyositis and dermatomyositis. *J Rheumatol*. Vol. 32, No. 1: pp. 58-64

Gerami, P., Schope, J.M., McDonald, L., Walling, H.W., & Sontheimer, R.D., (2006) A systematic review of adult-onset clinically amyopathic dermatomyositis (dermatomyositis sine myositis): a missing link within the spectrum of the idiopathic inflammatory myopathies. *J Am Acad Dermatol*. Vol. 54, No. 4: pp. 597-613

Ghirardello, A., Zampieri, S., Iaccarino, L., Tarricone, E., Bendo, R., Gambari, P.F., & Doria, A., (2005) Anti-Mi-2 antibodies. *Autoimmunity*. Vol. 38, No. 1: pp. 79-83

Grau, J.M., Miro, O., Pedrol, E., Casademont, J., Masanes, F., Herrero, C., Haussman, G., & Urbano-Marquez, A., (1996) Interstitial lung disease related to dermatomyositis. Comparative study with patients without lung involvement. *J Rheumatol*. Vol. 23, No. 11: pp. 1921-1926

Griggs, R.C., Askanas, V., DiMauro, S., Engel, A., Karpati, G., Mendell, J.R., & Rowland, L.P., (1995) Inclusion body myositis and myopathies. *Ann Neurol*. Vol. 38, No. 5: pp. 705-713

Hengstman, G.J., ter Laak, H.J., Vree Egberts, W.T., Lundberg, I.E., Moutsopoulos, H.M., Vencovsky, J., Doria, A., Mosca, M., van Venrooij, W.J., & van Engelen, B.G., (2006) Anti-signal recognition particle autoantibodies: marker of a necrotising myopathy. *Ann Rheum Dis*. Vol. 65, No. 12: pp. 1635-1638

Hengstman, G.J., Vree Egberts, W.T., Seelig, H.P., Lundberg, I.E., Moutsopoulos, H.M., Doria, A., Mosca, M., Vencovsky, J., van Venrooij, W.J., & van Engelen, B.G., (2006) Clinical characteristics of patients with myositis and autoantibodies to different fragments of the Mi-2 beta antigen. *Ann Rheum Dis*. Vol. 65, No. 2: pp. 242-245

Hirakata, M. & Nagai, S., (2000) Interstitial lung disease in polymyositis and dermatomyositis. *Curr Opin Rheumatol*. Vol. 12, No. 6: pp. 501-508.

Hoogendijk, J.E., Amato, A.A., Lecky, B.R., Choy, E.H., Lundberg, I.E., Rose, M.R., Vencovsky, J., de Visser, M., & Hughes, R.A., (2004) 119th ENMC international workshop: trial design in adult idiopathic inflammatory myopathies, with the exception of inclusion body myositis, 10-12 October 2003, Naarden, The Netherlands. *Neuromuscul Disord*. Vol. 14, No. 5: pp. 337-345

Kakugawa, T., Mukae, H., Saito, M., Ishii, K., Ishimoto, H., Sakamoto, N., Takazono, T., Fukuda, Y., Ooe, N., & Kohno, S., (2008) Rapidly progressive interstitial pneumonia associated with clinically amyopathic dermatomyositis successfully treated with polymyxin B-immobilized fiber column hemoperfusion. *Intern Med*. Vol. 47, No. 8: pp. 785-790

Kameda, H., Nagasawa, H., Ogawa, H., Sekiguchi, N., Takei, H., Tokuhira, M., Amano, K., & Takeuchi, T., (2005) Combination therapy with corticosteroids, cyclosporin A, and intravenous pulse cyclophosphamide for acute/subacute interstitial pneumonia in patients with dermatomyositis. *J Rheumatol*. Vol. 32, No. 9: pp. 1719-1726

Kang, E.H., Lee, E.B., Shin, K.C., Im, C.H., Chung, D.H., Han, S.K., & Song, Y.W., (2005) Interstitial lung disease in patients with polymyositis, dermatomyositis and amyopathic dermatomyositis. *Rheumatology (Oxford)*. Vol. 44, No. 10: pp. 1282-1286

Kourakata, H., Takada, T., Suzuki, E., Enomoto, K., Saito, I., Taguchi, Y., Tsukada, H., Nakano, M., & Arakawa, M., (1999) Flowcytometric analysis of bronchoalveolar lavage fluid cells in polymyositis/dermatomyositis with interstitial pneumonia. *Respirology*. Vol. 4, No. 3: pp. 223-228

Kurasawa, K., Nawata, Y., Takabayashi, K., Kumano, K., Kita, Y., Takiguchi, Y., Kuriyama, T., Sueishi, M., Saito, Y., & Iwamoto, I., (2002) Activation of pulmonary T cells in corticosteroid-resistant and -sensitive interstitial pneumonitis in dermatomyositis/polymyositis. *Clin Exp Immunol*. Vol. 129, No. 3: pp. 541-548

Kushi, H., Miki, T., Okamaoto, K., Nakahara, J., Saito, T., & Tanjoh, K., (2005) Early hemoperfusion with an immobilized polymyxin B fiber column eliminates humoral mediators and improves pulmonary oxygenation. *Crit Care*. Vol. 9, No. 6: pp. R653-661

Labirua, A. & Lundberg, I.E., (2010) Interstitial lung disease and idiopathic inflammatory myopathies: progress and pitfalls. *Curr Opin Rheumatol*. Vol. 22, No. 6: pp. 633-638

Lee, C.S., Chen, T.L., Tzen, C.Y., Lin, F.J., Peng, M.J., Wu, C.L., & Chen, P.J., (2002) Idiopathic inflammatory myopathy with diffuse alveolar damage. *Clin Rheumatol*. Vol. 21, No. 5: pp. 391-396

Love, L.A., Leff, R.L., Fraser, D.D., Targoff, I.N., Dalakas, M., Plotz, P.H., & Miller, F.W., (1991) A new approach to the classification of idiopathic inflammatory myopathy: myositis-specific autoantibodies define useful homogeneous patient groups. *Medicine (Baltimore)*. Vol. 70, No. 6: pp. 360-374

Marie, I., Hachulla, E., Cherin, P., Dominique, S., Hatron, P.Y., Hellot, M.F., Devulder, B., Herson, S., Levesque, H., & Courtois, H., (2002) Interstitial lung disease in polymyositis and dermatomyositis. *Arthritis Rheum*. Vol. 47, No. 6: pp. 614-622

Marie, I., Hatron, P.Y., Hachulla, E., Wallaert, B., Michon-Pasturel, U., & Devulder, B., (1998) Pulmonary involvement in polymyositis and in dermatomyositis. *J Rheumatol*. Vol. 25, No. 7: pp. 1336-1343

Miller, F.W., *Polymyositis and dermatomyositis.*, in *Cecil textbook of medicine. 22nd edn.*, A.D. Goldman L, Editor. 2004, Saunders: Philadelphia. p. 1680-1684.

Miyake, S., Ohtani, Y., Sawada, M., Inase, N., Miyazaki, Y., Takano, S., Miyasaka, N., & Yoshizawa, Y., (2002) Usefulness of cyclosporine A on rapidly progressive interstitial pneumonia in dermatomyositis. *Sarcoidosis Vasc Diffuse Lung Dis*. Vol. 19, No. 2: pp. 128-133

Miyazaki, E., Ando, M., Muramatsu, T., Fukami, T., Matsuno, O., Nureki, S.I., Ueno, T., Tsuda, T., & Kumamoto, T., (2005) Early assessment of rapidly progressive interstitial pneumonia associated with amyopathic dermatomyositis. *Clin Rheumatol*. Vol., No.: pp. 1-4

Mukae, H., Ishimoto, H., Sakamoto, N., Hara, S., Kakugawa, T., Nakayama, S., Ishimatsu, Y., Kawakami, A., Eguchi, K., & Kohno, S., (2009) Clinical differences between interstitial lung disease associated with clinically amyopathic dermatomyositis and classic dermatomyositis. *Chest*. Vol. 136, No. 5: pp. 1341-1347

Nawata, Y., Kurasawa, K., Takabayashi, K., Miike, S., Watanabe, N., Hiraguri, M., Kita, Y., Kawai, M., Saito, Y., & Iwamoto, I., (1999) Corticosteroid resistant interstitial pneumonitis in dermatomyositis/polymyositis: prediction and treatment with cyclosporine. *J Rheumatol*. Vol. 26, No. 7: pp. 1527-1533

Oddis, C.V., (2000) Current approach to the treatment of polymyositis and dermatomyositis. *Curr Opin Rheumatol*. Vol. 12, No. 6: pp. 492-497

Oddis, C.V., (2002) Idiopathic inflammatory myopathy: management and prognosis. *Rheum Dis Clin North Am*. Vol. 28, No. 4: pp. 979-1001

Sato, S., Hirakata, M., Kuwana, M., Suwa, A., Inada, S., Mimori, T., Nishikawa, T., Oddis, C.V., & Ikeda, Y., (2005) Autoantibodies to a 140-kd polypeptide, CADM-140, in Japanese patients with clinically amyopathic dermatomyositis. *Arthritis Rheum*. Vol. 52, No. 5: pp. 1571-1576

Sato, S., Hoshino, K., Satoh, T., Fujita, T., Kawakami, Y., & Kuwana, M., (2009) RNA helicase encoded by melanoma differentiation-associated gene 5 is a major autoantigen in patients with clinically amyopathic dermatomyositis: Association with rapidly progressive interstitial lung disease. *Arthritis Rheum*. Vol. 60, No. 7: pp. 2193-2200

Schnabel, A., Reuter, M., Biederer, J., Richter, C., & Gross, W.L., (2003) Interstitial lung disease in polymyositis and dermatomyositis: clinical course and response to treatment. *Semin Arthritis Rheum*. Vol. 32, No. 5: pp. 273-284

Selva-O'Callaghan, A., Labrador-Horrillo, M., Munoz-Gall, X., Martinez-Gomez, X., Majo-Masferrer, J., Solans-Laque, R., Simeon-Aznar, C.P., Morell-Brotard, F., & Vilardell-Tarres, M., (2005) Polymyositis/dermatomyositis-associated lung disease: analysis of a series of 81 patients. *Lupus*. Vol. 14, No. 7: pp. 534-542

Seo, Y., Abe, S., Kurahara, M., Okada, D., Saito, Y., Usuki, J., Azuma, A., Koizumi, K., & Kudoh, S., (2006) Beneficial effect of polymyxin B-immobilized fiber column (PMX) hemoperfusion treatment on acute exacerbation of idiopathic pulmonary fibrosis. *Intern Med*. Vol. 45, No. 18: pp. 1033-1038

Shinohara, T., Hidaka, T., Matsuki, Y., Ishizuka, T., Takamizawa, M., Kawakami, M., Kikuma, H., Suzuki, K., & Nakamura, H., (1997) Rapidly progressive interstitial lung disease associated with dermatomyositis responding to intravenous cyclophosphamide pulse therapy. *Intern Med*. Vol. 36, No. 7: pp. 519-523

Shoji, T., Bando, T., Fujinaga, T., Okubo, K., Yukawa, N., Mimori, T., & Date, H., (2010) Living-donor lobar lung transplantation for interstitial pneumonia associated with dermatomyositis. *Transpl Int*. Vol. 23, No. 5: pp. e10-11

Stonecipher, M.R., Jorizzo, J.L., White, W.L., Walker, F.O., & Prichard, E., (1993) Cutaneous changes of dermatomyositis in patients with normal muscle enzymes: dermatomyositis sine myositis? *J Am Acad Dermatol*. Vol. 28, No. 6: pp. 951-956

Suda, T., Fujisawa, T., Enomoto, N., Nakamura, Y., Inui, N., Naito, T., Hashimoto, D., Sato, J., Toyoshima, M., Hashizume, H., & Chida, K., (2006) Interstitial lung diseases associated with amyopathic dermatomyositis. *Eur Respir J*. Vol. 28, No. 5: pp. 1005-1012

Suzuki, Y., Hayakawa, H., Miwa, S., Shirai, M., Fujii, M., Gemma, H., Suda, T., & Chida, K., (2009) Intravenous immunoglobulin therapy for refractory interstitial lung disease associated with polymyositis/dermatomyositis. *Lung*. Vol. 187, No. 3: pp. 201-206

Takada, K., Kishi, J., & Miyasaka, N., (2007) Step-up versus primary intensive approach to the treatment of interstitial pneumonia associated with dermatomyositis/polymyositis: a retrospective study. *Mod Rheumatol*. Vol. 17, No. 2: pp. 123-130

Tansey, D., Wells, A.U., Colby, T.V., Ip, S., Nikolakoupolou, A., du Bois, R.M., Hansell, D.M., & Nicholson, A.G., (2004) Variations in histological patterns of interstitial pneumonia between connective tissue disorders and their relationship to prognosis. *Histopathology*. Vol. 44, No. 6: pp. 585-596

Targoff, I.N., (2008) Autoantibodies and their significance in myositis. *Curr Rheumatol Rep*. Vol. 10, No. 4: pp. 333-340

Tazelaar, H.D., Viggiano, R.W., Pickersgill, J., & Colby, T.V., (1990) Interstitial lung disease in polymyositis and dermatomyositis. Clinical features and prognosis as correlated with histologic findings. *Am Rev Respir Dis*. Vol. 141, No. 3: pp. 727-733

Tjiu, J.W., Lin, S.J., Wang, L.F., Shih, J.Y., Yu, C.J., Liang, C.W., & Chu, C.Y., (2004) Digital infarcts showing microangiopathy in adult dermatomyositis suggest severe pulmonary involvement and poor prognosis. *Br J Dermatol*. Vol. 150, No. 6: pp. 1214-1216

Troyanov, Y., Targoff, I.N., Tremblay, J.L., Goulet, J.R., Raymond, Y., & Senecal, J.L., (2005) Novel classification of idiopathic inflammatory myopathies based on overlap syndrome features and autoantibodies: analysis of 100 French Canadian patients. *Medicine (Baltimore)*. Vol. 84, No. 4: pp. 231-249

7

Myositis and Cancer

Sergio Prieto-González[1], Vladimir Lazo[1], Ernesto Trallero-Araguás[2], Albert Selva-O'Callaghan[2] and Josep M Grau[1]
[1]*Muscle Research Unit, Internal Medicine Department, Hospital Clínic, Barcelona, Universitat de Barcelona and CIBERER,*
[2]*Internal Medicine Department, Hospital Vall d'Hebrón, Barcelona, Spain*

1. Introduction

The idiopathic inflammatory myopathies (IIM), classically dermatomyositis (DM), polymyositis (PM), and inclusion body myositis (IBM), are acquired systemic autoimmune disorders defined by chronic muscle weakness and inflammation of unknown aetiology. The combination of clinical, laboratory, electromyographic, and histological features is the basis of diagnosis, as well as exclusion of several mimicking conditions (Bohan & Peter, 1975; Dalakas & Hohlfeld, 2003; Mann et al, 2010; Mastaglia & Phillips, 2002). IIM are the most common causes of acquired muscle disease in adults, but are still rare conditions with an estimated overall prevalence of 50 to 100 cases per million (Oddis et al., 1990; Prieto & Grau 2010; Wilson et al., 2008).

In recent years, taking into account additional clinical, immunological and histological features, new phenotypes among IIM, such as antisynthetase syndrome, autoimmune necrotizing myopathy, connective tissue disorder-associated myositis, or cancer-associated myositis (CAM), have been described (Cox et al., 2010; Dalakas, 2010; Dimachkie, 2011; Rider & Miller, 2011; Targoff, 2008).

The association between cancer and IIM has been widely reported in the medical literature, particularly in DM patients (Buchbinder et al., 2001; Sigurgeirsson et al., 1992). Cancer screening is a common practice in patients recently diagnosed with IIM, but there is not consensus about how, and how often screening should be performed. The aim of this chapter is to describe the epidemiological, clinical, laboratory, and histological reported features about CAM, to analyze the current potentially approach to preclude malignancy in IIM, and to provide an advisable algorithm in the diagnosis of occult cancer in myositis.

2. Background

The association between IIM and malignancy has been appreciated for nearly a century. From the first case reports in 1916 (Kankeleit, 1916; Stertz, 1916), large, retrospective studies and reviews examining this association have been subsequently published (Airio et al., 1995; Antiochos et al., 2009; Barnes & Mawr 1976; Buchbinder et al, 2001; Chow et al., 1995; Fardet et al., 2009; Hill et al., 2001; Huang et al., 2009; Madan et al., 2009; Sigurgeirsson et al., 1992;

Stockton et al., 2001; Wakata et al., 2002; Williams Jr., 1959; Zantos et al., 1994). Although the frequency in case reports showed a very wide range from 3 to 60%, population-based cohort studies have demonstrate that cancer is detected in approximately 30% of DM and 15% of PM patients, and both groups have increased cancer risks compared with the general population (Table 1) (Zampieri et al., 2010). In recent years, relevant progress has been made in understanding the link between cancer and myositis, providing accurate description about their temporal relationship and the rationale about their pathophysiological mechanisms.

Myositis patients number		**CAM number and (%)**		**Reference**
DM	PM	DM	PM	
392	396	94 (24)	58 (15)	Sigurgeisson (14)
618	914	198 (32)	137 (15)	Hill (22)
85	321	36 (42)	58 (18)	Buchbinder (13)
286	419	77 (27)	71 (17)	Stockton (21)
28	64	10 (36)	2 (3)	Wakata (23)
103	109	15 (15)	6 (6)	Chinoy (55)
1059	661	136 (13)	46 (7)	Huang (25)
121	NE	29 (24)	NE	Fardet (24)

CAM: cancer associated myositis; DM: dermatomyositis; PM: polymyositis; NE: not evaluated.

Table 1. Summary of reported CAM case series (adapted from Zampieri et al, 2010).

3. Other neuromuscular paraneoplastic conditions

Paraneoplastic syndromes (PS) are a group of conditions caused by an underlying immune response to cancer, thus not related to nutritional abnormalities, amyloid deposition, or adverse effects of treatment (Braik et al., 2010). Specific PS involving the neurological system (PNS) are rare, affecting 0,01% of patients with cancer and with overall incidence of about 1-10 per 10,000. Only Lambert-Eaton myasthenic syndrome (LEMS) is relatively common, affecting 1% of patients with small cell lung cancer. The most common forms of PNS are the paraneoplastic sensory neuronopathy (3-7 per 1,000), the paraneoplastic encephalitis (3 per 1,000), and the cerebellar degeneration (2 per 1,000). It is important to remark that these data may be underestimated because positive autoantibodies as a diagnostic criterium in these series were required (Graus & Dalmau, 2007; Honnorat & Antoine, 2007).

PNS may affect the central nervous system (CNS), the neuromuscular junction, and the peripheral nervous system. Cognitive disorders, personality changes, ataxia, cranial nerve paralysis, weakness, numbness, and jerks are the main described symptoms. Clinical and laboratory features of the most frequent PNS are described in Table 2. Onconeuronal antibodies are the basis of the PNS pathogenesis, produced by an immune cross reaction between tumor and CNS cells (Didelot & Honnorat, 2009). PNS may be classified into classical and non-classical disorders, being the first group more often associated with cancer (Table 3).

Paraneoplastic neurological syndromes			
PNS	**Clinical Presentation**	**Associated cancer**	**Antibodies**
LEMS	Lower limbs proximal muscle weakness	SCLC	Anti-VGCC, anti-SOX
Paraneoplastic cerebellar degeneration	Ataxia, diplopia, dysphagia, dysartria	Ovary, breast, SCLC, Hodgkin's disease	Anti-Yo, anti-Hu, anti-CV2, anti-Ma, anti-Tr
Opsoclonus-myoclonus	Dyskinetic shakes and myoclonic jerks of trunk and extremities	Neuroblastoma, breast, lung	Anti-Hu, anti-Ri
Sensory neuronopathy	Paresthesias/pain followed by ataxia	SCLC	Anti-Hu, anti-CV2
Limbic encephalitis	Mood changes, hallucinations, memory loss, seizures	SCLC, testicular	Anti-Hu, anti-CV2, anti -Ma, anti-amphiphysin

PNS: Paraneoplastic neurological syndrome; LEMS: Lambert-Eaton myasthenic syndrome; SCLC: smal cell lung cancer.

Table 2. Main features of most common PNS (modified from Braik et al., 2010; Didelot & Honnorat 2009; Graus et al., 2010).

Paraneoplastic neurological syndromes	
Classical	**Non-classical**
Encephalomyelitis	Optic neuritis
Limbic encephalitis	Cancer associated retinopathy
Subacute cerebellar degeneration	Melanoma associated retinopathy
Opsoclonus-myoclonus	Stiff person syndrome
Subacute sensory neuronopathy	Necrotising myelopathy
Chronic gastrointestinal pseudo-obstruction	Motor neuron diseases
Lambert-Eaton myasthenic syndrome	Acute sensorimotor neuropathy : - Guillain-Barré syndrome - Brachial neuritis
Dermatomyositis	Subacute/chronic sensorimotor neuropathies
	Neuropathy and paraproteinaemia
	Neuropathy with vasculitis
	Autonomic neuropathies
	Myasthenia gravis
	Acquired neuromyotonia
	Acute necrotising myopathy

PNS: Paraneoplastic neurological syndrome.

Table 3. Classical and non-classical PNS (modified from Graus et al., 2004)

The presence of a PNS may offer the possibility of early diagnosis of cancer, since PNS occurs in up to 50 to 80% of cases without any other malignancy signs. Diagnosis should be made in 3 steps:

1. To exclude other diagnosis: other conditions that may mimic PNS should be ruled out . These include: vascular diseases, connective tissue disorders, infections, nutritional disorders, adverse drug reactions, and exposure to toxins;
2. To search for cancer: comprehensive medical history, physical examination, laboratory, and imaging techniques should be performed;
3. To establish the diagnosis of PNS: this may require blood tests, imaging studies, electroencephalogram, nerve conduction studies, electromyography, and CSF examination. Onconeuronal antibodies may be positive in serum and/or CSF in 30% of patients (Braik et al., 2010). Table 4 summarizes the situations defined as definite or possible diagnosis of PNS.

PNS Diagnostic Criteria

Definite PNS	**Possible PNS**
1. Classical syndrome and cancer that develop within five years of the diagnosis of the neurological disorder.	1. Classical syndrome, no onconeuronal antibodies, no cancer but at high risk to have an underlying tumour.
2. Non-classical syndrome that resolves or significantly improves after cancer treatment without concomitant immunotherapy, provided that the syndrome is not susceptible to spontaneous remission.	2. Neurological syndrome (classical or not) with partially characterized onconeuronal antibodies and no cancer.
3. Non-classical syndrome with onconeural antibodies (well characterized or not) and cancer that develop within five years of the diagnosis of the neurological disorder.	3. Non-classical syndrome, no onconeuronal antibodies, and cancer present within two years of diagnosis.
4. Neurological syndrome (classical or not) with well characterized onconeural antibodies (anti-Hu, Yo, CV2, Ri, Ma2, or amphiphysin) and no cancer evidence.	

Well characterized onconeuronal antibodies included: Anti-Hu, Yo, CV2, Ri, Ma2, amphiphysin. Partially characterized onconeuronal antibodies: anti-Tr, ANNA3, PCA2, Zic4, mGluR1.

Table 4. PNS diagnostic criteria.

4. Myositis as paraneoplastic process

Taken into account the aforementioned epidemiological and clinical data, as well as temporal relationship, it is important to note the possibility that many cases of the IIM represent autoimmune paraneoplastic processes related to solid tumor oncogenesis, indicating an immune-mediated destruction of muscle and skin as response to cancer antigens. This observation has been extensively described in the autoimmune PNS, in which severe, immune-mediated neuronal damage occurs in the setting of solid tumours whose primary sites are outside of the central nervous system (Albert & Darnell, 2004). The serological hallmark of this associated group of disorders is the association of stereotypical autoantibody profiles with specific clinical phenotypes; furthermore, although the tumours are not neuronal in origin, they express high levels of protein antigens that are also highly expressed in neuronal tissue (Albert & Darnell, 2004; Furneaux et al., 1990).

With regard to CAM, the underlying pathogenetic molecular mechanisms are still unknown, but some findings leading to better understanding have been reported. It is published that some tumours (breast, lung adenocarcinoma, hepatocellular carcinoma), but not the corresponding normal tissues, do express high levels of myositis autoantigens (Casciola-Rosen et al., 2005); moreover, it has been reported that regenerating myoblasts overexpress myositis specific autoantigens in affected muscles from myositis patients, as well as tumor cells, indicating an immune response directed against cancer cells, cross-reacting with immature myoblasts in genetically predisposed individuals (Casciola-Rosen et al, 2005; Levine, 2006; Zampieri et al., 2010).

5. Cancer chronopathology

The temporal relationship between myopathy and cancer can widely vary. Malignancy may occur following the IIM diagnosis, be concurrently detected, or develop before. Despite this heterogeneous presentation, what is known is that cancer is usually recognized within 2-3 years of diagnosis of IIM, with most cases within 12 months.

6. Clinical, laboratory and pathological features

Older age, male sex, severe skin manifestations, such as cutaneous necrosis, distal muscle involvement, as well as dysphagia or diaphragmatic involvement are more frequent among patients with CAM. Specific capillaroscopic patterns and refractory or recurrent disease have also been related to this association (Andras et al., 2008; Chen et al., 2001; Fardet et al., 2009; Selva-O'Callaghan et al., 2010; Selva-O'Callaghan et al., 2002). Contrary to classical thought, case series suggest that cancer can also be present in the antisynthetase syndrome, indicating that the presence of antisynthetase antibodies does not rule out the CAM diagnosis (Buchbinder et al., 2001; Dugar et al., 2010; Legault et al., 2008; Mileti et al., 2009).

Among the laboratory parameters, the role of raised creatine kinase is controversial. It can be normal or slightly elevated, but highly elevations in CAM have been reported. Low levels of complement factor 4 have been published as a risk factor to occult cancer, whereas low baseline lymphocyte count and the presence of antinuclear antibodies have been reported as a protective features (Andras et al., 2008; Fardet et al., 2009).

Although no definite pathological features have been reported in CAM, the presence of a necrotizing myopathy, type of myopathy with severe necrosis with almost complete absence of inflammation (Amato & Barohn 2009; Dalakas 2011; Wegener et al., 2010), a higher number of fibers with internally located nuclei (Zampieri et al., 2010), and the identification of the neural cell adhesion molecules (Jensen & Berthold 2007; Zampieri et al., 2010) has been associated with cancer.

7. Screening approach

There is no doubt that an individually tailored screening for cancer in IIM patients is recommended according to age, sex, ethnicity, and subset of IIM, although, to date, there are no evidence-based recommendations. Moreover, continued surveillance is needed during the follow-up since cancer risk remains elevated for years after the diagnosis of IIM.

7.1 Standard work-up

An advisable approach include a careful history-taking and physical examination, blood tests with full blood count, erythrocyte sedimentation rate, routine biochemistry, chest RX, urinary cytology, fecal occult test, whole-body computed tomography scanning, and mammography, gynaecological examination, and pelvic ultrasonography in female patients, as well as prostate examination in men.

7.2 Immunoserological testing

Autoantibodies, including myositis-associated (MAA) and myositis-specific (MSA), are found in about 40% of patients with IIM. MAA include PM-Scl, Ku, snRNP, Ro60/SSA, Ro52, and La/SSB. MSA antibodies are highly specific for IIM, defining clinical and immunogenetics subsets of patients that may show different response to therapy and prognosis (Danko et al., 2009, 21; Love et al., 1991, 70; Rider & Miller, 2011), such as antisynthetases, anti-signal recognition particle (SRP), anti-Mi-2, and recently, anti-155/140. Classically, a negative association between the presence of antisynthetase antibodies was accepted, but, in recent years, scarce cases and small series of patients with antisynthetase syndrome and cancer have been published (Dugar et al., 2010; Legault et al., 2008; Mileti et al., 2009). Cancer relevance of anti-Mi-2 antibodies is unknown since only two studies have explored this issue with opposite results (Hengstman et al., 2006; O'Hanlon et al., 2006).

Anti p155, autoantibody against a 155kDa protein identified as transcriptional intermediary factor 1-γ (TIF1-γ), was first defined by Targoff in 2006 (Targoff et al., 2006) as an autoantibody associated with DM and CAM. The association between antip155 and malignancy has subsequently been confirmed by other investigators, reinforcing this link (Table 5) (Chinoy et al., 2009, 21; Fujikawa et al., 2009, 38; Gunawardena et al., 2008, 47; Kaji et al., 2007; Trallero-Araguas et al., 2010). The interest of antip155 autoantibody lies in its high negative predictive value or, in other words, its capacity to reasonable rule out the presence of occult cancer in patients with DM. An unpublished meta-analysis of the reported studies on this subject performed by the authors (Selva-O'Callaghan et al., 2010) to determine the overall accuracy of this autoantibody in DM reveals a specificity of 89% [95% CI 85-93] and sensitivity of 70% [95% CI 56-82], with a negative predictive value of 93% and a diagnostic odds ratio of 18 [95% 8-40], this means a 18-fold higher risk of cancer in patients with positive testing to p155.

N	CAM (Ab)*	No CAM (Ab)**	NPV	PPV	Reference
45	6 (6)	39 (8)	100	42,9	Targoff et al.
20	3 (3)	17 (3)	100	50	Gunawardena et al.
52	10 (5)	42 (2)	88,9	71,4	Kaji et al.
103	15 (8)	88 (11)	91,6	42,1	Chinoy et al.
30	5 (5)	25 (0)	100	100	Fujikawa et al.
65	14 (10)	51 (5)	92	66,7	Trallero-Araguás et al.

Ab, antibody; CAM, cancer-associated myositis; N, number of patients; NPV, negative predictive value; PPV, positive predictive value.

**Number of patients with CAM (number of those who are antibody-positive).*

***Number of patients without CAM (number of those who are antibody-positive).*

Table 5. Antip155 and CAM in DM (Selva-O'Callaghan et al., 2010).

7.3 Positron emission tomography

Positron emission tomography (PET) using [^{18}F] fluorodeoxyglucose (FDG), and more recently, combined FDG-PET/computed tomography (FDG-PET/CT), is one of the most sensitive imaging techniques to diagnose malignant disorders, successfully used in other paraneoplastic conditions (Hadjivassiliou et al., 2009; Patel et al., 2008). Our group performed a multicenter, prospective study including 55 consecutive DM/PM patients, diagnosed over a three-year period, to compare conventional cancer screening as mentioned above, with whole-body FDG-PET/CT (Selva-O'Callaghan et al., 2010). A sensitivity and specificity of both approaches were similar in excluding an occult malignancy, as well as false-positive and false-negative results; furthermore, a combination of two methods did not significantly increase the predictive value. From these results we suggest that FDG-PET/CT may be a good alternative to broad conventional malignancy screening, with the added advantage that a single imaging technique is more convenient for both the patient and the physician.

8. Clinical practice

Given the mentioned results of immunological (antip155 antibodies) and imaging (FDG-PET/CT) tests, we propose a reasonable approach for ruling out occult cancer in myositis (Fig.1) (Selva-O'Callaghan et al., 2010).

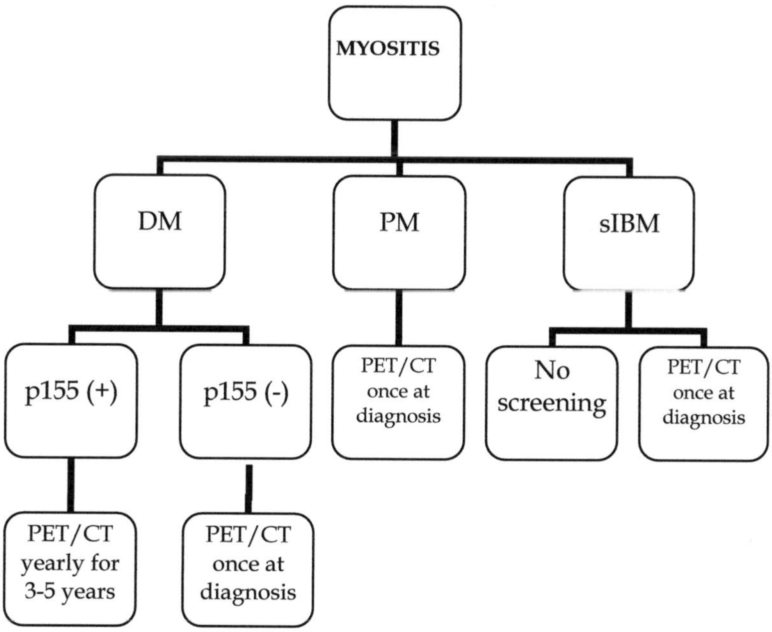

DM: dermatomyositis; PM: polymyositis; sIBM: sporadic inclusion body myositis, PET: positron emission tomography; CT: computed tomography.

Fig. 1. Algorithm for diagnosis of occult cancer in inflammatory myopathies (Selva-O'Callaghan et al., 2010).

After unequivocal diagnosis of IIM (especially in PM), a careful history-taking and physical examination, and standard laboratory testing should be performed in all patients.

- In IBM patients, given that the risk of cancer is extremely low, no screening or a single FDG-PET/CT is recommended.
- In PM patients, a population with moderate risk, yearly FDG-PET/CT for 3-5 years would be reasonable. Antip155 test is not useful because it is rarely present in this IIM subset.
- In DM patients, we recommend an initial antip155 determination. When the test is negative, a single FDG-PET/CT would be enough to preclude malignancy. However, in patients with DM and positive antip155 test, yearly FDG-PET/CT for, at least, 3-5 years is warranted.

Considering that test for detecting antip155 antibodies and FDG-PET/CT are available at only a few hospitals, as well as the high cost of the imaging technique, we propose a more straightforward alternative guideline to rule out cancer in myositis patients (Fig.2):

- In IBM patients, no screening or a single standard work-up (see above).
- In PM patients, yearly standard work-up for 3-5 years.
- In DM patients, yearly standard work-up for 3-5 years.

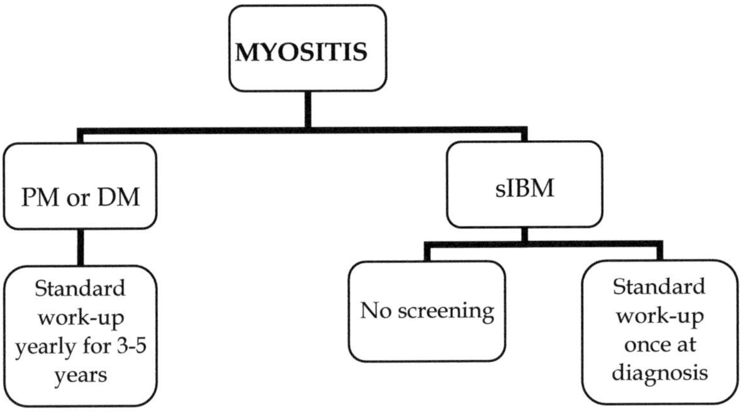

DM: dermatomyositis; PM: polymyositis; sIBM: sporadic inclusion body myositis.

Fig. 2. Alternative algorithm for diagnosis of occult cancer in inflammatory myopathies.

9. References

Airio, A., E. Pukkala, and H. Isomaki. 1995. Elevated cancer incidence in patients with dermatomyositis: a population based study. *J.Rheumatol.* 22, no. 7:1300-1303.

Albert, M. L. and R. B. Darnell. 2004. Paraneoplastic neurological degenerations: keys to tumour immunity. *Nat.Rev.Cancer.* 4, no. 1:36-44.

Amato, A. A. and R. J. Barohn. 2009. Evaluation and treatment of inflammatory myopathies. *J.Neurol.Neurosurg.Psychiatry.* 80, no. 10:1060-1068.

Andras, C., A. Ponyi, T. Constantin, Z. Csiki, E. Szekanecz, P. Szodoray, and K. Danko. 2008. Dermatomyositis and polymyositis associated with malignancy: a 21-year retrospective study. *J.Rheumatol.* 35, no. 3:438-444.

Antiochos, B. B., L. A. Brown, Z. Li, T. D. Tosteson, R. L. Wortmann, and W. F. Rigby. 2009. Malignancy is associated with dermatomyositis but not polymyositis in Northern New England, USA. *J.Rheumatol.* 36, no. 12:2704-2710.

Barnes, B. E. and B. Mawr. 1976. Dermatomyositis and malignancy. A review of the literature. *Ann.Intern.Med.* 84, no. 1:68-76.

Bohan, A. and J. B. Peter. 1975. Polymyositis and dermatomyositis (first of two parts). *N.Engl.J.Med.* 292, no. 7:344-347.

Braik, T., A. T. Evans, M. Telfer, and S. McDunn. 2010. Paraneoplastic neurological syndromes: unusual presentations of cancer. A practical review. *Am.J.Med.Sci.* 340, no. 4:301-308.

Buchbinder, R., A. Forbes, S. Hall, X. Dennett, and G. Giles. 2001. Incidence of malignant disease in biopsy-proven inflammatory myopathy. A population-based cohort study. *Ann.Intern.Med.* %19;134, no. 12:1087-1095.

Casciola-Rosen, L., K. Nagaraju, P. Plotz, K. Wang, S. Levine, E. Gabrielson, A. Corse, and A. Rosen. 2005. Enhanced autoantigen expression in regenerating muscle cells in idiopathic inflammatory myopathy. *J.Exp.Med.* 201, no. 4:591-601.

Chen, Y. J., C. Y. Wu, and J. L. Shen. 2001. Predicting factors of malignancy in dermatomyositis and polymyositis: a case-control study. *Br.J.Dermatol.* 144, no. 4:825-831.

Chinoy, H., J. A. Lamb, W. E. Ollier, and R. G. Cooper. 2009. An update on the immunogenetics of idiopathic inflammatory myopathies: major histocompatibility complex and beyond. *Curr.Opin.Rheumatol.* 21, no. 6:588-593.

Chow, W. H., G. Gridley, L. Mellemkjaer, J. K. McLaughlin, J. H. Olsen, and J. F. Fraumeni, Jr. 1995. Cancer risk following polymyositis and dermatomyositis: a nationwide cohort study in Denmark. *Cancer Causes Control.* 6, no. 1:9-13.

Cox, S., V. Limaye, C. Hill, P. Blumbergs, and P. Roberts-Thomson. 2010. Idiopathic inflammatory myopathies: diagnostic criteria, classification and epidemiological features. *Int.J.Rheum.Dis.* 13, no. 2:117-124.

Dalakas, M. C. 2010. Immunotherapy of myositis: issues, concerns and future prospects. *Nat.Rev.Rheumatol.* 6, no. 3:129-137.

Dalakas, 2011. Review: An update on inflammatory and autoimmune myopathies. *Neuropathol.Appl.Neurobiol.* 37, no. 3:226-242.

Dalakas, M. C. and R. Hohlfeld. 2003. Polymyositis and dermatomyositis. *Lancet.* %20;362, no. 9388:971-982.

Danko, K., A. Ponyi, A. P. Molnar, C. Andras, and T. Constantin. 2009. Paraneoplastic myopathy. *Curr.Opin.Rheumatol.* 21, no. 6:594-598.

Didelot, A. and J. Honnorat. 2009. Update on paraneoplastic neurological syndromes. *Curr.Opin.Oncol.* 21, no. 6:566-572.

Dimachkie, M. M. 2011. Idiopathic inflammatory myopathies. *J.Neuroimmunol.* 231, no. 1-2:32-42.

Dugar, M., S. Cox, V. Limaye, P. Blumbergs, and P. J. Roberts-Thomson. 2010. Clinical heterogeneity and prognostic features of South Australian patients with anti-synthetase autoantibodies. *Intern.Med.J.*

Fardet, L., A. Dupuy, M. Gain, A. Kettaneh, P. Cherin, H. Bachelez, L. Dubertret et al. 2009. Factors associated with underlying malignancy in a retrospective cohort of 121 patients with dermatomyositis. *Medicine (Baltimore).* 88, no. 2:91-97.

Fujikawa, K., A. Kawakami, K. Kaji, M. Fujimoto, S. Kawashiri, N. Iwamoto, T. Aramaki et al. 2009. Association of distinct clinical subsets with myositis-specific autoantibodies towards anti-155/140-kDa polypeptides, anti-140-kDa polypeptides, and anti-aminoacyl tRNA synthetases in Japanese patients with dermatomyositis: a single-centre, cross-sectional study. *Scand.J.Rheumatol.* 38, no. 4:263-267.

Furneaux, H. M., M. K. Rosenblum, J. Dalmau, E. Wong, P. Woodruff, F. Graus, and J. B. Posner. 1990. Selective expression of Purkinje-cell antigens in tumor tissue from patients with paraneoplastic cerebellar degeneration. *N.Engl.J.Med.* 322, no. 26:1844-1851.

Graus, F. and J. Dalmau. 2007. Paraneoplastic neurological syndromes: diagnosis and treatment. *Curr.Opin.Neurol.* 20, no. 6:732-737.

Graus, F., J. Y. Delattre, J. C. Antoine, J. Dalmau, B. Giometto, W. Grisold, J. Honnorat et al. 2004. Recommended diagnostic criteria for paraneoplastic neurological syndromes. *J.Neurol.Neurosurg.Psychiatry.* 75, no. 8:1135-1140.

Graus, F., A. Saiz, and J. Dalmau. 2010. Antibodies and neuronal autoimmune disorders of the CNS. *J.Neurol.* 257, no. 4:509-517.

Gunawardena, H., L. R. Wedderburn, J. North, Z. Betteridge, J. Dunphy, H. Chinoy, J. E. Davidson, R. G. Cooper, and N. J. McHugh. 2008. Clinical associations of autoantibodies to a p155/140 kDa doublet protein in juvenile dermatomyositis. *Rheumatology.(Oxford).* 47, no. 3:324-328.

Hadjivassiliou, M., S. J. Alder, E. J. Van Beek, M. B. Hanney, E. Lorenz, D. G. Rao, B. Sharrack, and W. B. Tindale. 2009. PET scan in clinically suspected paraneoplastic neurological syndromes: a 6-year prospective study in a regional neuroscience unit. *Acta Neurol.Scand.* 119, no. 3:186-193.

Hengstman, G. J., W. T. Vree Egberts, H. P. Seelig, I. E. Lundberg, H. M. Moutsopoulos, A. Doria, M. Mosca et al. 2006. Clinical characteristics of patients with myositis and autoantibodies to different fragments of the Mi-2 beta antigen. *Ann.Rheum.Dis.* 65, no. 2:242-245.

Hill, C. L., Y. Zhang, B. Sigurgeirsson, E. Pukkala, L. Mellemkjaer, A. Airio, S. R. Evans, and D. T. Felson. 2001. Frequency of specific cancer types in dermatomyositis and polymyositis: a population-based study. *Lancet.* 357, no. 9250:96-100.

Honnorat, J. and J. C. Antoine. 2007. Paraneoplastic neurological syndromes. *Orphanet.J.Rare.Dis.* 2:22.:22.

Huang, Y. L., Y. J. Chen, M. W. Lin, C. Y. Wu, P. C. Liu, T. J. Chen, Y. C. Chen et al. 2009. Malignancies associated with dermatomyositis and polymyositis in Taiwan: a nationwide population-based study. *Br.J.Dermatol.* 161, no. 4:854-860.

Jensen, M. and F. Berthold. 2007. Targeting the neural cell adhesion molecule in cancer. *Cancer Lett.* 258, no. 1:9-21.

Kaji, K., M. Fujimoto, M. Hasegawa, M. Kondo, Y. Saito, K. Komura, T. Matsushita et al. 2007. Identification of a novel autoantibody reactive with 155 and 140 kDa nuclear proteins in patients with dermatomyositis: an association with malignancy. *Rheumatology.(Oxford).* 46, no. 1:25-28.

Kankeleit, H. 1916. Über primäre nichteitrige polymyositis. *Dtshch.Arch.Klin.Med* 120:335-349.

Legault, D., J. McDermott, A. M. Crous-Tsanaclis, and G. Boire. 2008. Cancer-associated myositis in the presence of anti-Jo1 autoantibodies and the antisynthetase syndrome. *J.Rheumatol.* 35, no. 1:169-171.

Levine, S. M. 2006. Cancer and myositis: new insights into an old association. *Curr.Opin.Rheumatol.* 18, no. 6:620-624.

Love, L. A., R. L. Leff, D. D. Fraser, I. N. Targoff, M. Dalakas, P. H. Plotz, and F. W. Miller. 1991. A new approach to the classification of idiopathic inflammatory myopathy: myositis-specific autoantibodies define useful homogeneous patient groups. *Medicine (Baltimore).* 70, no. 6:360-374.

Madan, V., H. Chinoy, C. E. Griffiths, and R. G. Cooper. 2009. Defining cancer risk in dermatomyositis. Part II. Assessing diagnostic usefulness of myositis serology. *Clin.Exp.Dermatol.* 34, no. 5:561-565.

Mann, H. F., J. Vencovsky, and I. E. Lundberg. 2010. Treatment-resistant inflammatory myopathy. *Best.Pract.Res.Clin.Rheumatol.* 24, no. 3:427-440.

Mastaglia, F. L. and B. A. Phillips. 2002. Idiopathic inflammatory myopathies: epidemiology, classification, and diagnostic criteria. *Rheum.Dis.Clin.North Am.* 28, no. 4:723-741.

Mileti, L. M., M. E. Strek, T. B. Niewold, J. J. Curran, and N. J. Sweiss. 2009. Clinical characteristics of patients with anti-Jo-1 antibodies: a single center experience. *J.Clin.Rheumatol.* 15, no. 5:254-255.

O'Hanlon, T. P., L. G. Rider, G. Mamyrova, I. N. Targoff, F. C. Arnett, J. D. Reveille, M. Carrington et al. 2006. HLA polymorphisms in African Americans with idiopathic inflammatory myopathy: allelic profiles distinguish patients with different clinical phenotypes and myositis autoantibodies. *Arthritis Rheum.* 54, no. 11:3670-3681.

Oddis, C. V., C. G. Conte, V. D. Steen, and T. A. Medsger, Jr. 1990. Incidence of polymyositis-dermatomyositis: a 20-year study of hospital diagnosed cases in Allegheny County, PA 1963-1982. *J.Rheumatol.* 17, no. 10:1329-1334.

Patel, R. R., R. M. Subramaniam, J. N. Mandrekar, J. E. Hammack, V. J. Lowe, and J. R. Jett. 2008. Occult malignancy in patients with suspected paraneoplastic neurologic syndromes: value of positron emission tomography in diagnosis. *Mayo Clin.Proc.* 83, no. 8:917-922.

Prieto, S. and J. M. Grau. 2010. The geoepidemiology of autoimmune muscle disease. *Autoimmun.Rev.* 9, no. 5:A330-A334.

Rider, L. G. and F. W. Miller. 2011. Deciphering the clinical presentations, pathogenesis, and treatment of the idiopathic inflammatory myopathies. *JAMA.* 305, no. 2:183-190.

Selva-O'Callaghan, A., V. Fonollosa-Pla, E. Trallero-Araguas, X. Martinez-Gomez, C. P. Simeon-Aznar, M. Labrador-Horrillo, and M. Vilardell-Tarres. 2010. Nailfold capillary microscopy in adults with inflammatory myopathy. *Semin.Arthritis Rheum.* 39, no. 5:398-404.

Selva-O'Callaghan, A., J. M. Grau, C. Gamez-Cenzano, A. Vidaller-Palacin, X. Martinez-Gomez, E. Trallero-Araguas, E. Buendia-Navarro, and M. Vilardell-Tarres. 2010. Conventional cancer screening versus PET/CT in dermatomyositis/polymyositis. *Am.J.Med.* 123, no. 6:558-562.

Selva-O'Callaghan, A., T. Mijares-Boeckh-Behrens, R. Solans-Laque, M. Labrador-Horrillo, E. Romero-Merino, J. M. Sopena-Sisquella, and M. Vilardell-Tarres. 2002. The neural network as a predictor of cancer in patients with inflammatory myopathies. *Arthritis Rheum.* 46, no. 9:2547-2548.

Selva-O'Callaghan, A., E. Trallero-Araguas, J. M. Grau-Junyent, and M. Labrador-Horrillo. 2010. Malignancy and myositis: novel autoantibodies and new insights. *Curr.Opin.Rheumatol.* 22, no. 6:627-632.

Sigurgeirsson, B., B. Lindelof, O. Edhag, and E. Allander. 1992. Risk of cancer in patients with dermatomyositis or polymyositis. A population-based study. *N.Engl.J.Med.* 326, no. 6:363-367.

Stertz, G. 1916. Polymyositis. *Berl.Klin.Wochenschr.* 53:489.

Stockton, D., V. R. Doherty, and D. H. Brewster. 2001. Risk of cancer in patients with dermatomyositis or polymyositis, and follow-up implications: a Scottish population-based cohort study. *Br.J.Cancer.* 85, no. 1:41-45.

Targoff, I. N. 2008. Autoantibodies and their significance in myositis. *Curr.Rheumatol.Rep.* 10, no. 4:333-340.

Targoff, I. N., G. Mamyrova, E. P. Trieu, O. Perurena, B. Koneru, T. P. O'Hanlon, F. W. Miller, and L. G. Rider. 2006. A novel autoantibody to a 155-kd protein is associated with dermatomyositis. *Arthritis Rheum.* 54, no. 11:3682-3689.

Trallero-Araguas, E., M. Labrador-Horrillo, A. Selva-O'Callaghan, M. A. Martinez, X. Martinez-Gomez, E. Palou, J. L. Rodriguez-Sanchez, and M. Vilardell-Tarres. 2010. Cancer-associated myositis and anti-p155 autoantibody in a series of 85 patients with idiopathic inflammatory myopathy. *Medicine (Baltimore).* 89, no. 1:47-52.

Wakata, N., T. Kurihara, E. Saito, and M. Kinoshita. 2002. Polymyositis and dermatomyositis associated with malignancy: a 30-year retrospective study. *Int.J.Dermatol.* 41, no. 11:729-734.

Wegener, S., J. Bremer, P. Komminoth, H. H. Jung, and M. Weller. 2010. Paraneoplastic Necrotizing Myopathy with a Mild Inflammatory Component: A Case Report and Review of the Literature. *Case.Rep.Oncol.* 3, no. 1:88-92.

Williams, R. C., Jr. 1959. Dermatomyositis and malignancy: a review of the literature. *Ann.Intern.Med.* 50, no. 5:1174-1181.

Wilson, F. C., S. R. Ytterberg, J. L. St Sauver, and A. M. Reed. 2008. Epidemiology of sporadic inclusion body myositis and polymyositis in Olmsted County, Minnesota. *J.Rheumatol.* 35, no. 3:445-447.

Zampieri, S., M. Valente, N. Adami, D. Biral, A. Ghirardello, M. E. Rampudda, M. Vecchiato et al. 2010. Polymyositis, dermatomyositis and malignancy: a further intriguing link. *Autoimmun.Rev.* 9, no. 6:449-453.

Zantos, D., Y. Zhang, and D. Felson. 1994. The overall and temporal association of cancer with polymyositis and dermatomyositis. *J.Rheumatol.* 21, no. 10:1855-1859.

8

Orbital Myositis

Toshinobu Kubota
National Hospital Organization, Nagoya Medical Center Nagoya, Japan

1. Introduction

Orbital myositis is an inflammation of mainly the extraocular muscles. Orbital myositis has a sudden onset, and the clinical course can be acute or chronic. The ocular signs and symptoms of eyes with orbital myositis are periocular pain, eyelid swelling and redness, restricted ocular motility, and strabismus. Computed tomographic (CT) scans show indistinct swelling around one or more extraocular muscles, and fat-suppressed T2-weighted magnetic resonance (MR) images show localized inflammations. The exact etiology of the inflammation has not been determined, however some cases have been reported to be caused by infectious agents while other cases by autoimmunity. Spirochetotic (Lyme disease), viral (herpes zoster virus), and bacterial infections (Group A streptococcal pharyngitis) can cause orbital myositis. Autoimmune-related orbital myositis is associated with relatively specific diseases: giant cell myocarditis, Crohn disease, and linear scleroderma.

Orbital myositis must be differentiated from other diseases that also have extraocular muscular enlargements, e.g., thyroid-associated orbitopathy, lymphoproliferative disorders, metastatic orbital diseases, parasitic infection, systemic anti-neutrophil cytoplasmic antibody-related vasculitis, and inflammatory conditions triggered by medications and foreign bodies.

The first line of treatment of orbital myositis is systemic corticosteroids to which the inflammation responds well especially the acute type. However, there are corticosteroid-resistant chronic types, and immunosuppressive and biological agents can be used in these types.

2. Patients, signs and symptoms, and imaging studies

2.1 Patients

The etiology of orbital myositis has not been completely established. In some cases, the orbital myositis has a specific etiology, which is described in Section 3. Although idiopathic orbital myositis may occur at any age, it is most commonly present in middle-aged patients. Meta-analysis, including the largest published series (Siatkowski et al., 1994), showed that orbital myositis occured most frequently in young to middle-aged patients with a 1 male to 2 female patient ratio (Table 1; Scott & Siatkowski, 1997). However, a relatively large published case series (Lacey et al., 1999) and our study did not reveal a female predominance (Table 1).

It has also been reported that idiopathic orbital myositis can develop in pediatric patients. Pediatric cases of orbital myositis develop secondary to systemic conditions, e.g., streptococcal pharyngitis (Alshaikh et al., 2008; Belanger et al., 2010) and presumed allergic responses (Yan et al., 2006). There are cases of orbital myositis that develop after pregnancy (Hiraga et al., 2008; Mombaerts & Koornneef, 1997) and cases with a familial history (Jacob et al., 2007; Maurer & Zierz, 1999). However, these may be exceptional cases.

References	Patient number	Male/female ratio	Median or mean age (range)
Scott et al. 1997	190	0.5	37 (3-84) years old
Lacey et al. 1999	40	0.74	40 (not available) years old
Our study	43	1.0	47 (23-91) years old

Table 1. Epidemiology of patients with idiopathic orbital myositis.

2.2 Signs and symptoms

Idiopathic orbital myositis is characterized by a sudden onset of orbital inflammation, periocular pain, swelling and redness of the eyelids, proptosis, ptosis, and ocular motility restrictions (Figure 1 to 7). It must be differentiated from idiopathic orbital inflammation and orbital cellulitis, because the signs and symptoms are similar. However, idiopathic orbital myositis can sometimes have atypical signs and symptoms, viz., subacute/chronic onset or be a non-inflammatory condition. These cases with atypical signs and symptoms simulate orbital tumors, and they account for 7% of all cases (Rootman, 2003).

Idiopathic orbital myositis must also be differentiated from other diseases that have enlargements of the extraocular muscles as described in Sections 4.3 to 4.10.

Idiopathic orbital myositis can affect any extraocular muscles but rarely the superior and inferior oblique muscles (Figure 7; Kau et al., 2006; Stidham et al., 1998). It also rarely affects the levator palpebrae muscle (Figure 1; Almekhlafi & Fletcher. 2008). Ocular motility is typically restricted in the field of action of the affected extraocular muscles, and also in the direction opposite to its field of action (Figure 5; Kubota & Kano. 2007; Lacey et al., 1999; Siatkowski et al., 1994).

Idiopathic orbital myositis can have an acute or chronic/recurrent clinical course. Acute orbital myositis is generally resolved within 2 months after systemic steroid therapy (Figure 5 and 6). However, chronic/recurrent orbital myositis responds poorly to systemic steroid therapy, and the ocular motility is restricted for more than 2 months and often years (Figure 7).

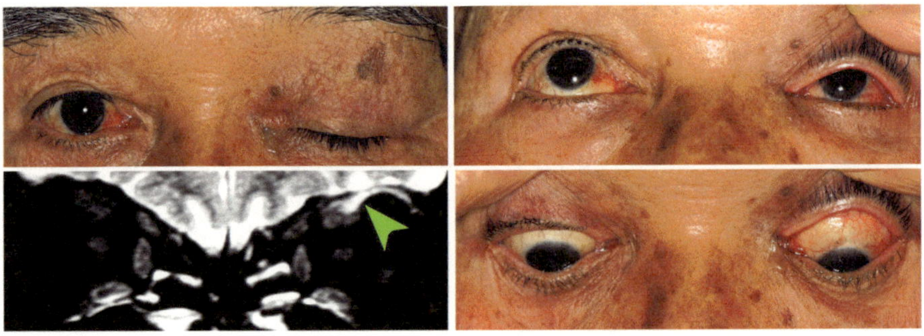

Fig. 1. Idiopathic orbital myositis of left levator palpebrae muscle.

External photograph of an 82-year-old man showing left ptosis but with normal ocular motility. Fat-suppressed T2-weighted MR image shows a hyperintense signal in the left levator palpebrae muscle (arrowhead). He recovered spontaneously.

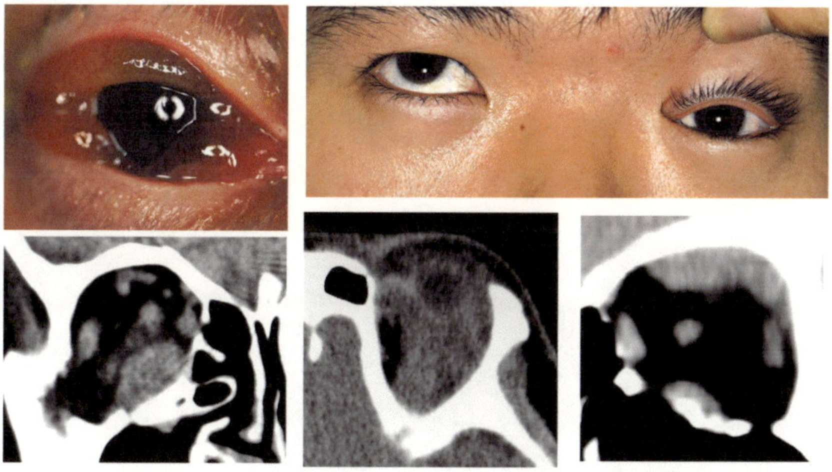

Fig. 2. External photographs of patients with idiopathic orbital myositis. Left. A 91-year-old woman showing unilateral chemosis and ptosis, and with ocular motility restrictions. Right. A 26-year-old man with ptosis, ocular motility restrictions, and periocular pain.

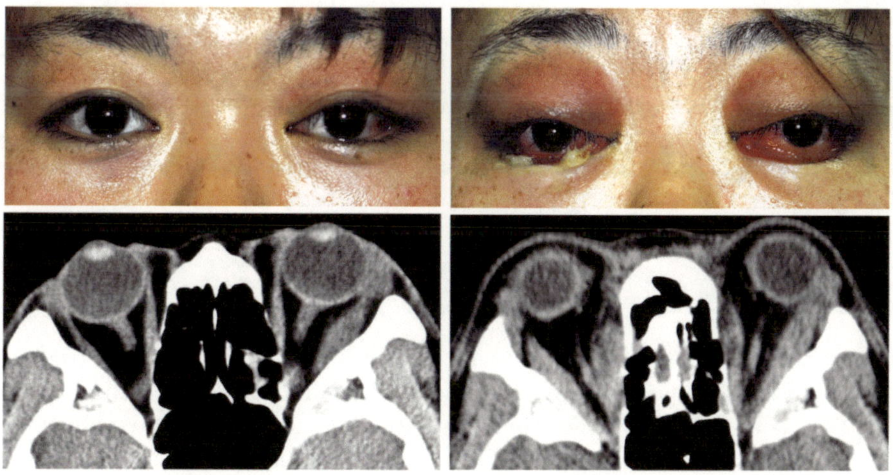

Fig. 3. External photographs of a patient with idiopathic orbital myositis. Left: A 32-year-old woman showing left upper eyelid swelling and redness. Right: Same patient after a bilateral recurrence while being treated with 5 mg maintenance dose of prednisolone and one week after 1000 mg intravenous methylprednisolone for 3 days.

2.3 Imaging studies

CT scans of eyes with idiopathic orbital myositis show indistinct swelling around one or more muscles with no specific pattern of which muscle is enlarged (Figure 2 to 6). On the other hand, the MR images of acute and chronic/recurrent type of orbital myositis have characteristic patterns. Fat-suppressed T2-weighted MR images showed inflammation of the extraocular muscles rather than the ocular adnexal structures (Ohnishi et al., 1994). Localized inflammation of the extraocular muscles in eyes with idiopathic orbital myositis at the active stage can be seen in Figures 4 to 7. The acute type of idiopathic orbital myositis has localized areas of hyperintense signals around the extraocular muscles and fascicle structures, whereas the chronic/recurrent type shows areas of hyperintense signals in the extraocular muscles (Kubota & Kano, 2007).

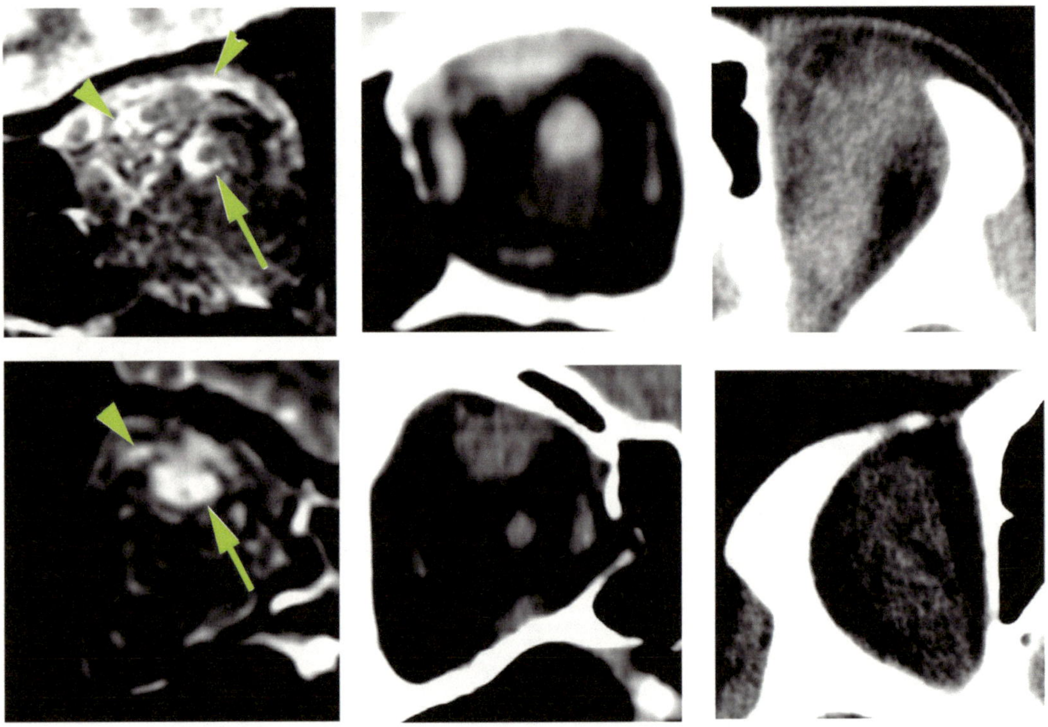

Fig. 4. Fat-suppressed T2-weighted MR image and coronal (middle) and axial (right) CT images recorded at the same time in a patient with idiopathic orbital myositis in the active phase. Top: Acute type of idiopathic orbital myositis. Fat-suppressed T2-weighted MR image shows a hyperintense signal in the fascicle structure (arrowhead) around the superior rectus muscle, and indistinct swelling around the superior rectus muscle in the CT image (Top center). An arrow points to the optic nerve for comparison to coronal CT scan at the posterior pole. Bottom: Chronic type of idiopathic orbital myositis. Fat-suppressed T2-weighted MR image shows a hyperintense signal of the superior rectus muscle (arrow) and the adjacent structures (arrowhead). Reproduced with permission from Kubota, T. & Kano, H. (2007) Assessment of inflammation in idiopathic orbital myositis with fat-suppressed T2-weighted magnetic resonance imaging. *American Journal of Ophthalmology,* Vol.143, No. 4, pp.718-720, ISSN:0002-9394

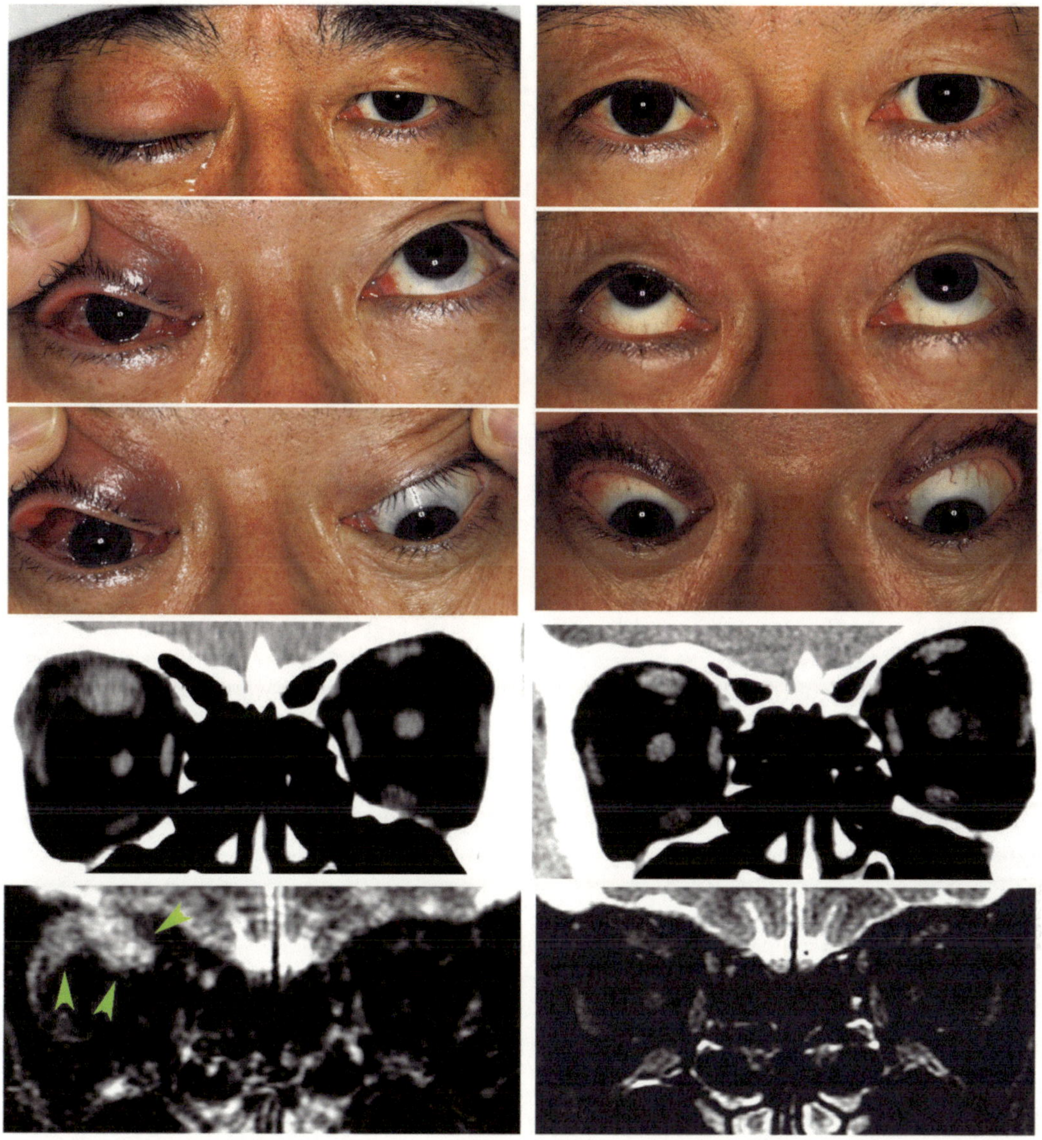

Fig. 5. Acute type of idiopathic orbital myositis. Left: External photographs of a 58-year-old man showing swelling of the right eyelid, ptosis, and ocular motility restrictions in the field of action and in the direction opposite to the field of action of the affected extraocular muscles. Severe engorgement of the conjunctival and episcleral vessels overlying the right eye. Fat-suppressed T2-weighted MR image at the active phase shows a hyperintense signal around the fascicular structures (arrowhead). Right: Same patient after 1000 mg intravenous methylprednisolone for 3 days (steroid pulse therapy). There is a complete recovery from signs and symptoms. MR images are normal.

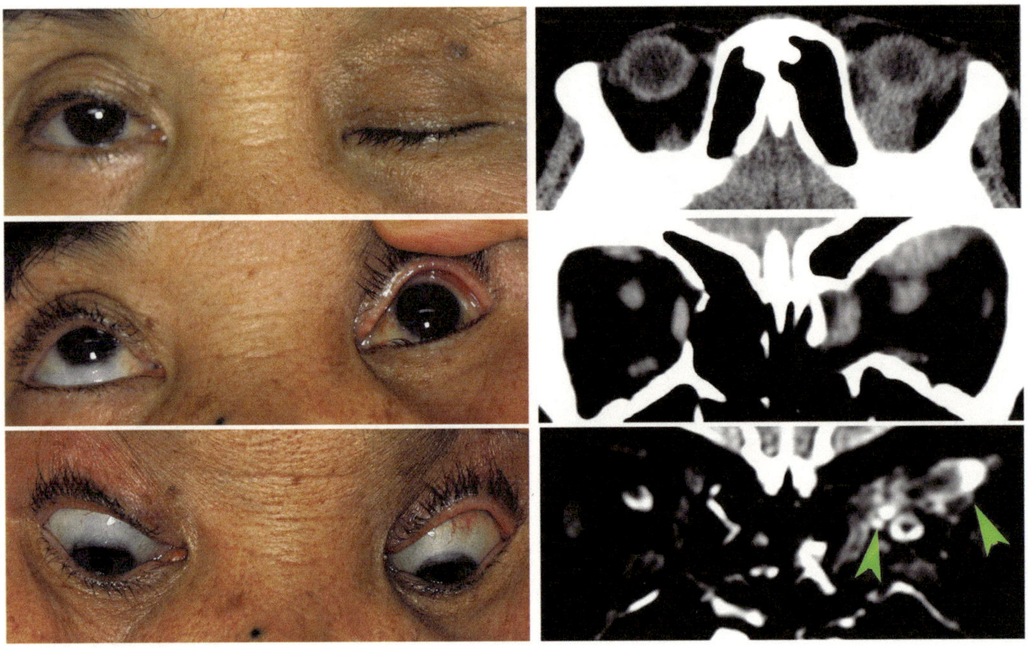

Fig. 6. Acute type of atypical idiopathic orbital myositis. Left: External photographs of a 65-year-old woman showing the left blepharoptosis, and also with ocular motility restrictions in the field of action of the affected extraocular muscles. Signs including subacute onset and non-inflammatory conditions indicate that this is atypical idiopathic orbital myositis. Right: CT images shows indistinct swelling around the superior rectus muscle of the left eye. Fat-suppressed T2-weighted MR image shows hyperintense signal around the fascicular structures (arrowhead). Following steroid pulse therapy, she completely recovered from the signs and symptoms.

3. Etiological factors

The cause of the orbital myositis is not known in most cases, however several cases with known etiology have been reported. Infectious and autoimmune-related factors that affect the extraocular muscles are described in this section.

3.1 Infectious agents causing orbital myositis

Cases of orbital myositis caused by infectious agents are rare. Spirochetes (Lyme disease), viruses (herpes zoster virus), and bacteria (Group A streptococcal pharyngitis) are microbes that can cause infectious orbital myositis. The signs and symptoms of each infectious agent are similar to those of idiopathic orbital myositis; acute onset, periocular inflammation, periocular pain, conjunctival hyperemia, eyelid swelling, diplopia, and restriction of ocular movements. Imaging studies show that the findings in eyes caused by the different infectious agent are also similar to those of idiopathic orbital myositis. The protocol of treatment depends on the sensitivity profile of each microbe.

Lyme disease is caused by the spirochete *Borrelia burgdorferi* and is mainly reported in the northern and western United States and also in Europe. Ticks transmit the spirochete which

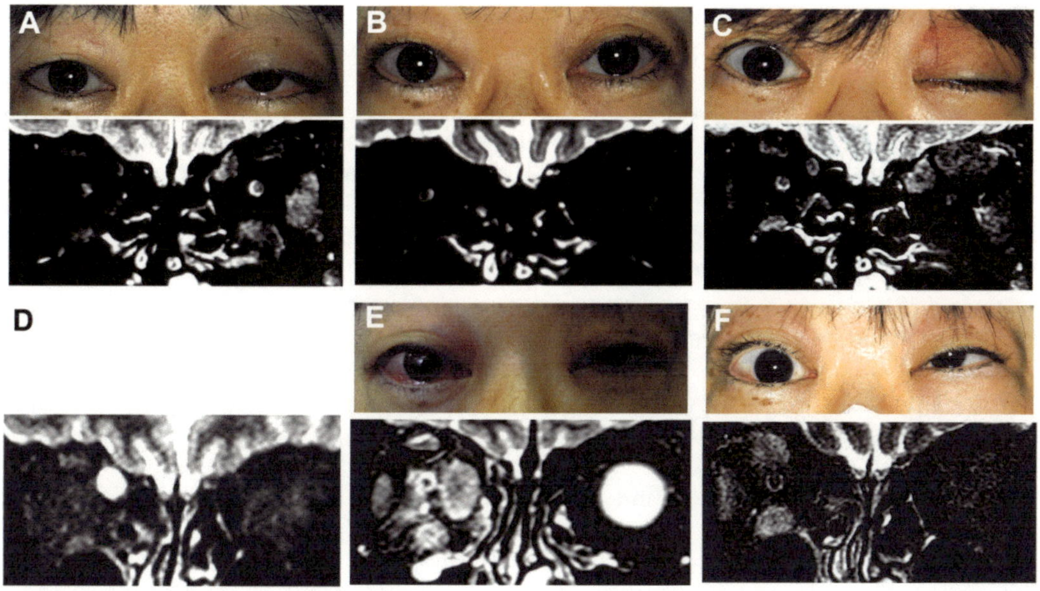

Fig. 7. Cronic/recurrent type of ipathic orbital myositis. A 46-year-old woman with left periocular inflammation and ocular motility restrictions was referred to our hospital because her myositis was refractory to high doses of prednisolone with a slow taper. A: Fat-suppressed T2-weighted MR image at the initial examination shows hyperintense signals in the left inferior and lateral rectus, and superior oblique muscles. B: Following steroid pulse therapy, there is a complete recovery of the signs and symptoms. C: and D: and E: She received high dose steroid (prednisolone 60mg) with a slow taper, however the myositis recurred three times during the tapering. Note that more than one muscle including the right superior oblique muscle was affected. F: She developed a strabisumus two years after the initial visit and had persistent ocular motility restrictions.

can affect different organ: the skin, nervous system, heart, joints, and muscles (Holmgren & Matteson, 2006; Muller-Felber et al., 1993; Pendse et al., 2006). The infection by *Borrelia burgdorferi* can be unilateral and more than one extraocular muscle can be infected. Lyme disease also has other ocular manifestations, dacroadenitis (Nieto et al., 2008), periocular inflammation (Carvounis et al., 2004; Holak et al., 2006), and neuro-ophthalmologic manifestations (Lesser et al., 1990; Pendse et al., 2006; Seidenberg et al., 1990). The diagnosis is based on the patients living in or visiting an endemic area, a skin rash, and a positive serologic test for *Borrelia burgdorferi*. Oral doxycycline is the best treatment, and steroids may also resolve the inflammation.

Herpes zoster is a rare cause of orbital myositis, but several cases have been extracted by a PubMed search (Badilla et al., 2007; Kawasaki & Borruat, 2003; Krasniaanski et al., 2004; Volpe et al., 1991). The signs and symptoms of orbital myositis associated with herpes zoster are similar to those of acute orbital myositis. The characteristic skin rash of herpes zoster may develop after the ocular adnexal inflammatory conditions (Kawasaki & Borruat, 2003). Herpes zoster can be unilateral and can affect more than one extraocular muscle. Acyclovir can improve the ocular manifestations, and cure the disease before progressing to the chronic clinical stage.

Orbital myositis following streptococcal pharyngitis is also a rare condition. Several cases have been reported based on a Pub Med search (Alshaikh et al., 2008; Belanger et al., 2010; Culligan et al., 2005; Purcell et al., 1981). The highest incidence of this type of orbital myositis is in infants and young adults. In general, the orbital myositis occurs two to six weeks after the development of streptococcal pharyngitis. The pathogenesis may have an immunocomprise factor rather than streptococcal A. Imaging studies show unilateral with single or multiple extraocular muscular enlargements. The orbital myositis following streptococcal pharyngitis responds to oral corticosteroids, and can be cured without progressing to the chronic stage.

3.2 Orbital myositis associated with autoimmunity

Cases of orbital myositis associated with autoimmunity are associated with relatively specific autoimmune diseases; giant cell myocarditis, Crohn disease, systemic lupus erythematosus, rheumatoid arthritis, and linear scleroderma.

Idiopathic giant-cell myocarditis is a rare and fatal disorder. Relatively young adults (mean age 43 years-old) are affected, and they usually die of heart failure and ventricular arrhythmia (Cooper et al., 1997). Nineteen percent of patients are associated with autoimmune disorders: Crohn disease, ulcerative colitis, and orbital myositis (Cooper et al., 1997). Five cases of orbital myositis associated with giant cell myocarditis have been published based on a Pub Med search (Kattah et al., 1990; Klein et al., 1989; Leib et al., 1994; Lind-Ayres et al., 2009; Stevens et al., 1996). The patients were 14-to 65-years-old and all were women. Their signs and symptoms are similar to those of patients with idiopathic orbital myositis, and patients present with periorbital pain, proptosis, ptosis, ocular motility restrictions, and swelling of the extraocular muscles including their tendons. Steroid treatments improve their signs and symptoms, but patients can develop cardiogenic episodes usually within a couple of months of onset of orbital myositis. Therefore, physicians should consider the possibility of idiopathic giant-cell myocarditis especially when a young woman is diagnosed with idiopathic orbital myositis.

Inflammatory bowel diseases, e.g., Crohn disease and ulcerative colitis, have ocular manifestations in 4% to 12% of the cases (Ghanchi et al., 2003). The signs and symptoms include scleritis, uveitis, neuro-ophthalmic, corneal and retinal complications, and orbital pseudotumor. Orbital inflammation is believed to be a true complication of inflammatory bowel disease (Ghanchi et al., 2003). Orbital inflammation rapidly responds to systemic steroids but a reduction of the steroid dose may lead to recurrences.

Scleroderma is a chronic autoimmune disease previously called the CREST syndrome and it has cutaneous manifestations that affect the arms and face. It is characterized by fibrosis, vascular alternations, and autoantibodies. The ocular manifestations involve the extraocular muscles which can appear atrophic (Suttorp-Schulten & Koornneef, 1990) or enlarged (Ramboer et al., 1997).

Several cases of orbital myositis associated systemic lupus erythematosus (Grimson et al, 1983; Serop et al., 1994) and rheumatoid arthritis have been published (Nabili et al., 2002; Panfilio et al., 2000).

4. Differential diagnosis

Orbital myositis is characterized by periocular and/or orbital inflammations and extraocular muscle enlargements. Various diseases must be differentiated from orbital myositis. First, periocular and/or orbital inflammations of idiopathic orbital inflammation and orbital cellulitis are similar to those of orbital myositis. Second, signs and symptoms of thyroid-associated orbitopathy have also similar to those of orbital myositis and it has high incidence among the orbital diseases. Finally, primary and secondary carcinoma, lymphoproliferative lesions, parasite infection, anti-neutrophil cytoplasmic antibody-mediated systemic vasculitis, some kind of drugs and foreign bodies can lead to extraocular muscle enlargements.

4.1 Idiopathic orbital inflammation

Idiopathic orbital inflammation is caused by unknown etiology, and inflammatory conditions are specific to the ocular adnexa: a lacrimal gland, an eye ball, extraocular muscles, and an optic nerve (Figure 8). This may be due to a number of different organ-specific immunologic disorders of more specific etiologies yet to be defined (Rootman, 2003). Imaging studies can differentiate each type. However, periocular type and idiopathic orbital myositis arising from superior or inferior extraocular muscles may often be difficult to differentiate between them.

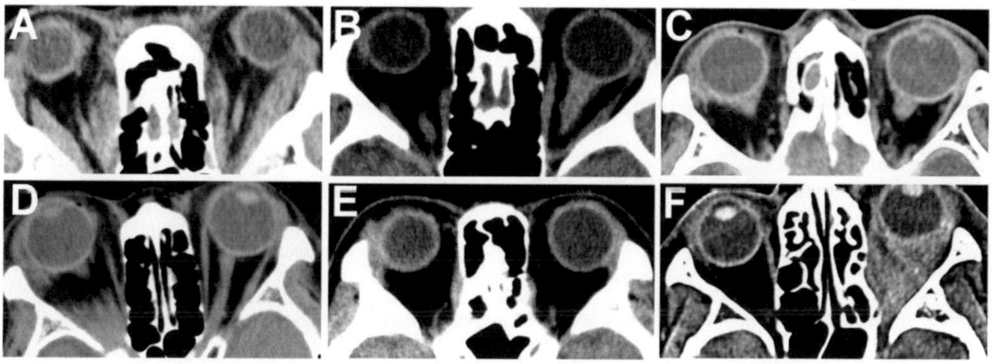

Fig. 8. CT images of each type of idiopathic orbital inflammation. A: orbital myositis, B: perioptic type, C: periocular type, D: apical type, E: lacrimal type, F: diffuse type

4.2 Orbital cellulitis

Orbital cellulitis is the inflammation caused by bacterial infections. It may be difficult to differentiate eye with orbital cellulitis from orbital myositis especially at early stage. Therefore, the diagnosis orbital myositis is often made following initial therapy for potential infectious etiology (Costa et al., 2009). In general, idiopathic orbital myositis characterizes a sudden onset. In addition, signs and symptoms reach their peak intensity at the initial onset. In contrast, orbital cellulitis characterizes an acute onset, but progressively develops signs and symptoms. Even though signs and symptoms resemble that of orbital myositis at active phase of orbital cellulitis (Figure 9), imaging studies may help a differential diagnosis between them. CT scans of idiopathic orbital myositis reveal extraocular muscle enlargements, whereas those of orbital cellulitis reveal fuzzy diffuse pattern in the orbit (Figure 9). However orbital cellulitis often progressive to massive lesions (Rootman, 2003). MR images of idiopathic orbital myositis reveal localized inflammations specific to affected extraocular muscles, whereas, those of orbital cellulitis reveal same signals in the vitreous body due to abscess formations that extend diffusely to the orbit (Figure 9).

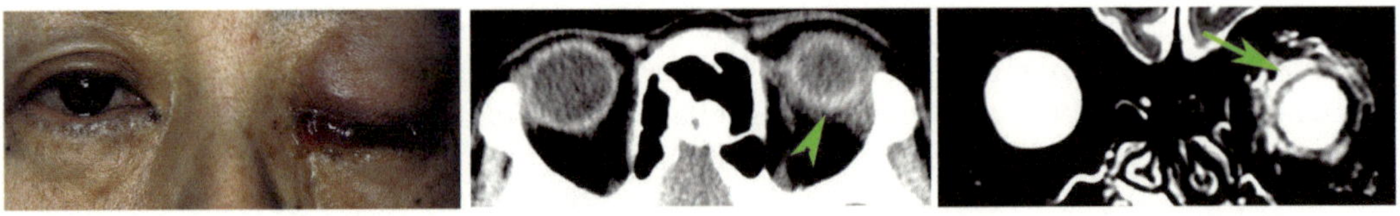

Fig. 9. Orbital cellulitis. A 60-year-old woman with orbital cellulitis had right upper lid swelling, chemosis, and ptosis at active phase. CT image shows fuzzy diffuse pattern in the orbit (arrowhead) and a lack of mass lesions. Fat-suppressed T2-weighted MR image shows high intensity signals that extend diffusely to the orbit (arrow). Compare the image with those of orbital myositis (Figure 1 to 7).

4.3 Thyroid-associated orbitopathy

Thyroid-associated orbitopathy is the most specific disease that shows extraocular muscle enlargements. The differential diagnosis thyroid-associated orbitopathy and orbital myositis are shown in Table 2. Patients with thyroid-associated orbitopathy had typically lack pain, have eyelid retraction with lagophthalmos, thyroid associated autoantibodies, and sparing of the extraocular muscle tendons on imaging (Figure 10). However, the signs and symptoms may overlap those of orbital myositis. For example, idiopathic orbital myositis without tendon involvement has been reported (Patrinely et al., 1989).

	Idiopathic orbital myositis	Thyroid-associated orbitopathy
Onset	Sudden, acute	Subacute, chronic
Periocular inflammatory signs	Frequent	Infrequent
Bilaterality	Infrequent	Frequent
Eyelid	Frequent ptosis	Frequent lid retraction
Extraocular movements	Limitation in the field of action and often in the direction opposite to the field of action of the affected extraocular muscles	Limitation in the direction opposite to the field of action of the affected extraocular
CT image	Indistinct swelling and frequent tendon involvement	Distinct swelling and infrequent tendon involvement
Fat-suppressed T2-weighted MR image	A hyperintense signal around fascicle structures in acute type or a hyperintense signal in the muscle in chronic type	A hyperintense signal in the muscle
Thyroid-associated autoantibodies	Negative	Frequently positive
Response to steroids	Dramatic with complete resolution in acute type and incomplete or recurrent in chronic type	Incomplete and slow

Table 2. Differential diagnosis of idiopathic orbital myositis versus thyroid-associated orbitopathy.

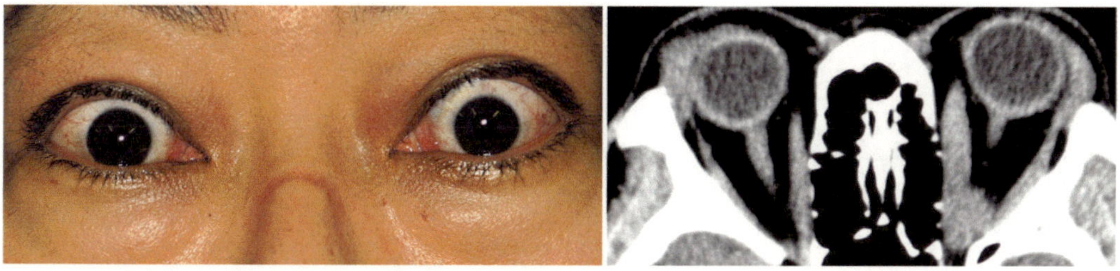

Fig. 10. Thyroid-associated orbitopathy. External photographs of a 44-year-old woman showing bilateral lid retraction, proptosis, and ocular motility restriction. CT image shows extraocular muscle enlargements without tendon involvement.

4.4 Primary and metastatic tumors

In a large cohort case series of orbital tumors and simulating lesions in the United States, Canada, and Japan, ocular adnexal lymphoid tumors accounted for approximately 10% to 18% of all cases (Garrity et al., 2007; Rootman, 2003; Shields et al., 2004; Shikishima, et al., 2006). Among malignant lymphomas, marginal zone B cell lymphomas made up the majority of the lymphomas arising from the ocular adnexa (Ferry et al., 2008). Among benign lymphoproliferative disorders, ocular adnexal IgG4-related related lymphoplasmacytic infiltrative disorder appeared to be a separate clinical entity that has unique clinical characteristics (Kubota et al., 2010). The signs and symptoms of them are frequently similar to those of atypical idiopathic orbital myositis (Figure 11 and 12). When patients have their sings and symptoms, physicians should consider either atypical idiopathic orbital myositis or ocular adnexal lymphoproliferative disorders. They should also consider an inicisional biopsy.

In the cohort case series studies, secondary or metastatic tumors account for approximately 20% to 40% of all cases (Garrity et al., 2007; Rootman, 2003; Shields et al., 2004; Shikishima, et al., 2006). Any malignant tumors in the body have a potential to metastasize to the extraocular muscles, and malignant tumor from the lung, breast, and thyroid ware found to predominate (Shikishima et al., 2006).

In imaging studies, the extraocular muscles in eyes with idiopathic orbital myositis appear indistinct and enlarged. On the other hand, metastatic tumors to the extraocular muscle appear sharply defined with irregular extraocular muscle enlargement (Figure 13). However, the images also resemble those of eyes with orbital myositis (Capone & Slamovis, 1990; Devine & Anderson, 1982; Slagle et al., 2009).

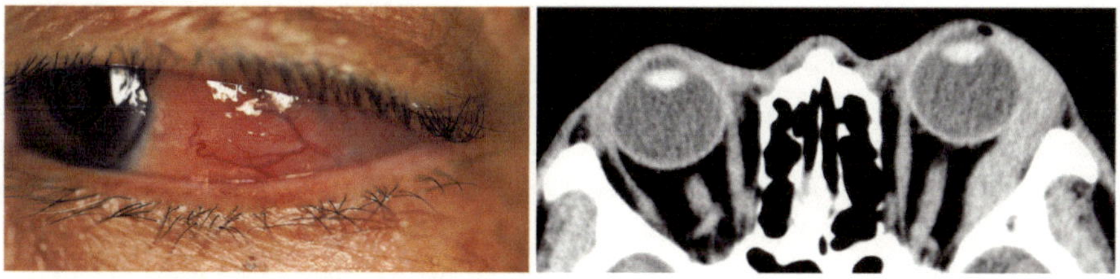

Fig. 11. Primary marginal zone B-cell lymphoma arising from left lateral rectus muscle. A 62-year-old man had periocular pain and ocular motility restrictions at initial visit. After steroid pulse therapy, he recovered from ocular symptoms but conjunctival mass lesions and extraocular muscle enlargements remained.

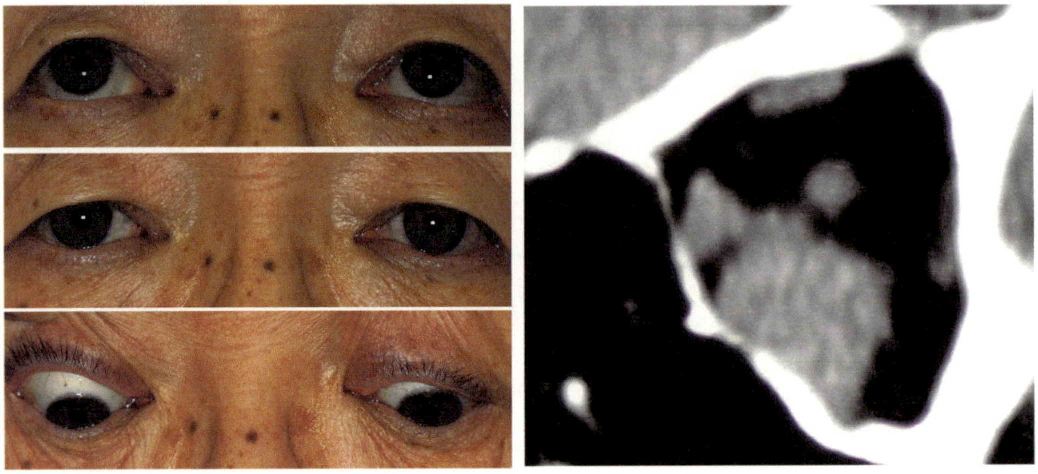

Fig. 12. Secondary follicular lymphoma. CT image of the orbit of a 57-year-old man with a history of follicular lymphoma had extraocular enlargements. Note that ocular motility is within normal limits despite of extraocular enlargements.

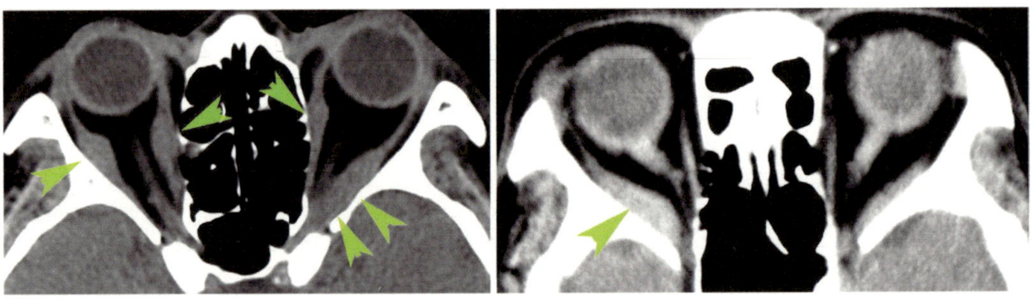

Fig. 13. Secondary carcinomas metastatic to extraocular muscles. Cases of breast carcinoma (left) and gastric carcinoma (Right) that metastasized to the orbit. Note that definitive and irregular enlargements of the extraocular muscle (arrowheads).

4.5 Parasitic infections

Two species of parasitic worms can infect the extraocular muscles; orbital sparganosis is reported mainly in eastern Asia and orbital cysticercosis mainly in India. Orbital sparganosis is caused by *Spirometra erinaceieuropaei* and can be acquired by drinking water containing copepods infected with the larval stage of the parasite. The orbit is a favorable site (Wiwanitkit, 2005; Yoon et al., 2004), and sparganosis can infect the extraocular muscles. (Figure 14; Kubota & Itoh, 2007). It is difficult to distinguish orbital myositis associated with sparganosis from idiopathic orbital myositis. A presumptive diagnosis of sparganosis can be made by finding a painful migratory subcutaneous nodule (Markell et al., 1999). An accurate diagnosis is made following the surgical removal and identification of the worm.

Orbital cysticercosis is caused by a parasitic *Cysticerucus cellulosae* infection which can infect the extraocular muscles. The host for *C. cellulosae* is the pig, and patients usually acquire the infection by eating undercooked pork. Imaging studies of orbital cysticercosis are characteristic, and the findings can differentiate of orbital cysticercosis from idiopathic orbital myositis (Angotti-Neto et al., 2007; Pushker et al., 2002; Rath et al., 2010)

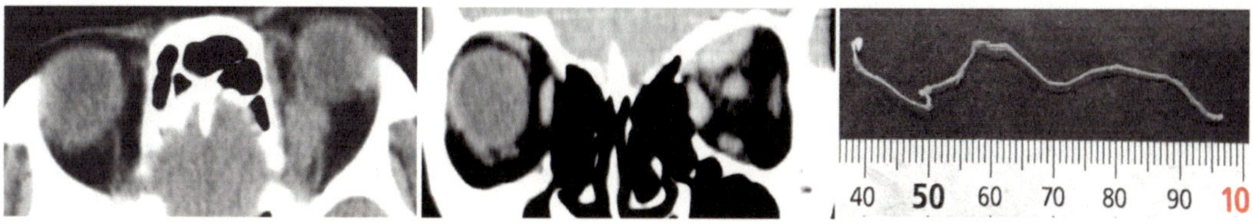

Fig. 14. Orbital axial and coronal CT images of a case of sparganosis at initial visit. Left and middle: Left superior rectus muscle is swollen. The images suggest orbital myositis. Right: Glistening and whitish larva about 7 cm long. Reproduced with permission from Kubota, T. & Itoh, M. (2007) Sparganosis associated with orbital myositis. *Japanese Journal of Ophthalmology*, Vol.51, No. 4, pp.311-312, ISSN:0021-5155

4.6 Anti-neutrophil cytoplasmic antibody (ANCA)-related vasculitis

Patients with systemic ANCA-related vasculitis, e.g., Churg-Strauss syndrome and Wegener granulomatosis, often also have pseudotumors in the ocular adnexae. The pseudotumors may resemble orbital myositis (Figure 15; Fujii et al., 2010; Takanashi et al., 2001). The ocular symptoms are often intolerable periocular pain that is markedly reduced following prednisolone plus cyclophosphamide.

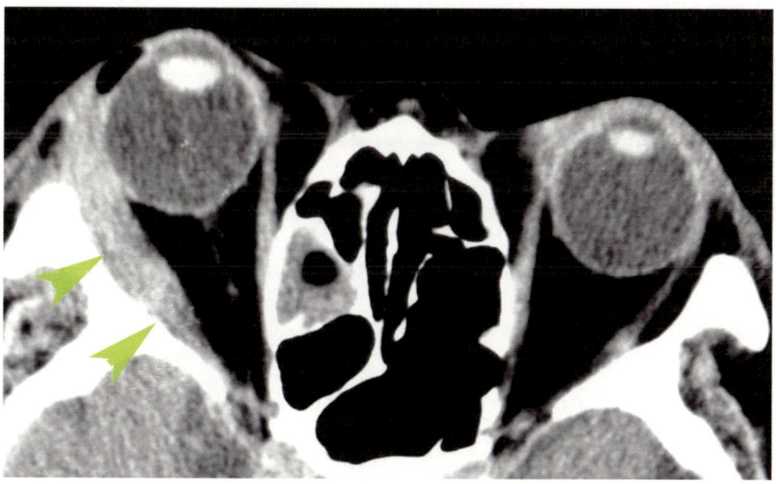

Fig. 15. Churg-Strauss syndrome. A 68-year-old man with Churg-Strauss syndrome had periocular pain and restrictions of ocular motility. CT image shows an apparent lateral rectus enlargement.

4.7 Orbital foreign body

Some foreign bodies may cause orbital inflammation. Polymethyl methacrylate (PMMA) is used by cosmetic surgeons in some countries, and can occasionally lead to serious ocular complications including orbital myositis (Figure 16; Kubota & Hirose, 2005; Sato et al., 2007; Silva & Curi, 2004)

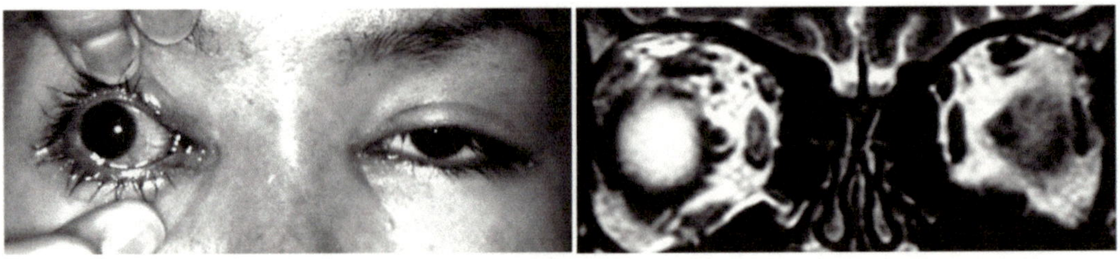

Fig. 16. Orbital inflammation associated with a foreign body. Left: A 29-year-old woman underwent cosmetic rhinoplastic surgery by a cosmetic surgeon. She developed ocular pain and a decrease of vision after the PMMA was injected. The right eye was displaced temporally leading to blepharoptosis. Her ocular motility was restricted. Right; T2-weighted MRI shows high signals from the right rectus muscles especially the medial rectus muscle. Reproduced with permission from Kubota T & Hirose H. (2005) Permanent loss of vision following cosmetic rhinoplastic surgery. *Japanese Journal of Ophthalmology*, Vol.49, No,6, pp.535-6, ISSN:0021-5155

4.8 Orbital inflammation triggered by drugs

Orbital inflammation including orbital myositis can be caused by bisphosphonates (Fraunfelder & Fraunfelder, 2003; Philips & Newman, 2008; Seth, et al., 2009; Sharma et al., 2008; Subramanian et al., 2003) and also by influenza vaccine (Thurairajan et al., 1997). Physicians should aware of these rare orbital conditions.

4.9 Arteriovenous shunting

Carotid cavernous fistulas leads to diffuse symmetric enlargement of most of the extraocular muscles and an enlargement of the superior ophthalmic vein (Figure 17).

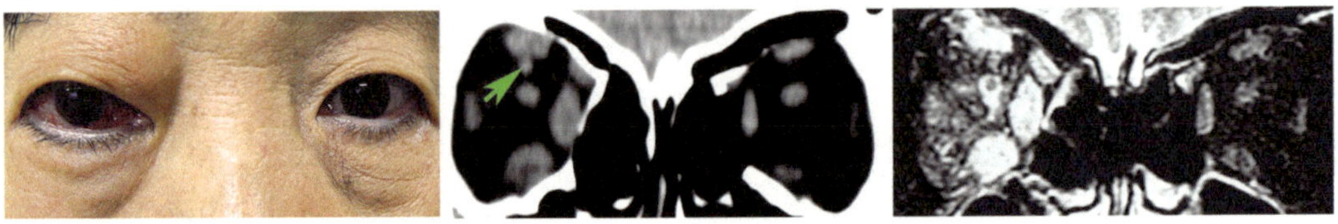

Fig. 17. Carotid cavernous fistulas. External photographs of a 65-year-old woman with swelling of the right eyelid and conjunctival injection. CT and MRI images show enlargements of the right superior, inferior, and medial rectus muscles and superior oblique muscles. In addition, an enlargement of the superior ophthalmic vein can also be seen (arrow).

4.10 Intramuscular hemangioma of the extraocular muscles.

Intramuscular hemangioma of the extraocular muscles is a rare clinical entity. Patients with intramuscular hemangioma of the extraocular muscles have isolated enlargement of extraocular muscles without pain and ocular motility restrictions (Kiratli et al., 2003). MR images show isointense T1-weight and hyperintense on T2-weight images, compared with extraocular muscles (Kiratli et al., 2003).

5. Treatments

Idiopathic orbital myositis is characterized by a variable natural course of evolution with spontaneous remission (Kubota & Kano, 2007; Slavin et al., 1982) to a corticosteroids-resistant progressive course. The first-line treatment is corticosteroids. It is believed that delayed diagnosis and treatment may lead to permanent dysfunction and both prompt therapy and a slow prolonged steroid taper can prevent ocular motility restrictions and recurrences (Costa et al., 2009; Scott & Siatkowski, 1997). In corticosteroids-resistant cases, the second-line treatment is done in a stepwise manner: first radiation, second immunosuppressive, and third biological agents.

5.1 Steroid treatment

It has been reported that oral NSAIDs are effective for idiopathic orbital myositis in a case series study (Mannor et al., 1997). However, in general the first-line treatment is corticosteroids. In the literature review, different initial doses ranging from 20 to 120 mg a day of oral prednisolone and 1000 mg intravenous methylprednisolone for 3 days have been used, and idiopathic orbital myositis frequently shifts toward recurrent and chronic course up to 75% despite the corticosteroids treatments (Costa et al., 2009).

5.2 Radiation therapy

Radiation therapy ranging from 16 to 30 Gy has been used for orbital myositis in corticosteroids-resistant cases or has been used as a corticosteroid-sparing method. In a review of radiation therapies patients with orbital myositis, approximately one-half of patients had a recurrence (Isobe et al., 2004).

5.3 Immunosuppressive therapy

Several case reports of immunosuppressive therapy for idiopathic orbital myositis have been published. Cyclosporine (Sanchez-Roman, et al. 1993), cyclophosphamide (Gunalp et al., 1996), and methotrexate (Kubota & Kano, 2007) have been use with variable results.

5.4 Biological agents

Therapy with tumor necrosis factor (TNF)-alpha inhibitor, such as infliximab is efficacious for immune-mediated inflammatory conditions, including rheumatoid arthritis and Crohn disease. Several published data showed that biological agents were successful in treating orbital myositis refractory to corticosteroids (Garrity et al., 2004; Miquel et al., 2008; Sahin et al., 2009) including orbital inflammatory disease (Kapadia & Rubin, 2006).

6. Conclusions

The etiology of orbital myositis is unknown. Orbital myositis associated with specific autoimmune disorders especially of giant cell myocarditis and Crohn disease may suggest a clue of pathogenesis of idiopathic orbital myositis, although the incidence of orbital myositis associated with autoimmune diseases is extremely low. Published case series studies have provided the best treatments by different initial doses of corticosteroids. But it appears to be difficult to evaluate the effectiveness for them using a meta-analysis. The acute and chronic/recurrent type of orbital myositis clearly respond differently to corticosteroids, therefore the type should be diagnosed before the treatment. Fat-suppressed T2-weighted

MR imaging may provide one of the predictive factors. Some orbital myositis refractory to corticosteroids can be effectively treated by immunosuppressive therapy and biologic agents. However, there is no randomized or comparison study and predictive factors for the effectiveness of different treatments.

7. References

Almekhlafi, MA. & Fletcher, WA. (2008) Levator palpebrae myositis. *Neurology,* Vol.71, No.15, pp.1202, ISSN: 0028-3878

Alshaikh, M., Kakakios, AM. & Kemp, AS. (2008) Orbital myositis following streptococcal pharngitis. *J Paediatr Child Health,* Vol.44, No. 4, pp.233-234, ISSN:1034-4810

Angotti-Neto, H., Goncalves, AC., Moura, FC. & Monteiro, ML. (2007) Extraocular muscle cysticerosis mimicking idiopathic orbital inflammation: case report. *Arq Bras Oftalmol,* Vol.70, No.3, pp.537-539, ISSN:0004-2749

Badilla, J. & Dolman, PJ. (2007) Orbital myositis involving the oblique muscles associated with herpes zoster ophthalmicus. *Ophthal Plast Reconstr Surg,* Vol.23, No.5, pp.411-413, ISSN:0740-9303

Belanger, C., Zhang, KS., Reddy, AK., Yen, MT. & Yen, KG. (2010) Inflammatory disorders of the orbit in childhood: a case series. *Am J Ophthalmol,* Vol. 150, No. 4, pp.460-463, ISSN:0002-9394

Camfield, PR., White, M., Warner, HA. & Lythgal, C. (1982) Orbital pseudotumor and Crohn disease. *J Pediatr,* Vol.101, No.1, pp.157-158, ISSN:0022-3476

Capone, A. Jr. & Slamovis, TL. (1990) Discrete metastasis of solid tumors to extraocular muscles. *Arch Ophthalmol,* Vol.108, No.2, pp.237-243, ISSN:0003-9950

Carvounis, PE., Mehta, AP., & Geist, CE. (2004) Orbital myositis associated with Borrelia burgdorferi (Lyme disease) infection. *Ophthalmology,* Vol.111, No. 5, pp.1023-1028, ISSN:0161-6420

Cheng, S., & Vu, P. (2009) Recurrent orbital myositis with radiological feature mimic thyroid eye disease in a patient with Crohn's disease. *Orbit,* Vol.28, No. 6, pp.368-370, ISSN:0167-6830

Cooper, LT. Jr., Berry, GJ. & Shabetai, R. (1997) Idiopathic giant-cell myocarditis—natural history and treatment. Multicenter Giant Cell Myocarditis study Group Investigators. *N Engl J Med,* Vol.236, No. 26, pp.1860-1866, ISSN:0028-4793

Costa, RM., Dumitrascu, OM. & Gordon, LK. (2009) Orbital myositis: diagnosis and management. *Curr Allergy Asthma Rep,* Vol.9, No. 4, pp.316-323, ISSN:1529-7322

Culligan, B. (2005) Orbital myositis following streptococcal pharyngitis in a pediatric patient. *Optmetry.* Vol. 76, No. 4, pp.250-258, ISSN:1558-1527

Culver, EL., Salmon, JF., Frith, P. & Travis, SPL. (2008) Recurrent posterior scleritis and orbital myositis as extra-intestinal manifestations of Crohn's disease: Case report and systemic literature review. *J Crohns colitis,* Vol.2, No.4, pp.337-342, ISSN:1873-9946

Divine, RD. & Anderson, RL. (1982) Metastatic small cell carcinoma masquerading as orbital myositis. *Ophthalmic surg,* Vol.13, No.6, pp.483-487, ISSN:0022-023X

Ferry, JA., Fung, CY., Zukerberg, L. Lucarelli, MJ. Hasserjian ,RP. Preffer, FI. & Harris, NL. (2007) Lymphoma of the ocular adnexa: a study of 353 cases. Am J Surg *Pathol,* Vol.31, No.2, pp.170-184, ISSN:0147-5185

Fraunfelder, FW. & Fraunfelder, FT. (2003) Bisphosphonates and ocular inflammation. *N Engl J Med,* Vol.348, No.12, pp.1187-1188, ISSN:0028-4793

Fujii ,T., Norizuki, M., Kobayashi, T., Yamamoto, M. & Kishimoto, M. (2010) A case of eosinophilic orbital myositis associated with CSS. *Mod Rheumatol*, VoI.20, No. 2, pp.196-199, ISSN:1439-7595

Garrity, JA., Coleman, AW., Matteson, EL., Eggenberger, ER. & Waitzman, DM. (2004) Treatment of recalcitrant idiopathic orbital inflammation (chronic orbital myositis) with infliximab. *Am J Ophthalmol*, VoI.138, No.6, pp.925-930, ISSN:0002-9394

Garrity, JA., Henderson, JW. & Cameron, JD. eds. (2007) *Henderson's orbital tumors.* (4th edition), Lippincott Williams and Wilkins, ISBN:978-0-7817-3896-9, Philadelphia Pennsylvania

Ghanchi, FD. & Rembacken ,BJ. (2003) Inflammatory bowel disease and eye. *Surv Ophthalmol*, VoI.48, No6, pp.663-676, ISSN:0039-6257

Grimson, BS. & Simons, KB. (1983) Orbital inflammation, myositis, and systemic lupus erythematosus. *Arch Ophthalmol*, VoI.101, No. 5, pp.736-738, ISSN:0003-9950

Gunalp, I., Gunduz, K. & Yazar, Z. (1996) Idiopathic orbital inflammatory disease. *Acta Ophthalmol Scand,* VoI.74, No.2, pp.191-193, ISSN:1395-3907

Hiraga, A., Uzawa, A. & Kamitsukasa, I. (2008) Orbital myositis after delivery. *Clin Neurol Neurosur,* VoI.110, No. 3, pp.316-317, ISSN:0303-8467.

Holak, H., Holak, N., Huzarska, M. & Holak, S. (2006) Tick inoculation in an eyelid region: report on five cases with complication of the orbital myositis associated with Lyme borreliosis. *Klin Oczna,* VoI.108, No.4-6, pp.220-224, ISSN:0023-2157

Holmgren, AR. & Matteson, EL. (2006) Lyme myositis. *Arthritis Rheum,* VoI.54, No.8, pp.2697-2700, ISSN:0004-3591.

Isobe, K., Uno, T., Kawakami, H., Ueno, N., Kawata, T., Abe, H., Minowa ,K., Yamamoto, S. & Ito, H. (2004) Radiation therapy for idiopathic orbital myositis: two case and literature review. *Radiat Med,* VoI. 22, No.6, pp.429-431, ISSN:0288-2043

Jacob, M., Ollagnon Roman, E. & Vighetto, A. (2007) Familial orbital myositis. *J Neurol,* VoI. 254, No.5, pp.666-667, ISSN: 0340-5354

Kapadia, MK. & Rubin, PA. (2006) The emerging use of TNF-alpha inhibitors in orbital inflammatory disease. *Int Ophthalmol Clin,* VoI.46, No.2, pp.165-181, ISSN:0020-8167

Kattah, JC., Zimmerman, LE., Kolsky, MP., Chrousos, G., Chavis, R., Jaffe, G. & Manz, HJ. (1990) Bilateral orbital involvement in fatal giant cell polymyositis. *Ophthalmology,* VoI. 97, No. 4, pp.520-525, ISSN:0161-6420

Kau, HC., Kao, SC., Peng, CH., Hsu ,WM. & Tsai, CC. (2006) Methylprednisolone pulse therapy in patient with isolated superior oblique myositis. *Eye(Lond),* VoI.20, No.9, pp.1106-1109, ISSN:0950-222X

Kawasaki, A. & Borruat, FX. (2003) An unusual presentation of Herpes zoster ophthalmicus: orbital myositis preceding vesicular eruption. *Am J Ophthalmol,* VoI.136, No. 3, pp.574-575, ISSN:0002-9394

Kiratli, H., Bilgic, S., Caglar, M. & Soylemezoglu, F. (2003) Intramuscular hemangiomas of extraocular muscles. *Ophthalmology,* VoI.110, No. 3, pp.564-568, ISSN:0161-6420

Klein, BR., Hedges, TR. 3rd, Dayal, Y. & Adelman, LS. (1989). Orbital myositis and giant myocarditis. *Neurology,* VoI.39, No.7, pp.988-990, ISSN:0028-3878

Knox, DL., Schachat, AP. & Mustonen, E. (1984) Primary, secondary and coincidental ocular complications of Crohn's disease. *Ophthalmology,* VoI.91, No.2, pp.163-173, ISSN:0161-6420

Krasnianski, M., Sievert, M., Bau, V. & Zierz, S. (2004) External ophthalmoplegia due to ocular myositis in a patient with ophthalmic herpes zoster. *Neuromuscul Disord,* VoI. 14, No.7, pp.438-441, ISSN:0960-8966

Kubota, T. & Hirose, H. (2005) Permanent loss of vision following cosmetic rhinoplastic surgery. *Jpn J Ophthalmol*, Vol.49, No.6, pp.535-536, ISSN:0021-5155

Kubota, T. & Itoh, M. (2007) Spargnosis associated with orbital myositis. *Jpn J Ophthalmol*, Vol.51, No. 4, pp.311-312, ISSN:0021-5155

Kubota, T. & Kano, H. (2007) Assessment of inflammation in idiopathic orbital myositis with fat-suppressed T2-weighted magnetic resonance imaging. *Am J Ophthalmol*, Vol.143, No.4, pp.718-720, ISSN:0002-9394

Kubota, T. Moritani, S. Katayama, M. & Terasaki, H. (2010) Ocular adnexal IgG4-related lymphoplasmacytic infiltrative disorder. *Arch Ophthalmol*, Vol.128, No.5, pp.577-584, ISSN:0003-9950.

Lacey ,B. Chang, W. & Rootman, J. (1999) Nonthyroid causes of extraocular muscle disease. *Surv Ophthalmol*, Vol.44, No.3, pp.187-213, ISSN:0039-6257

Leib, ML., Odel, JG. & Cooney, MJ. (1994) Orbital polymyositis and giant cell myocarditis. *Ophthalmology*, Vol.101, No.5, pp.950-954, ISSN:0161-6420

Lesser, RL., Kornmehl, EW., Pachner, AR., Kattah, J., Hedges, TR. 3rd, Newman, NM., Ecker, PA. & Glassman, MI. (1990) Neuro-ophthalmologic manifestations of Lyme disease. *Ophthalmology*, Vol.97, No.6, pp.699-706, ISSN:0161-6420

Lind-Ayres, MR., Abramowsky, C. & Mahle, WT. (2009) Pediatric giant cell myocarditis and orbital myositis. *Pediatr Cardiol*, Vol.30, No. 4, pp.510-512, ISSN:0172-0643

Maalouf ,T., Angioi, K. & George, JL. (2001) Recurrent orbital myositis and Crohn's diseas. *Orbit*, Vol.20, No.1, pp.75-80, ISSN:0167-6830

Mannor, GE., Rose, GE., Moseley, IF. & Write, JE. (1997) Outcome of orbital myositis. Clinical features associated with recurrence. *Ophthalmology*, Vol.104, No. 3, pp.409-413, ISSN:0161-6420

Markell, EK., John, DT. & Krotoski, WA. (1999) The cestodes, *Markell and Voge's Medical parasitology* (8 edition), pp.238-240, WB Saunders co, ISBN: 0-7216-7634-0, Philadelphia

Maurer, I. & Zierz ,S. (1999) Recurrent orbital myositis: report of a familial incidence. *Arch Neurol*, Vol.56, No.11, pp.1407-1409, ISSN:0003-9942

Miquel, T., Abad, S., Badelon, I., Vignal, C., Warzocha, U., Larroche, C., Morax, S. & Dhote, R. (2008) Successful treatment of idiopathic orbital inflammation with infliximab: an alternative to conventional steroid sparing agents. *Ophthal Plast Reconstr Surg*, Vol.24, No.5, pp.415-417, ISSN:0740-9303

Mombaerts, I. & Koornneef, L. (1997) Current status in the treatment of orbital myositis. *Ophthalmology*, Vol.104, No.3, pp.402-408, ISSN:0161-6420

Muller-Felber, W., Reimers, CD., de Koning, J., Fischer, P., Pilz, A. & Ponqratz, DE. (1993) Myositis in Lyme borreliosis: an immunohistochemical study of seven patients. *J Neurol Sci*, Vol.118, No.2, pp.207-212, ISSN:0022-510X

Nabili, S., McCarey, DW., Browne, B. & Capell, HA. (2002) A case of orbital myositis associated with rheumatoid arthritis. *Ann Rheum Dis*, Vol.61, No.10, pp.938-939, ISSN:0003-4967

Nieto, JC., Kim, N. & Lucarelli, MJ. (2008) Dacroadenitis and orbital myositis associated with lyme disease. *Arch Ophthalmol*, Vol.126, No.8, pp.1165-1166, ISSN:0003-9950

Ohnishi, T., Noguchi, S., Murakami, N., Tajiri, J., Harao, M., Kawamoto, H., Hoshi, H., Jinnouchi, S., Futami, S. & Nagamachi, S., et al. (1994) Extraocular muscles in Graves ophthalmopathy: usefulness of T2 relaxation time measurements. *Radiology*, Vol.190, No. 3, pp.857-862. ISSN:0033-8419

Panfilio, CB. Hernandez-Cossio, O. & Hernandez-Fustes, OJ. (2000) Orbital myositis and rheumatoid arthritis: case report. *Arq Neuropsiquiat,* Vol.58, No.1, pp.174-177, ISSN:0004-282X

Patrinely, JR., Osborn, AG., Anderson, RL. & Whiting, AS. (1989) Computed tomographic features of nonthyroid extraocular muscle enlargement. *Ophthalmology,* Vol. 96, No. 7, pp.1038-1047, ISSN:0161-6420

Pendse, S., Bilyk, JR. & Lee, MS. (2006) The ticking time bomb. *Surv Ophthalmol,* Vol.51, No. 3, pp.274-279, ISSN:0039-6257

Phillips, PM. & Newman, SA. (2008) Orbital inflammatory disease after intravenous infusion of zoledronate for treatment of metastatic renal cell carcinoma. *Arch Ophthalmol,* Vol.126, No. 1, pp.137-139, ISSN:0003-9950

Purcell, JJ jr. & Taulbee, WA. (1981) Orbital myositis after upper respiratory tract infection. *Arch Ophthalmol,* Vol.99, No.3, pp.437-438, ISSN:0003-9950

Pushker, N., Bajaj, MS. & Betharia, SM. (2002) Orbital and adnexal cysticercosis. *Clin Experiment Ophthalmol,* Vol.30, No. 5, pp.323-333, ISSN:1442-6404

Ramalho, J. & Castillo, M. (2008) Imaging of orbital myositis in Crohn's disease. *Clin Imaging,* Vol.32, No. 3, pp.227-229, ISSN:0899-7071

Ramboer, K., Demaerel, PH., Baert, AL., Casteels, I. & Dralands, G. (1997) Linear scleroderma with orbital involvement: follow-up and magnetic resonance imaging. *Br J Ophthalmol,* Vol.80, No10, pp.930-932, ISSN:0007-1161

Rath, S., Honavar, SG., Naik, M., Anand, R., Agarwal, B., Krishnaiah, S. & Sekhar, GC. (2010) Orbital cysticercosis: clinical manifestations, diagnosis, management, and outcome. *Ophthalmology,* Vol.117, No. 3, pp.600-605.e1, ISSN:0161-6420

Rootman, J. (2003) *Disease of the orbit. A multidisciplinary approach.* (2nd edition), Lippincott Williams and Wilkins, ISBN:0-7817-1512-1, Philadelphia Pennsylvania

Roulez, FM., Dangoisse, C., Dufour, D. & Meire, FM. (2007) Orbital myositis in a child with linear scleroderma en coup de saabre. *J Pediatr Ophthalmol Strabismus,* Vol. 44, No. 5, pp.264-266, ISSN:0191-3913

Sahlin, S., Lignell, B., Williams, M., Dastmalchi, M. & Orrego, A. (2009) Treatment of idiopathic sclerosing inflammation of the orbit (myositis) with infliximab. *Acta Ophthalmol,* Vol.87, No.8, pp.906-908, ISSN:1755-375X

Sanchez-Roman, J., Varela-Aquilar, JM., Bravo-Ferrer, J., Sequeiros Madueno, E. & Fernandez de Bobadilla, M. (1993) Idiopathic orbital myositis: treatment with cyclosporine. *Ann Rheum Dis,* Vol.52, No.1, pp.84-85, ISSN:0003-4967

Sato, MT., Oliveira e Cruz, GA., Neto Hde, O., Moreira,AT. & Salles, MV. (2007) Extraocular muscle myositis. *Ophthalmology,* Vol.114, No. 3, pp.623-624, ISSN:0161-6420

Scott, IU. & Siatkowski, RM. (1997) Idiopathic orbital myositis. *Curr Opin Rheumatol,* Vol.9, No.6, pp.504-512, ISSN:1040-8711

Seidenberg, KB. & Leib, ML. (1990) Orbital myositis with Lyme disease. *Am J Ophthalmol,* Vol.109, No.1, pp.13-16, ISSN:0002-9394

Serop, S., Vianna, RN., Claeys, M. & De Laey, JJ. (1994) Orbital myositis secondary to systemic lupus erythematosus. *Acta Ophthalmol,* Vol.72, No. 4, pp.520-523, ISSN:0001-639X

Seth, A., Anderson, DP., Albiani, DA. & Barton, JJ. (2009) Orbital inflammation snd optic neuropathy with zoledronic acid for metastatic prostate cancer. *Can J Ophthalmol,* Vol.44, No.4, pp.467-468, ISSN:0008-4182

Sharma, NS., Ooi, JL., Masselos, K., Hooper, MJ. & Francis, IC. (2008) Zoledronic acid infusion and orbital inflammatory disease. *N Engl J Med,* Vol. 359, No.13, pp.1410-1411, ISSN:0028-4793

Shields, JA., Shields, CL. & Scartozzi, R. (2004) Survey of 1264 patients with orbital tumors and simulating lesions: The 2002 Montgomery Lecture, part 1. *Ophthalmology*, Vol.111, No. 5, pp.997-1008, ISSN:0161-6420

Shikishima, K., Kawai, K. & Kitahara, K. (2006) Pathological evaluation of orbital tumors in Japan: analysis of a large case series and 1379 cases reported in the Japanese literature. *Clin Experiment Ophthalmol*, Vol.34, No. 3, pp.239-244, ISSN:1442-6404

Siatkowski, RM., Capo, H., Byrne, SF., Gendron, EK., Flynn, JT., Munoz, M. & Feuer, WJ. (1994) Clinical and echographic findings in idiopathic orbital myositis. *Am J Ophthalmol*, Vol. 118, No.3, pp.343-350, ISSN: 0002-9394

Silva, MT. & Curi, AL. (2004) Blindness and total ophthalmoplegia after aesthetic polymethymethacrylate injection: case report. *Arq Neuropsiquiat*,. Vol.62, No.3B, pp.873-874, ISSN:0004-282X

Slagle, WS., Eckermann, DR., Musick, AN. & Slagle, AM. (2009) Adenocarcinoma metastasis causing discrete extraocular muscle enlargement. *Optometry*, Vol.80, No.7, pp.367-374, ISSN:1558-1527

Slavin, ML. & Glaser, JS. (1982) Idiopathic orbital myositis: report of six cases. *Arch Ophthalmol*, Vol.100, No. 8, pp.1261-1265, ISSN:0003-9950

Stevens, AW., Grossman, ME. & Barr, ML. (1996) Orbital myositis, vitiligo, and giant cell myocarditis. *J Am Acad Dermatol*, Vol.35, No. 2 Pt2, pp.310-312, ISSN:0190-9622

Stidham, DB., Sondhi, N., Plager, D. & Helveston, E. (1998) Presumed isolated inflammation of the superior oblique muscle in idiopathic orbital myositis. *Ophthalmology*, Vol.105, No.12, pp.2216-2219, ISSN:0161-6420

Subramanian, PS., Kerrison, JB., Calvert, PC. & Miller, NR. (2003) Orbital inflammatory disease after pamidronate treatment for metastatic prostate cancer. *Arch Ophthalmol*, Vol.121, No. 9, pp.1335-1336, ISSN:0003-9950

Suttorp-Schulten, MS. & Koornneef, L. (1990) Linear scleroderma associated with ptosis and motility disorders. *Br J Ophthalmol*, Vol.74, No.11, pp.694-695, ISSN:0007-1161

Takanashi, T., Uchida, S., Arita, M., Okada, M. & Kashii, S. (2001) Orbital inflammatory pseudotumore and ischemic vasculitis in Churg-Strauss syndrome: report of two cases and review of the literature. *Ophthalmology*, Vol.108, No.6, pp.1129-1133, ISSN:0160-6420

Thurairajan, G., Hope-Ross, MW., Situnayake, RD. & Murray, PI. (1997) Polyarthropathy, orbital myositis and posterior scleritis: an unusual adverse reaction to influenza vaccine. *Br J Rheumatol*, Vol.36, No.1, pp.120-123, ISSN:0263-7103

Volpe, NJ. & Shore, JW. (1991) Orbital myositis associated with herpes zoster. *Arch Ophthalmol*, Vol.109, No.4, pp.471-472, ISSN:0003-9950

Weinstein, JM., Koch, K. & Lane, S. (1984) Orbital pseudotumor in Crohn's colitis. *Ann Ophthalmol*, Vol.16, No.3, pp.275-278, ISSN:0003-4886

Wiwanitkit, V. (2005) A review of human sparganosis in Thailand. *Int J Infect Dis*, Vol.9, No.6, pp.312-316, ISSN:1201-9712

Yan, Qiu, H., Wu ,Z. & Li Y. (2006) Idiopathic orbital inflammatory pseudotumor in Chinese children. *Orbit*, Vol.25, No.1, pp.1-4, ISSN:0167-6830

Young, RS., Hodes, BL., Cruse, RP., Koch, KL. & Garovoy, MR. (1981) Orbital pseudotumor and Crohn disease. *J Pediatr*, Vol.99, No.2, pp.250-252, ISSN:0022-3476

Yoon, KC., Seo, MS., Park, SW. & Park, YG. (2004) Eyelid sparganosis. *Am J Ophthalmol*, Vol.138, No.5, pp.873-875, ISSN:0002-9394

9

Myouclear Breakdown in Sporadic Inclusion Body Myositis

Satoshi Nakano[1,2] and Hirofumi Kusaka[2]
[1]*Osaka City general Hospital*
[2]*Kansai Medical University*
Japan

1. Introduction

Sporadic inclusion body myositis (s-IBM) is categorized as a form of the idiopathic autoimmune inflammatory myopathies and it is common myopathy in the elderly. Unlike polymyositis which preferentially shows proximally-dominant skeletal muscle involvement, s-IBM displays a unique distribution of muscle atrophy and weakness: patients with s-IBM often have severely atrophic muscles in the forearm flexors and quadriceps femoris. Unlike other inflammatory myopathies, this disorder is usually unresponsive to therapy and has a slowly progressive course. The pathological findings define the diagnosis of s-IBM. They include: 1) mononuclear cell infiltration surrounding and invading non-necrotic muscle fibers; 2) Congo-red positive inclusions; and 3) vacuoles lined by basophilic materials called rimmed vacuoles. The pathogenesis of s-IBM remains undetermined.

In s-IBM muscle biopsy, electron microscopy shows myonuclear abnormalities, such as filamentous inclusions and rare nuclear envelope breakdown. Based on such observation, it has been proposed that the myonuclear change is closely associated with the pathogenesis. Also, several studies have indicated that a focal cytoplasmic deposits of nucleus-proper and nucleus-oriented proteins in s-IBM abnormal muscle fibers. Recently, elemental components of the nucleus, such as nuclear envelope proteins (e.g., emerin and lamin A/C), histone H1, or DNA have been detected on vacuolar membranes or within vacuoles. The results strongly support the theory that myonuclear breakdown results in rimmed vacuoles.

In this chapter, we first present figures that show abnormal localization of nuclear proteins associated with MAP kinase in s-IBM muscle fibers. The results suggest that inhibition of nuclear transport during myogenesis. We next describe abnormal localization of histone H1 in s-IBM with some comments on a unique character of histone H1 among several histones as a transcriptional regulator and a player in the DNA damage response. Lastly, our recent investigation of DNA damage is included. Our studies in s-IBM support the theory that nuclear damage is closely associated with its etiology.

2. Background

2.1 History

The term "inclusion body myositis (IBM)" was proposed in 1971. As some of the patients who had been diagnosed as having IBM in earlier studies were young, and the pathology showed no inflammation (Yunis and Samaha 1971), the diagnosis of these patients could be "hereditary inclusion body myopathy (h-IBM)" or "myofibrillar myopathy" according to the current definition. Sporadic inclusion body myositis (s-IBM) is now considered as a form of idiopathic inflammatory myopathies which include polymyositis and dermatomyositis (Dalakas 2006, Needham and Mastaglia 2008). The diagnosis of s-IBM was initially done based on the presence of unique tubulofilamentous inclusions in the nucleus and cytoplasm under electron microscopic study in patients who had been usually diagnosed as having chronic polymyositis. Later, it became recognized as a common form of inflammatory myopathy in the elderly, which shows slowly progressive, frequent involvement of distal muscles, male predominance, and resistance of corticosteroid therapy (Lotz et al 1989). The characteristic histopathological findings are nuclear and cytoplasmic tubulofilamentous inclusions and vacuoles lined by basophilic materials (rimmed vacuoles) (Carpenter et al 1978). In 1991, Mendel et al. identified Congo-red positive inclusions in s-IBM muscle fibers, which subsequently were shown to be composed of β-amyloid (Askanas et al 1992). In 1995, the diagnostic criteria for s-IBM were proposed (Griggs et al 1995). According to it, the pathological diagnosis of s-IBM necessitates 1) mononuclear cell infiltration surrounding and invading non-necrotic muscle fibers; 2) Congo-red positive inclusions in light microscope or tubulofilaments of about 15-18 nm in diameter in electron microscopic study; and 3) rimmed vacuoles. Each of these findings alone is not specific to s-IBM. Collection of inflammatory cells surrounding and invading non-necrotic muscle fibers is found in polymyositis. Detection of congophilic inclusions is one of the hallmarks of myofibrillar myopathy (Selcen and Engel 2010). In distal myopathy with rimmed vacuoles (DMRV)/hereditary inclusion body myopathy (h-IBM), the presence of rimmed vacuoles is diagnostic, but the muscle tissue shows no inflammatory exudates (Nonaka et al 1998). The definite diagnosis of s-IBM needs all of the three findings.

The muscle biopsy studies have provided important information about the pathological mechanism of each change in s-IBM. By analyzing subtypes of cells infiltrating to muscle tissue or immunological molecular ligand-receptor relationships have indicated almost identical immunological mechanism of s-IBM to that of polymyositis. In s-IBM and polymyositis, cytotoxic CD8-positive T-cells invade MHC-I-expressing muscle fibers (Dalakas 2006). In both, myeloid dendritic cells were frequently surrounded and sometimes invading non-necrotic fibers. The radiation of myeloid dendritic cells in dense collections of inflammatory exudates containing T cells suggests local intramuscular antigen presentation in s-IBM and polymyositis (Greenberg et al 2007a).

Concerning to congophilic inclusions, they are generally thought to be composed of β-amyloid and its related proteins as detected in the brain of neurodegenerative diseases (Askanas and Engel 2008), although their exact nature remains to be determined (Greenberg 2009). Congophilic inclusions are more conspicuous in myofibrillar myopathy than s-IBM. However, the congo-red positive inclusions in myofibrillar myopathy may not correspond to amyloid fibrils, but Z-line derived, degenerating products of myofibrils based on ultrastructural studies (Selcen and Engel 2010).

2.2 Our study of phosphorylated proteins and nuclear components in s-IBM

We first examined phosphorylation systems and found cytoplasmic and perinuclear deposition of nucleus-oriented and nucleus-proper proteins in s-IBM muscle fibers. The results suggest that inhibited nuclear transport of some enzymes involved in myogenesis.

As for rimmed vacuoles, some studies have shown that they are positive for autophagic/lysosome markers, suggesting that rimmed vacuoles are autophagic vacuoles

(Kumamoto et al 2004). But autophagic vacuoles in muscle, such as those found in acid maltase deficiency are not rimmed (Dubowitz and Sewry 2007).

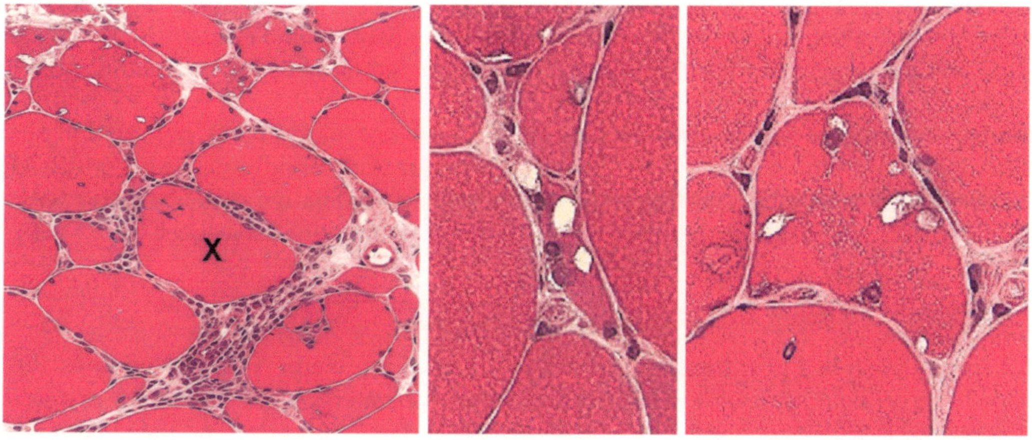

Fig. 1. H&E stained cryostat sections of muscle biopsy in a patient with s-IBM. Mononuclear cells surround a non-necrotic fiber (X). Vacuoles with thin blue membranes are seen. Some vacuoles contain fluffy inclusions.

The peripheries of rimmed vacuoles are often lined by basophilic materials in Hematoxyline and Eosin (H&E) staining (figure 1). Several studies have suggested that rimmed vacuoles are product of nuclear breakdown. If vacuoles are nuclear origin, the basophilic substances should be some nuclear components. As histones represent basophilic nuclear proteins, we examined histones in s-IBM by immunnohistochemistry. The study has shown that some of the basophilic materials are indeed positive for histone H1, supporting nuclear breakdown in s-IBM (Nakano et al 2008).

3. The detection of phosphorylated proteins in s-IBM

3.1 Phosphorylated neurofilament protein epitopes in s-IBM

Some investigators consider that the ectopic deposition of proteins of neurodegenerative diseases is the central event in the pathogenesis of s-IBM (Askanas and Engel 2008). Others have tried to connect the inflammation and the amyloid deposition, suggesting that ectopic proteins may be induced by inflammatory cytokines (Schmidt et al 2008), which in turn provokes autophagy/lysosomal system (Lunemann et al 2007). There is, however, controversy against the real identity of the congophilic inclusions (Greenberg 2009). Some studies showed the rarity or absent reactivity for β-amyloid in patients with otherwise clinically and pathologically typical s-IBM (Sherriff et al 1995, Nalbantoglu et al 1994). The results may raise doubts over the significance of the neurodegenerative protein deposition in the pathogenesis of s-IBM. One of the authors (S Nakano), as a muscle pathologist, also found only small amounts of β-amyloid positive inclusions in s-IBM. Nonetheless, we often detected SMI-31 positive inclusions in a significant proportion of s-IBM vacuolated fibers. The antibody named SMI-31 was originally made as an antibody for the lysine-serine-proline (KSP) repeats of the neurofilament proteins in which the serine is phosphorylated, and it can also attach to other proteins, such as microtubule associated protein 2, containing

the same epitope (Nukina et al 1987). As SMI-31antibody cross-reacts with tau, it was suggested that the antibody SMI-31 could combine with tau and that tubulofilaments in s-IBM might paired-helical filaments as found in the brain with Altzheimer's disease (Askanas et al 1994), although several other antibodies for tau failed to localize the inclusions (Mirabella et al 1996). We also found the gap between the results with SMI-31 and some antibodies against phosphorylated tau. It suggested existence of some other proteins containing KSP (in which S is phosphorylated) sequence.
Moreover, using several antibodies against tau, western blot studies indicated that an electrophorectic profile of a doublet within the range of 60-62 kDa isoforms, which was different from tauopathies of the central nervous system (Maurage et al 2004) and SMI-31 did not react tau in the first place, but some other nuclear proteins (Salajegheh et al 2009b).

3.2 Phosphorylation is a dynamic process significantly involved in signal transduction

Phosphorylation is a post-translational modification of a protein. A phosphate molecule is added to a serine or threonine residue by serine/threonine kinases and removed by specific phosphatases. The phosphorylation modification is dynamic processes and they play central roles in controlling protein function and thereby intracellular signal transduction (Hunter and Karin 1992). Phosphorylation of a tyrosine residue is another post-translational protein modification that also has significant roles in the signal transduction. As we hypothesized that the SMI-31-positive inclusions in s-IBM could indicate perturbation of the signal transduction system, we initially examined s-IBM muscle biopsy materials using antibody against phosphorylated tyrosine. Figure 2 indicates the results displaying inclusions of substances containing phosphorylated tyrosine. Western blotting studies using muscle homogenates disclosed several positive bands, one of which corresponds to ERK2, a protein kinase belonging to the MAP kinases (Nakano et al 1998). The results led us to study MAP kinase cascades.

4. Studies of mitogen-activated protein kinase (MAPK) cascades in s-IBM

4.1 MAPK cascades

The enzymes belonging to MAPK family play pivotal roles in intracellular signal transduction that transduces extracellular signals to the nucleus (Hill and Treisman 1995, Robinson and Cobb 1997). Growth factors, hormones and cytokines induce an intracellular signaling cascade that leads to the activation of MAPK kinases 1 and 2 (MKK1/2), which successively phosphorylate and activate ERK1 and ERK2. In a similar fashion, stresses and pro-inflammatory cytokines provoke signal transduction cascades, activating other MKKs. These MKKs then phosphorylate and activate p38 MAPK and c-Jun N-terminal kinase (JNK) (Figure 3) (Reffas and Schlegel 2000). The complex phosphorylation systems provide for a delicately tuned, prompt regulation of signals at each level of the cascade, with cross-talks with other intracellular transduction systems. Finally, activated MAPKs phosphorylate several cytoplasmic proteins associated with signal transduction, migrating into the nucleus, within which MAPKs phosphorylate and regulate transcription factors. Activated MAPKs are dephosphorylated and inactivated by phosphatases, such as MAP kinase phosphatases (MKPs) that are specialized for the deactivation of MAPKs (Keyse 2000).

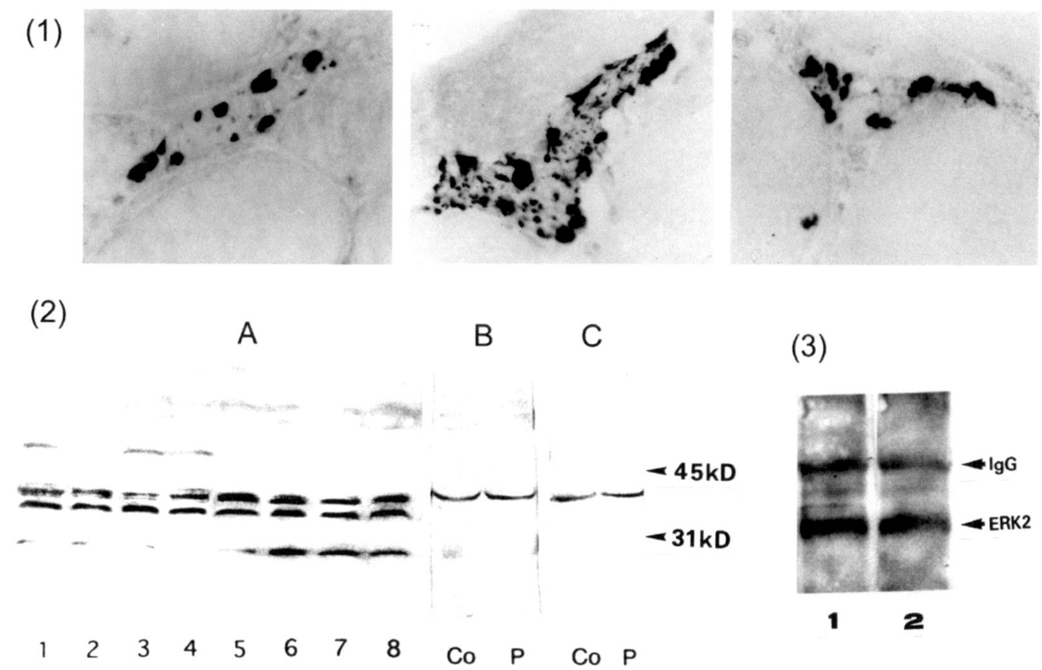

Fig. 2. Phophotyrosine study in s-IBM. (1) Localization of phosphotyrosine-containing proteins in s-IBM using anti-phosphotyrosine antibody showing positive deposits in vacuolated fibers. (2) Resolution of phosphotyrosine-containing proteins on immunoblots of muscle homogenates separated by SDS-PAGE. (A) Lanes 1-4: normal controls; 5-8: s-IBM. (B) Immunoblots with anti-ERK2 antibody. Co-migration of about 40 kD protein in A with ERK2. (C) Immunoblots with anti active form of ERK1/2. Co: a control; P: an s-IBM patient. Apart from 40 kD bands, bands of 38 kD in all cases, 27 kD in s-IBM are present. (3) Immunoprecipitation with anti-phosphotyrosine antibody followed by immunoblotting. After separation of the immunoprecipitates on SDS-PAGE, the membrane was immunoblotted with anti-ERK2 antibody (lane 1), and anti-acitive form of ERK (lane2). Both lanes show positive bands at approximately 40 kD of ERK2

Activated ERK1/2 phosphorylates various cytoplasmic molecules and traverse the nuclear envelope into the matrix, phosphorylating a transcription factor called Elk-1 (Figure 3) (Force and Bonventre 1998). The phosphorylated form of Elk-1 in the association with serum response factor (SRF), binds to the serum response element (SRE) of the promoter region of immediate early genes, including c-fos (Treisman, 1994). In stress-activated cascades, p38 MAPK and c-Jun N-terminal protein kinase (JNK), two subclasses of the MAPK family, take the equivalent position to ERK in the ERK cascade (Kyriakis and Avruch 1996).

4.2 Deposits of ERK is found in s-IBM vacuolated fibers

To start investigating the MAPK cascades, we examined ERK, p38 MAPK and JNK as well as two of their nuclear substrates by immunohistochemistry (Nakano et al 2001). The results showed that more than 60% of vacuolated fibers in s-IBM displayed very strong immunoreactive deposits of ERK that appeared round or irregular inclusions.

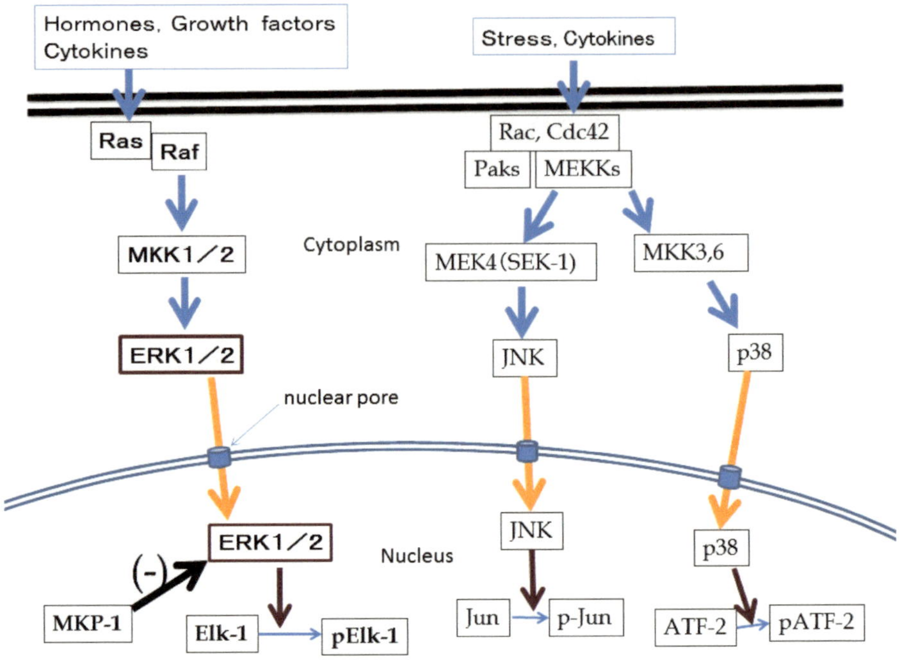

Fig. 3. MAPK cascades.

In contrast, no or few deposits positive for p38 or JNK were observed in vacuolated fibers. In control subjects, diffuse and moderate ERK, p38 and JNK immunoreactivity was found in regenerating fibers and in some degenerating fibers. As for the substrates, we immunolocalized phosphorylated Elk-1 (pElk-1) as is phosphorylated by ERK. There were strong pElk-1–immunopositive deposits in s-IBM. The localization of pElk-1 was identical with those of ERK-positive deposits, which had been confirmed in a double immunofluorescence study. The relationship between the pElk-1–positive deposits and those of SMI-31-positive deposits in vacuolated fibers in immunofluorescence study showed colocalization of pElk-1 and SMI-31-positive deposits. The substrate of JNK (c-Jun) was negative.

ERK, JNK and p38 are involved in muscle fiber maturation. In studies of muscle cell cultures, ERK, more specifically ERK2, is required in muscle fiber terminal differentiation (Li and Johnson 2006), and ERK positively regulated the activity of MyoD (a myogenic transcription factor), when the high JNK activity of myoblasts was downregulated (Gredinger et al 1998). Also, p38 may play a positive role in muscle fiber differentiation earlier than ERK via another myogenic transactivation factor, MEF2 (Zetser et al 1999, Lluís et al 2006). Regenerating fibers consist of replicating myoblasts and differentiating myotubes (Banker and Engel 2004). Thus, the increases of MAPKs in regenerating fibers in diseased muscles may correlate with the findings of the cell culture studies. Because SRF, the partner of activated Elk-1 in the nucleus, is also necessary for muscle fiber differentiation (Soulez et al 1996), ERK is probably involved in myogenesis via phosphorylation of Elk-1.

Another group has examined several MAPKs in s-IBM (Li et al 2000a). Their results also showed abnormal expression of ERK (more specifically ERK2), but not JNK or p38 in s-IBM. Moreover, immuno-histochemical analysis using antibodies against phosphoserine showed accumulations of phosphoserine-containing protein deposits in s-IBM vacuolated fibers. Western blots of muscle lysates demonstrated a 35 kD phosphoprotein. They concluded that the hyperexpression of 35kD protein may represent cytoskeletal by-products due to ERK activation and that the abundant expression of phosphoserine-containing protein in s-IBM implies that hyperphosphorylated myofibrillar proteins may be involved in the primary disease process.

4.3 ERK- or Elk-1–positive deposits are often perinuclear in s-IBM muscle fibers

With nuclear DNA staining, we found that ERK- or pElk-1–positive deposits were often detected on the external surface of the nuclei, although they were sometimes present also in the cytoplasm unrelated to the nuclear localization. There were sometimes overlaps of the positive deposits and nuclei. In rare fibers, protrusions of the positive deposits into nuclei were observed. A quantitative study of the relationship between ERK-positive deposits and nuclei in ERK-positive fibers showed that 78.2% of the nuclei were closely associated with the deposits; 3.2% of the nuclei had ERK-positive deposits occupying more than half of their area, and 75.0% of the nuclei were touched, penetrated, or partially covered by the deposits. The nuclear transcription factor pElk-1 displayed similar cytoplasmic aggregation and perinuclear localization. There was cytoplasmic and perinuclear inclusions of ERK in vacuolated fibers, but not of JNK or p38. JNK and p38, however, showed strong activity in regenerating fibers as ERK (Nakano et al 2001).

During muscle fiber differentiation, ERK is the last MAPK that becomes activated (Gredinger et al 1998, Zetser 1999). Therefore, the abnormality that causes ERK deposition may occur in the last phase of differentiation, when JNK and p38 activities have decreased.

4.4 Analysis of MKKs and MAP kinase phosphatases

4.4.1 MAP kinase kinases(MKKs)

ERK appeared to be up-regulated in vacuolated fibers in IBM and ERK is activated by MKK1/2 in the phosphorylation cascade triggered by extracellular stimuli (Fig. 3.). We therefore next tested MKK1/2 in s-IBM (Nakano et al 2003). Whereas in normal muscle fibers, weak immunoreactivity of MKK1/2 was observed, strong immunoreactivity of MKK1/2 was found in some of the regenerating or degenerating muscle fibers. In IBM, vacuolated fibers showed no or mild cytoplasmic immunoreactivity for MKK1/2, even fibers with ERK-positive inclusions. We then tested MKK3 and MKK4 to reject the possibility that other MKK might induce ERK in IBM, although MKK3 and MKK4 actually activate p38 MAPK or JNK, but not ERK (Fig. 3.) (Reffas and Schlegel 2000). Regenerating/degenerating fibers showed positive immunoreaction for these MKKs, vacuolated fibers in IBM were negative for MKK3 or MKK4.

Concerning to the increased MKKs in regenerating/degenerating fibers, growth factors promoting myogenesis (Groungs 1999) or cytokines locally produced or ischemic stresses in the affected tissue in inflammatory myopathies (Lundberg et al 1997) could induce them. As a proportion of vacuolated fibers also showed some positivity for MKK1/2, comparable myogenic factors or other extracellular signals might induce ERK cascade in vacuolated fibers in IBM. However, the intensity of the immunoreaction of MKK1/2 in vacuolated fibers was weaker than those regenerating/degenerating fibers in control specimens and the reaction did not form inclusions. The results exclude a possibility that a specific extracellular signal induces the increase of ERK protein.

4.4.2 MKPs

The study of MAP kinase phosphatases (MKPs), i.e., enzymes that deactivate MAPKs, was done with MKP-1, MKP-2 and MKP-3 (Nakano et al 2003). In MKP-1 analysis, some regenerating/degenerating fibers showed strong nuclear staining with moderate cytoplasmic positivity of MKP-1. In IBM, vacuolated fibers or some other structurally abnormal fibers contained inclusions that were strongly immunoreactive for MKP-1. The MKP-1-positive inclusions were colocalized with ERK in dual fluorescence study. Inclusions of MKP-2 with less conspicuous than MKP-1 were found in some vacuolated fibers. Although diffusely increased Immunoreactivity of MKP-3 was found in some regenerating fibers, MKP-3 was negative in vacuolated fibers.

MKP-1 expression increases during the early stage of myogenesis, and regulates ERK at the stage of muscle specific gene expression (Bennett and Tonks 1997, Shi et al 2010). The findings indicating that regenerating fibers showed increased expression of MKP-1 are consistent with the experimental results. In ERK phosphorylation cascade, MKP-1 serves as a negative regulator of ERK (Robinson and Cobb 1997). Moreover, MKPs make a tight complex with their substrates when catalyzed. Thus, it is highly probable that MKP-1 is induced to inactivate ERK in s-IBM vacuolated fibers.

4.5 Conclusion of MAPK cascades study: abnormal deposition of nuclear proteins involved in myogenesis

Nuclear migration of ERK is necessary for myogenic gene expression (Gredinger et al 1998). Based on the results of our MAPK cascade study, we hypothesize an inhibition of protein transport from the cytoplasm into the nucleus. In s-IBM muscle fibers, normal levels of activation of ERK phosphorylation cascade may proceed down to MKK1/2, the activations of which occur on the plasma membrane or in the cytoplasm, triggered by myogenic or other stimulation in s-IBM-vacuolated fibers. Moreover, frequent perinuclear accumulation of ERK protein in vacuolated fibers suggests that the nuclear translocation of ERK is inhibited. Due to aggregation of ERK, the ERK protein might accumulate in the cytoplasm and become unable to move across the nuclear envelope. Otherwise, due to impaired nuclear transmigration of ERK protein, it could deposit in the cytoplasm and perinuclear region. Activated ERK phosphorylates its nuclear substrates probably immediately after its synthesis and forms complexes in the cytoplasm. The abnormal activation of ERK could induce MKP-1. These enzyme-substrate complexes further congregate together in the cytoplasm. The protein complexes might grow to the "aggresomes" in the perinuclear region to process the aggregates with extralysosomal protein degradation system (Johnston et al 1999). Some of the components of aggresomes were indeed found in s-IBM muscle fibers (Ferrer et al 2005).

Nuclear transport of ERK is a mediated process. This process is required for the induction of many cellular responses, yet the molecular mechanisms that regulate ERK nuclear translocation are not fully understood (Lidke et al 2010). In s-IBM, presence of specific antibodies against the nucleus has been shown (Dalakas et al 1997). Sera from patients with s-IBM and other idiopathic inflammatory myopathies sometimes contain antibodies against nuclear enzymes and components (Brouwer et al 2001). Furthermore, several autoimmune-diseases are associated with autoantibodies against chaperone proteins as well as well-known anti-nuclear antibodies (Corrigall et al 2001). In experiment, injection of antibodies against a heat shock cognate protein 70 that assists nuclear transport results in cytoplasmic accumulation of several nuclear proteins in human cell cultures (Imamoto et al 1992). Inhibition of carrier proteins or nuclear pore proteins involved in the nuclear transport results in the cytoplasmic and perinuclear accumulation of the cargo proteins (Görlich and Mattaj 1996). It is, therefore, suggested that a certain autoimmune mechanism could affect molecules involved in nuclear transport of ERK and induce cytoplasmic accumulation of ERK and its associated proteins in vacuolated fibers in IBM. Apart from autoimmune mechanism, nuclear envelope dysfunction could be aggravated by reactive oxygen species induced by inflammatory cytokines and by aging, as we will discuss them later.

Lack of proper nuclear migration of ERK inhibits MyoD expression (Gredinger et al 1998). Furthermore, forced induction of MKP-1 during myotube formation prevents myoblast fusion when the expression of the myosin heavy chain has occurred (Bennett and Tonks 1997). It is suggested that in s-IBM, there is an altered program of myogenesis due to abnormal aggregation of nuclear proteins that are associated with the differentiating process of muscle. The aggregation in turn may induce the protein degradation system, such as proteasmal pathways (Ferrer et al 2004) and autophagy (Kumamoto et al 2004), both of which are increased in s-IBM muscle fibers.

Our earlier report has shown CDK5-positive deposits in vacuolated fibers in s-IBM. A high proportion of the CDK5-positive deposits were perinuclear, as ERK. CDK5 co-localized with SMI-31 reactive deposits as ERK (Nakano et al 1999). CDK5, like ERK, belongs to the proline-directed kinases which can phosphorylate serine or threonine followed by proline sequences. CDK5 transiently appears in the nucleus during the terminal differentiation and promotes the process (Lazaro et al 1997). Thus, two protein kinases ERK and CDK5, both normally activated and translocated into the nucleus during the terminal phase of differentiation, accumulate in the cytoplasm and around the nuclei in s-IBM vacuolated fibers. We therefore hypothesize that the induction of ERK and CDK5 is part of the intrinsic program of muscle fiber differentiation, and one possibility is that the abnormally high concentration of these enzymes results from their aggregation in the cytoplasm and inability to enter the nucleus.

5. Nuclear abnormality in s-IBM: history

Several studies have shown distinct myonuclear alterations in s-IBM before establishing its nosology. In ultrastructural study, filamentous inclusions were sometimes detected in myonuclei as well as in the cytoplasm (Chou 1967). These inclusions in rare occasion appeared to be released from nuclei into the cytoplasm with breaks in the nuclear membrane. In s-IBM, but not in controls, myonuclei accumulate an unidentified a single stranded DNA-binding protein (Nalbantoglu et al 1994). Most of the sites of binding were myonuclei, whereas some were rimmed vacuoles. The figures suggest that rimmed vacuoles probably result from nuclear breakdown. Recent studies added valosin-containing protein (VCP) (Greenberg et al 2007b) and TDP-43 (Salajegheh et al 2009) to the list of proteins localized in both nuclear and rimmed vacuoles, supporting the hypothesis that nuclear breakdown results in rimmed vacuoles.

As our phosphoprotein study suggested the nuclear alterations in s-IBM vacuolated fibers, we thought to identify elemental components in rimmed vacuoles. If rimmed vacuoles originate from the nucleus, the basophilic components associated with them should be some components of the nucleus. Histones are representative of the basophilic substances, which prompted us to investigate histones in s-IBM.

While our preparation of papers with histone H1, another group showed existence of nuclear membrane protein emerin and lamin A/C within rimmed vacuoles (Greenberg et al 2006)

6. Immunolocalization study of histones in sporadic inclusion body myositis (s-IBM)

6.1 Histones and dynamic function of histone H1

In inactive chromatin, the DNA is combined to histones and forms nucleosomes. A nucleosome is an octamer of four pairs of the core histones H2A, H2B, H3 and H4. Double-stranded DNA twines around nucleosomes. Histone H1 binds to the linker DNA that connects the individual nucleosomes. Among histones, histone H1 shows dynamic behavior to regulate chromatin folding and gene expression, while core histones are integral components of chromatin fibers (Bustin et al 2005). The H1 binding to linker DNA is essential for the generation of the highly condensed chromatin structure and plays a pivotal role in gene regulation (Brown 2003). H1 is rich in arginine and lysine residues, which makes it highly basic (Woodcock et al 2006).

6.2 Histone H1, but not core histones (H2A, H2B, H3 and H4), are associated with rimmed vacuoles

Figure 4 displays the results in triple-fluorescence study of histone H1, emerin (a nuclear envelope protein associated with inner nuclear membrane) and DAPI (a marker of nuclear DNA). After the fluorescence studies, the same sections are stained with H&E as shown in the right column. The figures clearly show rimmed vacuole are products of nuclear degeneration. They reveal several modes of nuclear alterations. 1) H1-positive rings or deposits are associated with the nuclear membrane protein and DNA. Strong vacuolar H1-positive reaction colocalized with a DNA ring is detected inside or on emerin-positive reaction in a proportion of vacuoles. The figures suggest swelling or ballooning of nuclei with scarce nuclear matrix proteins. 2) H1-positive reaction that appeared to be leaking beyond emerin-positive lines is found in some other vacuoles. The cytoplasmic release of H1 is also observed in some morphologically intact nuclei (Nakano et al 2008). The H&E after the fluorescence study showed that H1 or emerin-positive products in vacuoles often appeared to correspond to the basophilic lines in H&E. A region of cytoplasmic H1-positive reaction usually corresponded to basophilic lakes around vacuoles or nuclei in H&E. The results indicated that release of H1 occurs even in an early phase of nuclear breakdown. In contrast, although regenerating fibers show increased H1 reactivity in their large and vesicular nuclei, H1-positive products fall within these nuclei. Calculation indicated that approximately 60% of vacuolated fibers contained H1-positive rings or other H1-positive remnants (Nakano et al 2008). Conversely, immunohistochemistry of histones H2A, H2B, H3 and H4 showed rare vacuoles harbored positive deposits. The comparative study with immunofluorescence and subsequent H&E staining suggested that histone H1 and other nuclear proteins comprise basophilic granules in rimmed vacuoles.

6.3 Cytoplasmic release of histone H1 suggests DNA double strand breaks

Cytoplasmic release of H1, but not other histones, has been observed in a type of apoptosis in an experimental study of cultured human cells: apoptosis induced by stimuli causing DNA double strand breaks such as X-ray irradiation, but not other apoptotic stimuli,

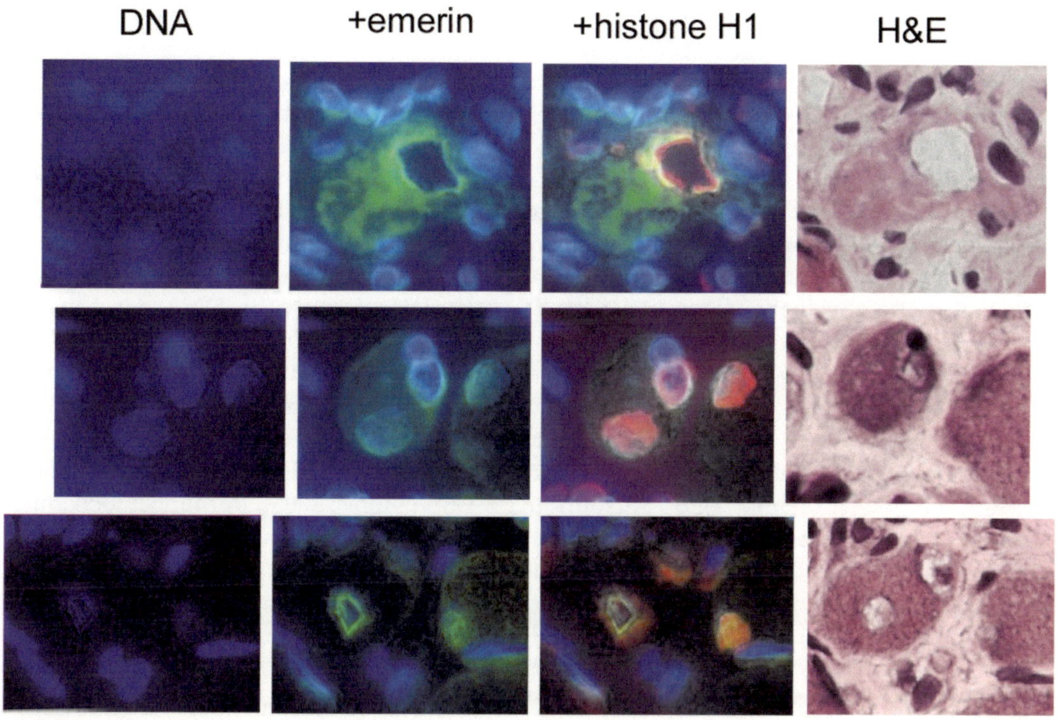

Fig. 4. Triple fluorescence studies in s-IBM vacuolated fibers. Blue: nuclear DNA; Green: emerin; Red: histone H1. Vacuoles usually appear to be more accentuated in H&E, probably due to dehydration process. The background green colour is purposely heightened to visualize muscle fibers.

releases histone H1 into the cytoplasm (Konishi et al 2003). Therefore, the cytoplasmic H1 release in s-IBM might indicate that some apoptotic stimuli causing DNA double strand breaks induce the s-IBM pathology. Apoptotic process exemplified by TUNEL revealed that it may scarcely operate in s-IBM muscle fibers (Hutchinson 1998). Nevertheless, several studies displayed some players of apoptosis in s-IBM muscle fibers (Behrens et al 1997, Li and Dalakas 2000b)

7. DNA double strand breaks (DSB) in s-IBM

7.1 The DNA damage responses

The primary structure of DNA is constantly exposed to cellular metabolites and extracellular DNA-damaging agents. These alterations can affect the cell to transcription of the genes. Other lesions induce potentially harmful mutations. Consequently, the DNA repair process must be constantly activated to respond to the damages in the DNA structure. Defects of the repair processes may cause genomic instability. To repair damage to one of the two paired molecules of DNA, there are many excision repair mechanisms that remove the damaged nucleotide and replace it with an undamaged nucleotide complementary to that found in the undamaged DNA strand. The examples of these are base excision repair, nucleotide excision repair, and DNA mismatch repair.

DNA double strand breaks (DSB), in which both strands in the double helix are severed, are particularly serious to the cell because they can lead to genome rearrangements. DSB are produced by reactive oxygen species, ionizing radiation, chemicals that generate reactive oxygen species and replication error. DSB are also a normal result of V(D)J recombination and immunoglobulin class-switching process. DSB are repaired either by homologous recombination (HR) or nonhomologous end-joining (NHEJ) mechanism (O'Driscol and Jeggo 2006). HR plays only in replicating cells, while NHEJ functions in both cells in the cell cycle and those terminally differentiated. Mature muscle cells are terminally differentiated cells, that is, the cells withdraw from the cell replication cycle. Terminally differentiated cells do not possess a replication-associated DNA repair mechanism (HR mentioned above). This lack makes the terminally differentiated cells particularly sensitive to DNA damage (Lee and McKinnon 2007). In a muscle cell culture study, the exposure of differentiated myocytes to hydrogen peroxide, which induces reactive oxygen species, resulted in the accumulation of foci of DSB. It is exemplified by immunolocalization of phosphorylated histone H2AX (γ-H2AX) (Narciso et al 2007). The detection of γ-H2AX is a sensitive marker of DSB (Nakamura 2006). Histone H2AX that is a variant of histone H2A is rapidly phosphorylated at Ser 139 in the chromatin region surrounding a DSB (Kinner 2008). Immunocytochemical staining of γ-H2AX has been broadly applied to reveal DNA damage caused by cancer and other cellular stresses (Nakamura 2006, Kinner 2008).

DSB is different from the apoptotic DNA fragmentation that has been residually detected in the s-IBM muscles (Hutchinson 1998). In DSB, DNA breaks are induced directly and randomly by radiation or other genotoxic agents, whereas apoptotic DNA fragmentation occurs at a late stage of programmed cell death, when endonucleases sever DNA strands at regular lengths, making a ladder formation in Southern blotting.

DNA-PK is an enzyme involved in the initial step of the DSB repair process NHEJ, which does not require DNA replication, and therefore NHEJ is the major DNA repair mechanism in terminally differentiated cells (O'Driscoll and Jeggo 2006, Mahaney et al 2009). DNA-PK consists of a catalytic subunit (DNA-PKcs) and two regulatory subunits (Ku70 and Ku80). The binding of hetero-duplexes of Ku70 and Ku80 to DSB sites initiates the repair process (Mari et al 2006, Weterings and Chen 2007).

We immunolocalized γ-H2AX in s-IBM and we also tested DNA-PK to see whether the repair mechanism is defective or not (Nishii et al 2011). In the study, vacuolar peripheries often showed strong immunoreactivity to γ-H2AX and the three components of DNA-PK (DNA-PKcs, Ku70, and Ku80). The percentage of positive nuclei for γ-H2AX was significantly higher in vacuolated fibers than non-vacuolated fibers in s-IBM, or fibers in polymyosits suggesting that nuclear breakdown occurs along with the accumulation of DSB in muscle cells in s-IBM. Moreover, a triple fluorescence study of Ku70, emerin, and DNA suggested impaired nuclear incorporation of Ku70. Nuclear translocation of Ku proteins is important for DBS repair, and a deficiency in nuclear translocation caused hypersensitivity against X-ray irradiation due to the lack of DBS repair in a cell culture study (Okui et al 2002). Therefore, we hypothesized that defects in Ku70 nuclear import accelerate DSB formation in s-IBM.

Despite DSB was the highest in s-IBM vacuolated fibers, DSB was sometimes found to be increased in myonuclei without nuclear breakdown. Therefore, additional factors may be involved in the nuclear breakdown detected in s-IBM. We consider that a dysfunction of nuclear envelope may explain all the alterations in s-IBM: 1) nuclear fragility; 2) DNA double-strand breaks; and 3) impaired nuclear transport in s-IBM.

Impaired DSB results growth arrest, senescence, and apoptosis (Rossetto et al 2010). Our earlier examination showed aberrant expressions of proteins associated with myogenic differentiation. In s-IBM, the accumulation of DSB could result in arrest of muscle fiber maturation.

8. Possible mechanism of nuclear breakdown

Nuclear envelope dysfunction can cause both mechanical fragility of the nucleus and DNA damage. Lamins are proteins of nuclear intermediate filaments that comprise the lamina, the meshwork supporting inner nuclear membranes. Mutations in the genes that encode lamins and emerin cause Emery-Dreifuss muscular dystrophy and a number of different diseases collectively called laminopathies (Capell and Collins 2006). In several laminopathies, blebbing of the nuclei in cultured fibroblasts can be seen, and it is hypothesized that such mutations result in fragile and mechanically unstable nuclei (Goldman et al 2004). Indeed, emerin mutations can cause myopathy with rimmed vacuoles (Paradas et al 2005, Fidziańska et al 2004). Besides structural integrity, the lamina is also involved in various other processes, such as replication and gene transcription, which are intimately associated with DNA damage repair. Accordingly, impaired DNA repair has been found in several laminopathies. Fibroblasts possessing a laminopathy mutation show an excessive amount of un-repaired DNA damage, as exemplified by γ-H2AX immunohistochemistry (Liu et al 2005). 3) Furthermore, lamins are important in the spatial rearrangement of nuclear pore complexes and therefore nuclear protein transport. Nuclear protein import is reduced in cells expressing lamin A mutants (Busch et al 2009). We repeatedly detected figures suggestive of impaired nuclear import of proteins, as has been described in our phosphorylated protein study.

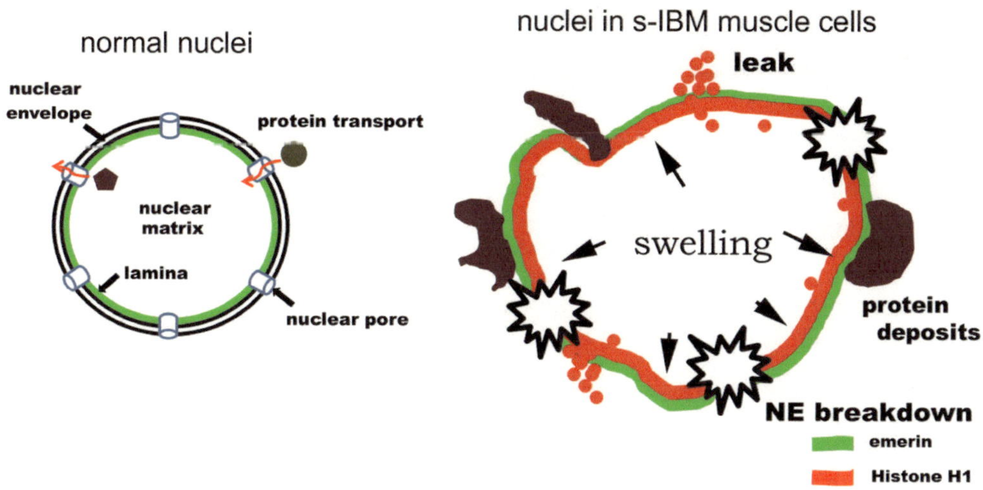

Fig. 5. Simplified schema of normal nuclei and nuclei in s-IBM muscle fibers. In s-IBM, nuclear proteins deposits occur in perinuclear regions due to inhibition of nuclear import, whereas histone H1 is released from nnclei. Finally, the nuclear envelopes break down to form rimmed vacuoles.

To summarize, dysfunctional lamins can explain the nuclear breakdown, accumulation of DSB, and impaired nuclear transport observed in s-IBM. As discussed in the section about perinuclear deposition of protein kinases, autoimmune mechanism could operate in the dysfunction of nuclear envelope. In addition, aging might increase the nuclear vulnerability and DNA damage. Nuclear pore complexes are not turned over in differentiated cells, and age-related alterations in nuclear pore complexes have been shown. Leaking of nuclear matrix proteins is dramatically accelerated during aging and that a subset of nucleoporins (components of nuclear pores) is oxidatively damaged in old cells (D'Angelo et al 2009). Moreover, several studies have indicated an age-dependent decline in DNA repair capacity (Gorbunova et al 2007). We suspect that these age-associated changes in nuclear envelope function and DNA repair mechanisms may predispose the muscles of the elderly to s-IBM pathology.

9. Similarity of s-IBM and DMRV/h-IBM

We found inclusions of a set of nucleus-oriented or nucleus-proper proteins in distal myopathy with rimmed vacuoles (DMRV)/hereditary inclusion body myopathy (h-IBM), a disorder in which the muscle biopsy displays rimmed vacuoles in muscle fibers as in s-IBM (Fig. 6) (Nakano et al 1999, 2001, 2003, 2008).

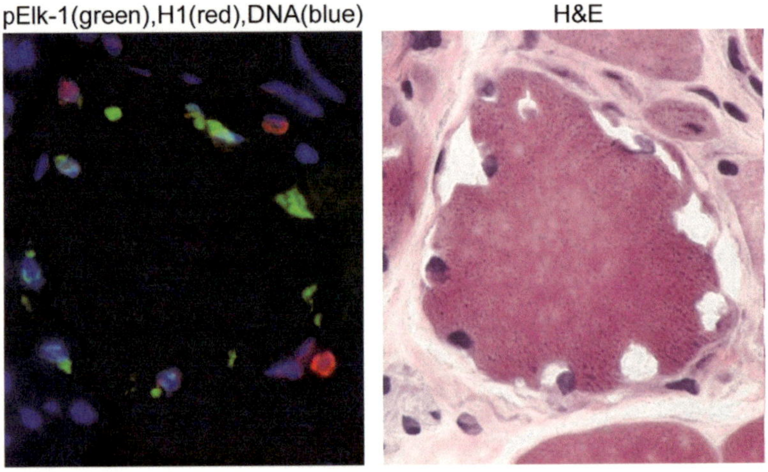

Fig. 6. Immunohistochemistry of pElk-1 and histone H1 in DMRV/h-IBM. Many pElk-1-positive deposits are seen in vacuoles .

Muscle pathology of DMRV/s-IBM shows rimmed vacuoles and tubulofilaments like s-IBM, but it lacks inflammation. The mutated gene for this autosomal recessive disease has been identified to be involved in glycosylation, named UDP-N-acetylglucosamine 2-epimerase/N-acetylmannosamine kinase (GNE) (Eisenberg et al 2001, Nishino et al 2002). Remarkably, N-acetylglucosamine, the substrate of this enzyme is also a substrate of UDP-N-acetylglucosamine:polypeptide β-N-acetylglucosaminyl transferase (OGT), the enzyme that adds O-linked-β-N-acetylglucosamine (O-GlcNAc) to a protein. A thousand of proteins including transcription factors, cytoskeletal proteins, kinases and nuclear pore proteins are modified with O-GlcNAc (Zachara and Hart 2004). O-GlcNAc is a highly dynamic process and acts as a modulator of protein function, in a manner analogous to protein phosphorylation. Moreover, there is a complex crosstalk between O-GlcNAc modification and phosphorylation. The two post-translational modifications often regulate in an opposite manner by competitive attachment to the same serine/threonine residue, but they sometimes function co-operatively by binding at different sites of the same molecule (Zeidan 2010). In DMRV/h-IBM as well as in s-IBM, abnormal expression of proteins concerning to phosphorylation could be related to perturbation of the O-GlcNAc modification of proteins.

10. Conclusion

We have examined myonuclear dysfunction s-IBM. Similar degenerative mechanism may exist in DMRV/h-IBM that shows almost identical pathology and nuclear breakdown concerning to muscle fiber degeneration (Nonaka et al 1998). To reveal how GNE enzyme dysfunction affects myonuclei in this disorder may contribute to unveil the etiology of s-IBM. In addition, myofibrillar myopathy is a genetic disorder in which mutations of several Z-line associated proteins have been identified. Muscle biopsy studies have found congophilic inclusions (Selcen and Engel 2010). Players involved in excessive protein processing have been detected in s-IBM and myofibrillar myopathy (Ferrer et al 2004, 2005). Moreover, the disorder sometimes accompanies rimmed vacuoles (Shinde et al 2008). The comparative study of s-IBM and myofibrillar myopathy may also be helpful.

Concerning to the relationship between inflammation and nuclear breakdown, some immunological mechanism could operate in nuclear envelope dysfunction. Otherwise, nuclear aging and decrease of DNA repair capacity due to aging could induce the nuclear degeneration.

11. Acknowledgment

This work was supported in part by Grant-in-Aids from the Japan Society for the Promotion of Science and from the Ministry of Health, Labour, and Welfare for Research on intractable diseases.

12. References

Askanas V, Engel WK, Alvarez RB. Light and electron microscopic localization of beta-amyloid protein in muscle biopsies of patients with inclusion-body myositis. Am J Pathol. 1992 Jul;141(1):31-6.

Askanas V, Engel WK, Bilak M, Alvarez RB, Selkoe DJ. Twisted tubulofilaments of inclusion body myositis muscle resemble paired helical filaments of Alzheimer brain and contain hyperphosphorylated tau. Am J Pathol 1994;144:177–187.

Askanas V, Engel WK. Inclusion-body myositis: muscle-fiber molecular pathology and possible pathogenic significance of its similarity to Alzheimer's and Parkinson's disease brains. Acta Neuropathol. 2008 Dec;116(6):583-95.

Banker B, Engel AG. Basic reactions of muscle. In: Engel AG, Franzini–Armstrong C, ed. Myology. 2nd ed. New York, NY: McGraw-Hill, 1994: 832–888.

Behrens L, Bender A, Johnson MA, Hohlfeld R. Cytotoxic mechanisms in inflammatory myopathies. Co-expression of Fas and protective Bcl-2 in muscle fibres and inflammatory cells. Brain. 1997 Jun;120 (Pt 6):929-38.

Bennett A, Tonks NK. Regulation of distinct stages of skeletal muscle differentiation by mitogen-activated protein kinases. Science 1997;278:1288-1291.

Brouwer R, Hengstman GJ, Vree Egberts W, Ehrfeld H, Bozic B, Ghirardello A, Grøndal G, Hietarinta M, Isenberg D, Kalden JR, Lundberg I, Moutsopoulos H, Roux-Lombard P, Vencovsky J, Wikman A, Seelig HP, van Engelen BG, van Venrooij WJ. Autoantibody profiles in the sera of European patients with myositis. Ann Rheum Dis 2001;60:116-123.

Brown DT. Histone H1 and the dynamic regulation of chromatin function. Biochem Cell Biol 2003;81:221-227.

Busch A, Kiel T, Heupel WM, Wehnert M, Hübner S. Nuclear protein import is reduced in cells expressing *O*-GlcNAc nuclear envelopathy-causing lamin A mutants. Exp Cell Res 2009;315:2373-2385.

Bustin M, Catez F, Lim JH. The dynamics of histone H1 function in chromatin. Mol Cell 2005;17:617-620.

Capell BC, Collins FS. Human laminopathies: nuclei gone genetically awry. Nat Rev Genet 2006;7:940-952.

Carpenter S, Karpati G, Wolfe L. Virus like filaments and phospholipid accumulations in a case of chronic myopathy. J Neuropathol Exp Neurol. 1971 Jan;30(1):136-7.

Carpenter S, Karpati G, Heller I, Eisen A. Inclusion body myositis: a distinct variety of idiopathic inflammatory myopathy. Neurology. 1978 Jan;28(1):8-17.

Chou SM. Myxovirus-like structures in a case of human chronic polymyositis. Science. 1967 Dec 15;158(807):1453-5.

Corrigall VM, Bodman-Smith MD, Fife MS, Canas B, Myers LK, Wooley P, Soh C, Staines NA, Pappin DJ, Berlo SE, van Eden W, van Der Zee R, Lanchbury JS, Panayi GS. The human endoplasmic reticulum molecular chaperone BiP is an autoantigen for rheumatoid arthritis and prevents the induction of experimental arthritis. J Immunol 2001;166:1492-1498.

Dalakas M, Illa I, Gallardo E, Juarez C. Inclusion body myositis and paraproteinemia: Incidence and immunopathologic correlations. Ann Neurol 1997;41:100-104.

Dalakas MC. Sporadic inclusion body myositis--diagnosis, pathogenesis and therapeutic strategies. Nat Clin Pract Neurol 2006;2:437-447.

D'Angelo MA, Raices M, Panowski SH, Hetzer MW. Age-dependent deterioration of nuclear pore complexes causes a loss of nuclear integrity in postmitotic cells. Cell. 2009 Jan 23;136(2):284-95.

Dubiwitz V, Sewry CA. Metabolic myopathies I: Glycogenosis. Muscle biopsy. 3rd ed., Sanders/Elsevier 2007: pp 453-468

Eisenberg I, Avidan N, Potikha T, Hochner H, Chen M, Olender T, Barash M, Shemesh M, Sadeh M, Grabov-Nardini G, Shmilevich I, Friedmann A, Karpati G, Bradley WG, Baumbach L, Lancet D, Asher EB, Beckmann JS, Argov Z, Mitrani-Rosenbaum S. The UDP-N-acetylglucosamine 2-epimerase/N-acetylmannosamine kinase gene is mutated in recessive hereditary inclusion body myopathy. Nat Genet. 2001 Sep;29(1):83-7.

Ferrer I, Carmona M, Blanco R, Moreno D, Torrejón-Escribano B, Olivé M. Involvement of clusterin and the aggresome in abnormal protein deposits in myofibrillar myopathies and inclusion body myositis. Brain Pathol. 2005;15(2):101-8.

Ferrer I, Martín B, Castaño JG, Lucas JJ, Moreno D, Olivé M. Proteasomal expression, induction of immunoproteasome subunits, and local MHC class I presentation in myofibrillar myopathy and inclusion body myositis. J Neuropathol Exp Neurol. 2004 May;63(5):484-98.

Fidziańska A, Rowińska-Marcińska K, Hausmanowa-Petrusewicz I. Coexistence of X-linked recessive Emery-Dreifuss muscular dystrophy with inclusion body myositis-like morphology. Acta Neuropathol 2004;107:197-203.

Force T, Bonventre JV. Growth factors and mitogen-activated protein kinases. Hypertension 1998; 31: 152–161.

Goldman RD, Shumaker DK, Erdos MR, et al. Accumulation of mutant lamin A causes progressive changes in nuclear architecture in Hutchinson-Gilford progeria syndrome. Proc Natl Acad Sci U S A 2004;101:8963-8968.

Gorbunova V, Seluanov A, Mao Z, Hine C. Changes in DNA repair during aging. Nucleic Acids Res 2007;35:7466-7474.

Görlich D, Mattaj IW. Nucleocytoplasmic transport. Science 1996; 271: 1513–1518.

Gredinger E, Gerber AN, Tamir Y, Tapscott SJ, Bengal E. Mitogen-activated protein kinase pathway is involved in the differentiation of muscle cells. J Biol Chem 1998;273:10436-10444.

Greenberg SA, Pinkus JL, Amato AA. Nuclear membrane proteins are present within rimmed vacuoles in inclusion-body myositis. Muscle Nerve 2006;34:406-416.

Greenberg SA, Pinkus GS, Amato AA, Pinkus JL. Myeloid dendritic cells in inclusion-body myositis and polymyositis. Muscle Nerve. 2007a Jan;35(1):17-23.

Greenberg SA, Watts GD, Kimonis VE, Amato AA, Pinkus JL. Nuclear localization of valosin-containing protein in normal muscle and muscle affected by inclusion-body myositis. Muscle Nerve. 2007b Oct;36(4):447-54.

Greenberg SA. How citation distortions create unfounded authority: analysis of a citation network. BMJ. 2009 Jul 20;339:b2680.

Griggs RC, Askanas V, DiMauro S, Engel A, Karpati G, Mendell JR, Rowland LP. Inclusion body myositis and myopathies. Ann Neurol 1995;38:705–713.

Grounds M. Muscle regeneration: molecular aspects and therapeutic implications. Curr Opin Neurol 1999;12:353-543.

Hartlerode AJ, Scully R. Mechanisms of double-strand break repair in somatic mammalian cells. Biochem J. 2009 Sep 25;423(2):157-68.

Hill C, Treisman R. Transcriptional regulation by extracellular signals: mechanisms and specificity. Cell 1995; 80: 199–211.

Hunter T, Karin M. The regulation of transcription by phosphorylation. Cell.1992 Aug 7;70(3):375-87.

Hutchinson DO. Inclusion body myositis: abnormal protein accumulation does not trigger apoptosis. Neurology. 1998 Dec;51(6):1742-5.

Imamoto N, Matsuoka Y, Kurihara T, Kohno K, Miyagi M, Sakiyama F, Okada Y,Tsunasawa S, Yoneda Y. Antibodies against 70-kD heat shock cognate protein inhibit mediated nuclear import of karyophilic proteins. J Cell Biol 1992; 119: 1047-1061

Johnston JA, Ward CL, Kopito RR. Aggresomes: a cellular response to misfolded proteins. J Cell Biol 1998; 143:1883-1898.

Keyse S. Protein phosphatases and the regulation of mitogen-activated protein kinase signalling. Curr Opin Cell Biol 2000;12:186-192.

Kinner A, Wu W, Staudt C, Iliakis G. Gamma-H2AX in recognition and signaling of DNA double-strand breaks in the context of chromatin. Nucleic Acids Res 2008;36:5678-5694.

Konishi A, Shimizu S, Hirota J, Takao T, Fan Y, Matsuoka Y, Zhang L, Yoneda Y, Fujii Y, Skoultchi AI, Tsujimoto Y. Involvement of histone H1.2 in apoptosis induced by DNA double-strand breaks. Cell 2003;114:673-688

Kumamoto T, Ueyama H, Tsumura H, Toyoshima I, Tsuda T. Expression of lysosome-related proteins and genes in the skeletal muscles of inclusion body myositis. Acta Neuropathol. 2004 Jan;107(1):59-65.
Kyriakis J, Avruch J. Mammalian mitogen-activated protein kinase signal transduction pathways activated by stress and inflammation. Physiol Rev 2001;81:807-869.
Lazaro J, Kitzmann M, Poul MA, Vandromme M, Lamb NJ, Fernandez A. Cyclin dependent kinase 5, cdk5, is a positive regulator of myogenesis in mouse C2 cells. J Cell Sci 1997; 110: 1251–1260.
Lee Y, McKinnon PJ. Responding to DNA double strand breaks in the nervous system. Neuroscience 2007;145:1365-1374.
Li J, Johnson SE. ERK2 is required for efficient terminal differentiation of skeletal myoblasts. Biochem Biophys Res Commun. 2006 Jul 14;345(4):1425-33.
Li M, Dalakas MC. The muscle mitogen-activated protein kinase is altered in sporadic inclusion body myositis. Neurology. 2000a Apr 25;54(8):1665-70.
Li M, Dalakas MC. Expression of human IAP-like protein in skeletal muscle: a possible explanation for the rare incidence of muscle fiber apoptosis in T-cell mediated inflammatory myopathies. J Neuroimmunol. 2000b Jul 1;106(1-2):1-5.
Lidke DS, Huang F, Post JN, Rieger B, Wilsbacher J, Thomas JL, Pouysségur J, Jovin TM, Lenormand P. ERK nuclear translocation is dimerization-independent but controlled by the rate of phosphorylation. J Biol Chem. 2010 Jan 29;285(5):3092-102.
Liu B, Wang J, Chan KM, Tjia WM, Deng W, Guan X, Huang JD, Li KM, Chau PY, Chen DJ, Pei D, Pendas AM, Cadiñanos J, López-Otín C, Tse HF, Hutchison C, Chen J, Cao Y, Cheah KS, Tryggvason K, Zhou Z. Genomic instability in laminopathy-based premature aging. Nat Med 2005;11:780-785.
Lluís F, Perdiguero E, Nebreda AR, Muñoz-Cánoves P. Regulation of skeletal muscle gene expression by p38 MAP kinases. Trends Cell Biol. 2006 Jan;16(1):36-44.
Lotz BP, Engel AG, Nishino H, Stevens JC, Litchy WJ. Inclusion body myositis. Observations in 40 patients. Brain. 1989 Jun;112 (Pt 3):727-47."
Lundberg I, Ulfgren A, Nyberg P,Andersson U, Klarreskog L. Cytokine production in muscle tissue of patients with idiopathic inflammatory myopathies. Arth Rheum 1997;40:865-874.
Lünemann JD, Schmidt J, Schmid D, Barthel K, Wrede A, Dalakas MC, Münz C. Beta-amyloid is a substrate of autophagy in sporadic inclusion body myositis. Ann Neurol. 2007 May;61(5):476-83.
Mahaney BL, Meek K, Lees-Miller SP. Repair of ionizing radiation-induced DNA double-strand breaks by non-homologous end-joining. Biochem J 2009;417:639-650.
Maurage CA, Bussière T, Sergeant N, Ghesteem A, Figarella-Branger D, Ruchoux MM, Pellissier JF, Delacourte A. Tau aggregates are abnormally phosphorylated in inclusion body myositis and have an immunoelectrophoretic profile distinct from other tauopathies. Neuropathol Appl Neurobiol. 2004 Dec;30(6):624-34.
Mari PO, Florea BI, Persengiev SP, Verkaik NS, Brüggenwirth HT, Modesti M, Giglia-Mari G, Bezstarosti K, Demmers JA, Luider TM, Houtsmuller AB, van Gent DC. Dynamic assembly of end-joining complexes requires interaction between Ku70/80 and XRCC4. Proc Natl Acad Sci U S A 2006;103:18597-18602.
Mendell JR, Sahenk Z, Gales T, Paul L. Amyloid filaments in inclusion body myositis. Novel findings provide insight into nature of filaments. Arch Neurol. 1991 Dec;48(12):1229-34.
Mirabella M, Alvarez RB, Bilak M, Engel WK, Askanas V. Difference in expression of phosphorylated tau epitopes between sporadic inclusion-body myositis and

hereditary inclusion-body myopathies. J Neuropathol Exp Neurol. 1996 Jul;55(7):774-86.

Nakamura A, Sedelnikova OA, Redon C, Pilch DR, Sinogeeva NI, Shroff R, Lichten M, Bonner WM. Techniques for gamma-H2AX detection. Methods Enzymol 2006;409:236-250.

Nakano S, Akiguchi I, Nakamura S, Satoi H, Kawashima S, Kimura J. Aberrant expression of cyclin-dependent kinase 5 in inclusion body myositis. Neurology 1999; 53: 1671-1676.

Nakano S, Kawashima S, Satoi H, et al. Active form of ERK2 is a major phosphorylated protein in vacuolated fibers in sporadic inclusion body myositis. Muscle & Nerve 1998; S130. Abstract.

Nakano S, Shinde A, Ito H, Ito H, Kusaka H. MAP kinase phosphatase-1 is induced in abnormal fibers in inclusion body myositis. Neurology. 2003 Aug 12;61(3): 322-6.

Nakano S, Shinde A, Kawashima S, Nakamura S, Akiguchi I, Kimura J. Inclusion body myositis:expression of extracellular signal-regulated kinase and its substrate. Neurology. 2001 Jan 9;56(1):87-93.

Nakano S, Shinde A, Fujita K, Ito H, Kusaka H. Histone H1 is released from myonuclei and present in rimmed vacuoles with DNA in inclusion body myositis. Neuromuscul Disord 2008;18:27-33.

Nalbantoglu J, Karpati G, Carpenter S. Conspicuous accumulation of a single-stranded DNA binding protein in skeletal muscle fibers in inclusion body myositis. Am J Pathol 1994;144:874-882.

Narciso L, Fortini P, Pajalunga D, et al. Terminally differentiated muscle cells are defective in base excision DNA repair and hypersensitive to oxygen injury. Proc Natl Acad Sci U S A 2007;104:17010-17015.

Needham M, Mastaglia FL. Sporadic inclusion body myositis: a continuing puzzle. Neuromuscul Disord 2008;18:6-16.

Nishii M, Nakano S, Nakamura S, Wate R, Shinde A, Kaneko S, Kusaka H. Myonuclear breakdown in sporadic inclusion body myositis is accompanied by DNA double strand breaks. Neuromuscul Disord. 2011 May;21(5):345-52.

Nishino I, Noguchi S, Murayama K, et al. Distal myopathy with rimmed vacuoles is allelic to hereditary inclusion body myopathy. Neurology 2002;59:1689-1693.

Nonaka I, Murakami N, Suzuki Y, Kawai M. Distal myopathy with rimmed vacuoles. Neuromuscul Disord 1998; 8: 333–337.

Nukina N, Kosik KS, Selkoe DJ. Recognition of Alzheimer paired helical filaments by monoclonal neurofilament antibodies is due to crossreaction with tau protein. Proc Natl Acad Sci USA 1987; 84: 3415–3419.

O'Driscoll M, Jeggo PA. The role of double-strand break repair - insights from human genetics. Nat Rev Genet 2006;7:45-54.

Okui T, Endoh D, Kon Y, Hayashi M. Deficiency in nuclear accumulation of G22p1 and Xrcc5 proteins in hyper-radiosensitive Long-Evans Cinnamon (LEC) rat cells after X irradiation. Radiat Res 2002;157:553-561.

Paradas C, Márquez C, Gallardo E, et al. X-linked Emery-Dreifuss muscular dystrophy and vacuoles: an immunohistochemical characterization. Muscle Nerve 2005;32:61-65.

Reffas S, Schlegel W. Compartment-specific regulation of extracellular signal-regulated kinase (ERK) and c-Jun N-terminal kinase (JNK) mitogen-activated protein kinases (MAPKs) by ERK-dependent and non-ERK-dependent inductions of MAPK phosphatase (MKP)-3 and MKP-1 in differentiating P19 cells. Biochem J 2000;352:701-708.

Robinson M, Cobb MH. Mitogen-activated protein kinase pathways. Curr Opin Cell Biol 1997;9:180-186.

Rossetto D, Truman AW, Kron SJ, Côté J. Epigenetic modifications in double-strand break DNA damage signaling and repair. Clin Cancer Res. 2010 Sep 15;16(18): 4543-52.

Salajegheh M, Pinkus JL, Taylor JP, et al. Sarcoplasmic redistribution of nuclear TDP-43 in inclusion body myositis. Muscle Nerve 2009a;40:19-31.

Salajegheh M, Pinkus JL, Nazareno R, Amato AA, Parker KC, Greenberg SA. Nature of "Tau" immunoreactivity in normal myonuclei and inclusion body myositis. Muscle Nerve. 2009b Oct;40(4):520-8.

Schillace R Scott JD. Organization of kinases, phosphatases, and receptor signaling complexes. J Clin Invest 2000;103:767-772.

Schmidt J, Barthel K, Wrede A, Salajegheh M, Bähr M, Dalakas MC. Interrelation of inflammation and APP in sIBM: IL-1 beta induces accumulation of beta-amyloid in skeletal muscle. Brain. 2008 May;131(Pt 5):1228-40.

Selcen D, Engel AG. Myofibrillar Myopathy. 2005 Jan 28 [updated 2010 Jul 27]. In: Pagon RA, Bird TD, Dolan CR, Stephens K, editors. GeneReviews [Internet]. Seattle (WA): University of Washington, Seattle; 1993-. Available from http://www.ncbi.nlm.nih.gov/bookshelf/br.fcgi?book=gene&part=mfm

Sherriff FE, Joachim CL, Squier MV, Esiri MM. Ubiquitinated inclusions in inclusion-body myositis patients are immunoreactive for cathepsin D but not beta-amyloid. Neurosci Lett. 1995 Jul 14;194(1-2):37-40

Shi H, Scheffler JM, Pleitner JM, Zeng C, Park S, Hannon KM, Grant AL, Gerrard DE. Modulation of skeletal muscle fiber type by mitogen-activated protein kinase signaling. FASEB J. 2008 Aug;22(8):2990-3000.S

Shinde A, Nakano S, Sugawara M, Toyoshima I, Ito H, Tanaka K, Kusaka H. Expression of caveolar components in primary desminopathy. Neuromuscul Disord.2008 Mar;18(3):215-9.

Soulez M, Rouviere CG, Chafey P, et al. Growth and differentiation of C2 myogenic cells are dependent on serum response factor. Mol Cell Biol 1996; 11: 6065–6074.

Treisman R. Ternary complex factors: growth factor regulated transcriptional activators. Curr Opin Genet Dev 1994; 4: 96–101.

Weterings E, Chen DJ. DNA-dependent protein kinase in nonhomologous end joining: a lock with multiple keys? J Cell Biol 2007;179:183-186.

Woodcock CL, Skoultchi AI, Fan Y. Role of linker histone in chromatin structure and function: H1 stoichiometry and nucleosome repeat length. Chromosome Res 2006;14:17-25.

Zachara NE, Hart GW. O-GlcNAc a sensor of cellular state: the role of nucleocytoplasmic glycosylation in modulating cellular function in response to nutrition and stress. Biochim Biophys Acta. 2004 Jul 6;1673(1-2):13-28.

Zeidan Q, Hart GW. The intersections between O-GlcNAcylation and phosphorylation: implications for multiple signaling pathways. J Cell Sci. 2010 Jan 1;123(Pt 1):13-22.

Zetser A, Gredinger E, Bengal E. p38 mitogen-activated protein kinase pathway promotes skeletal muscle differentiation. J Biol Chem 1999; 274: 5193–5200.

10

Immunoglobulin Treatment in Polymyositis and Dermatomyositis

Maria Giovanna Danieli[1], Lucia Pettinari[1], Romina Moretti[1], Francesco Logullo[2] and Armando Gabrielli[1]
[1]*Clinica Medica, Dipartimento di Scienze Mediche e Chirurgiche,*
[2]*Clinica Neurologica, Università Politecnica delle Marche & Ospedali Riuniti, Ancona*
Italy

1. Introduction

Polymyositis (PM) and dermatomyositis (DM) are systemic autoimmune diseases of unknown aetiology in which the skeletal muscles are the main targets (Bohan & Peter, 1975). Despite the improvement obtained in recent years with new therapeutic options, their prognosis remains poor, with higher rates of morbidity and mortality (Dalakas, 1991, 2001). Due to the rarity of the disease, few well-designed studies have been published and, to the best of our knowledge, only five randomised controlled trials have been carried out (Choy, 2002). A low incidence of the disease, a characteristic relapsing/remitting or chronic and persistently active course, a lack of agreed standardised criteria for diagnosis and for assessment of disease activity makes it difficult to carry out and to compare studies. Conventional first line therapy is based on glucocorticoids and their use in many patients requires long-term use to control disease. Many patients suffer from the side effects of glucocorticoids while others can be refractory to first-line therapy. Thus, there is often the need to add immunosuppressive or immunomodulatory agents both to improve the disease's response and to reduce the risk of long-term complications linked to glucocorticoids (Choy, 2009).
Among the treatment options, the use of intravenous immunoglobulin is still matter of debate.
In this chapter we describe the use of intravenous immunoglobulin in inflammatory myopathies, revising the literature and reporting our experience. Most of the patients with polymyositis or dermatomyositis receive an immunosuppressant such as azathioprine, methotrexate, cyclosporine A or mycophenolate mofetil. We decided to verify if the use of intravenous immunoglobulin as add-on treatment with cyclosporine A or mycophenolate mofetil could improve the outcome or reduce the rate of side effects that are usually linked to the immunosuppressant. The subcutaneous administration of immunoglobulin could be considered as an alternative to intravenous immunoglobulin. In primary immunodeficiency, subcutaneous immunoglobulin has been demonstrated to be linked to a lower incidence of adverse reactions, with reliable efficacy and improvement in the quality of life of treated subjects. We have been the first to publish a series of seven patients with immune-mediated myopathies treated with subcutaneous immunoglobulin. Here we present data relating to a larger series. Finally, our intention is to review the data related to the mechanisms of action

of immunoglobulin in immune-mediated diseases, in particular underlining the different proposed mechanism of intravenous and subcutaneous immunoglobulin.

2. Intravenous immunoglobulin in inflammatory myopathies

2.1 Background

Intravenous immunoglobulin is a therapeutic preparation of pooled polyspecific IgG obtained from the plasma of a large number of healthy individuals. The preparations were commercialized in the early 1980s to replace intramuscular preparations of polyspecific IgG, which were the only available substitutive therapy at that time for patients with primary or secondary immunodeficiencies. For patients with primary immunodeficiencies, intravenous immunoglobulin (or subcutaneous immunoglobulin) remains the treatment option of choice.

Despite the large number of autoimmune diseases treated with intravenous immunoglobulin, guidance on the clinical usage is limited to only three conditions: idiopathic thrombocytopenic purpura, Guillian-Barrè syndrome and Kawasaki disease (rev. in Elovaaraa et al., 2008). In other neurological conditions, such as chronic inflammatory demyelinating polyradiculoneuropathy, multifocal motor neuropathy, and in acute exacerbations and short-term treatment of severe myasthenia gravis, their use is codified (Elovaaraa et al., 2008).

Because of the costs, finite supply and time required for the patient receiving intravenous therapy, there is a need to rationalize and prioritize the disorders for which, based on currently available evidence, intravenous immunoglobulin is adopted. In France, the Comité d'Evaluation et de Diffusion des Innovations Technologiques (CEDIT) -Intravenous Immunoglobulin Expert Group, aims to identify scientifically validated uses and issue recommendations regarding the usage of intravenous immunoglobulin (Mouthon, 2006). Guidelines for the use of immunoglobulin have also been developed in the United Kingdom (UK Department of Health, 2009), Canada (Mydlarski, 2006; Feasby et al., 2007), Australia (Australian Health Minister, 2009) and elsewhere.

For most of the diseases, intravenous immunoglobulin is not always used as a first-line therapy. It may be administered as a steroid-sparing agent and in certain conditions may represent an alternative to other available therapeutic approaches, such as immunosuppressants, plasma exchange or monoclonal antibodies. Intravenous immunoglobulin is also often employed to treat diseases that are refractory to other treatments or where conventional therapies result in unacceptable side effects. Combination therapy of intravenous immunoglobulin with immunosuppressants has been applied successfully in several conditions, including autoimmune vasculitis, and chronic inflammatory myopathies (Hartung et al., 2009; Harvey, 2005).

In 1987, Roifman et al. described the first patient with refractory polymyositis successfully treated using intravenous immunoglobulin, whereas in 1991 Lang et al. were the first to highlight the beneficial use of intravenous immunoglobulin in the treatment of dermatomyositis. Several additional papers have since been published. However, a review of the available literature about the use of intravenous immunoglobulin in inflammatory myopathies shows the lack of randomised controlled trials due to the difficulty of conducting high quality randomised controlled trials in rare diseases. Despite the different significance and rationale regarding the use of intravenous immunoglobulin treatment in polymyositis and dermatomyositis, the majority of studies reported the use in mixed populations of patients with both diseases. Moreover, in most studies, intravenous immunoglobulin has been used in association with other drugs, such as immunosuppressants. It is thus difficult to evaluate optimal strategies and efficacy: safety ratio in inflammatory myopathies. Here we present a brief revision of the most relevant studies on the use of intravenous immunoglobulin in inflammatory myopathies. The application in combined treatment with immunosuppressant is analysed in Paragraphs 3 and 4.

2.2 Mechanisms of action of intravenous immunoglobulin

Intravenous immunoglobulin was first introduced in the middle of the twentieth century for the treatment of primary immunodeficiencies. In 1981, Paul Imbach noticed an improvement of immune-mediated thrombocytopenia in patients receiving intravenous immunoglobulin for immunodeficiencies (Imbach et al., 1981). This opened a new era for the treatment of autoimmune conditions with intravenous immunoglobulin. Since then, intravenous immunoglobulin has become an important treatment option in an ever-increasing number of autoimmune diseases (Arson et al., 2009; Kivity et al., 2010; Mimouni et al., 2011) and, more recently, for the treatment of tumor metastases (Damianovich et al., 2009). Immune dysregulation and loss of self-tolerance are the keystones of autoimmunity (Agmon-Levin et al., 2011). There is a large body of evidence that intravenous immunoglobulin has the ability to modulate immune reaction at several cellular levels (T and B cells, macrophages), interfere with antibody production and degradation, modulate the complement cascade, and effect the cytokine network. Despite success in clinical application, the precise mechanism of action is not yet clear, but several non-mutually exclusive mechanisms have been proposed to explain the beneficial effects of intravenous immunoglobulin.

To understand how intravenous immunoglobulin reverses inflammation in autoimmune disease, it is helpful to consider how immunoglobulin G (IgG) auto-antibodies cause inflammation. IgG molecules are the most abundant antibody class in the sera of humans; they are a family of molecules consisting of four subclasses which vary in their serum prevalence and capacity to trigger effector functions, such as binding to cellular Fc-receptors for IgG or activating the complement pathway. They seem to have the unique feature of initiating pro- and anti-inflammatory reactions: they are the primary mediators of protective humoral immunity against pathogens, but they can also be pathogenic. Acting as cytotoxic molecules or as immune complexes, IgG auto-antibodies are the principal mediators of autoimmune diseases. This pro-inflammatory activity mainly depends on the presence of cellular Fc-receptors for IgG.

Aschermann et al. (2010) proposed a possible explanation based on the interaction interference of cellular Fc-receptors on IgG (FCγR), and the complement components of the Fc-fragment which could prevent the auto-antibodies-mediated FCγR activation by blocking FCγ and FCγR interaction. Anthony et al. (2008) describe a model wherein sialylated IgG Fc protein interacts with a currently unidentified sialic acid-specific receptor on specific regulatory macrophages in the marginal zone of spleen. This consequently enhances the expression of the Fcγ receptor IIB on effector macrophages, highlighting that Fcγ receptor has a critical role in mediating the therapeutic effects of intravenous immunoglobulin. The mechanisms by which high doses of pooled, monomeric IgG provide anti-inflammatory activity have been the subject of much speculation, stemming from the fact that IgG can form many different binding interactions through both their antigen binding and Fc domains. In some cases, antigen binding alone might be sufficient to mediate the anti-inflammatory effects attributed to intravenous immunoglobulin, for example, by blocking interactions between a pro-inflammatory ligand and its receptor or by neutralizing its ability to elicit an inflammatory response.

Moreover, due to their presence in natural auto-antibodies against the receptors sialic acid binding immunoglobulin (Ig)-like lectin (Siglec)-8 and Siglec-9 that mediate cell death, anti-proliferative effects and inhibition of cellular activities, intravenous immunoglobulin may exert anti-inflammatory properties by increasing the concentration of natural anti-Siglec autoantibodies in blood and tissues (Von Gunten et al., 2008). Due to the content of anti-Siglec-8, the usefulness of intravenous immunoglobulin can be hypothesised in hypereosinophilic syndrome or in Churg-Strauss syndrome, because of the documented death's induction by natural antibodies against Siglec-8 and Siglec-9 present in intravenous immunoglobulin in both eosinophils and neutrophils in a concentration-dependent manner. In a controlled trial regarding Churg-Strauss syndrome it was documented that all patients in the intravenous immunoglobulin group were in remission with a significantly favourable outcome, compared to controls, which remained after three years. (Danieli et al., 2004).

It is possible that not all IgG in intravenous immunoglobulin is effective and in all probability the involved mechanisms vary from one disease to another. The different molecular and cellular pathways involved could explain the wide spectrum of diseases in which intravenous immunoglobulin could exert its immunomodulatory and anti-inflammatory properties. Particular intravenous immunoglobulin activities are also believed to be related to the sialylation of IgG through which they become functional in restricted subset of diseases such as inflammatory-ones (Seite et al., 2008).

Due to the method of preparation, the content of immunoglobulin product is variable, including natural antibodies and natural auto-antibodies that play a major role in its activity (Seite et al., 2008; Vani et al., 2008; Schwartz-Albiez et al., 2009). Other relevant supposed mechanisms of action take account of modulation of idiotype-anti-idiotype dimers network by binding idiotypic determinants of auto-antibodies; activation, differentiation and effector functions of T and of antigen-presenting cells; modulation of B cells via the antigen receptor; and interferences with activation of complement and the cytokine network (Seite et al., 2008).

In regard to inflammatory muscle diseases, which have different clinical, histological, and immunopathological features, the mechanism of action may be different according to the properties of individual diseases. The cause of polymyositis and dermatomyositis is unknown, but an immune-mediated pathogenesis is strongly implicated.

As illustrated by Dalakas (2006) intravenous immunoglobulin is thought to work by inhibiting complement consumption and intercepting membrane attack complexes, suppressing cytokines, adhesion molecules and fibrogenetic factors, and altering biologically relevant immunoregulatory or tissues remodelling genes. Resolution of the aberrant immunopathological parameters, including interception of complement activation products and down-regulation of T cells, intercellular adhesion molecule-1 (ICAM-I), vascular cell adhesion molecule (VCAM), transforming growth factor (TGF)-b and major histocompatibility complex (MHC)-I molecules, was also noted.

Dermatomyositis is histologically characterised by complement-mediated microangiopathy beginning with complement activation in the periphery that eventually leads to the formation of membrane attack complexes, which are deposited on the capillaries causing destruction of endomysial capillaries. A number of cytokines and chemokines are thought to be in involved in the process. These molecules may also be responsible for the up-regulation of the major histocompatibility complex (MHC) class I antigen and signal trasducer and activator of transcription (STAT) 1 expression on the perifascicular's muscle fibre. The actual effectiveness of intravenous immunoglobulin was demonstrated by Dalakas (2006) in a double-blind placebo-controlled study. His results demonstrated the improvement in muscle cytoarchitecture, down-regulation of cytokine and adhesion molecules, effect on complement activation and MAC formation and the improvement of the muscle microvasculature. Down-regulation of intercellular adhesion molecule-1 (ICAM-I) more than likely has an effect on the exit of activated T cells from the capillaries toward the muscle fibres, reducing inflammatory cells infiltrate. Another possible effect is the down-regulation of TGF-β and TGF-β mRNA, which induces chronic inflammation and fibrosis if in excess, as seen in the tissue of patients with dermatomyositis, where it is in generally up-regulated. Consequently, intravenous immunoglobulin facilitated neovascularisation and normalisation of the capillaries and muscle fibres.

In polymyositis the muscle injury appears to be T-cells mediated and directed against unknown antigens expressed on the sarcolemma of the muscle fibres. A severe perturbation of peripheral blood T cell TCR repertories was displayed, characterized by the presence of antigen specific T-cell with killer/effector phenotype (Mizuno et al., 2004). Thus, CD8+ cytotoxic T cells clonally expand and lead to muscle fibres necrosis via perforin pathway, according to the observed rearrangement of T-cell-receptor genes among autoinvasive T cells and expression of co-stimulatory molecules, adhesion molecules and cytokines (Dalakas, 2010).

With intravenous immunoglobulin it is thus possible to restore immunoregulation and normal immune homeostasis (Gurcan et al., 2010; Seite et al., 2008).

2.3 Intravenous immunoglobulin in dermatomyositis

With regard to dermatomyositis, a Cochrane review article looking at randomised controlled studies (Choy, 2009) identified only the pioneering trial of Dalakas (1993) in 15 patients with treatment-resistant disease which compared monthly infusions of 2 g/kg of immunoglobulin for three months in association with pre-existing low-dose glucocorticoids to placebo. The study demonstrated a statistically significant improvement in muscle strength measured by mean scores on the neuromuscular symptom scale ($P = .035$) and the modified Medical Research Council scale (from 76.6 to 84.6; $P = .018$; with a mean difference of 9.50 (95% confidence interval (CI) 4.33 to 14.67) in the treated group. Even though the trial measured muscle strength after only three months, the improvements, even in cutaneous manifestations, lasted for several weeks. This trial remains the fundamental work demonstrating that intravenous immunoglobulin is a beneficial strategy in dermatomyositis. The successful use of intravenous immunoglobulin has also been highlighted in other studies that show the improvement of 75% to 92% of adults using this treatment modality for refractory disease (Gelfand, 1989; Mastaglia, 1998; Marie, 2001). A recent work by Gottfried et al. (2000) indicated that remission was documented in particular in patients with predominant cutaneous symptoms, absence of autoantibodies, without accompanying neoplasia.

Based on expert consensus, Feasby et al. (2007) conclude that intravenous immunoglobulin is recommended, in combination with prednisone, for patients with dermatomyositis who have not satisfactorily responded to glucocorticoids. Intravenous immunoglobulin is recommended, in association with immunosuppressants, as a steroid-sparing option or as the first-line treatment in life-threatening disease (Feasby et al., 2007). With regards to treatment dose and duration, the reported dose is usually 2g/kg, given for two/five days in adult patients. In a single treatment course the maximum dose should be 2g/kg. In patients responding to this treatment, every attempt should be made to determine the minimum effective dose and the use of intravenous immunoglobulin should be continued only if there are objective measures of sustained effectiveness.

2.4 Intravenous immunoglobulin in polymyositis

The application of intravenous immunoglobulin in polymyositis has not yet been assessed with a randomised trial. Their efficacy was highlighted by Cherin et al. in 1991 with a study of 20 patients with chronic and refractory polymyositis or dermatomyositis showing clinical improvement of fifteen patients (75%) and biochemical improvement in all of them (Cherin, 1991). The subsequent follow-up, with an increased series including 35 patients with refractory dermatomyositis or polymyositis, presented pooled data confirming the improvement of patients treated with this regime (Cherin & Herson, 1994). The authors documented a significant improvement in mean muscle power ($P = 0.01$) with a reduction in mean steroid dose ($P = 0.05$) and a decrease in creatine kinase levels ($P = 0.01$). The same group presented data on the only published non-randomised controlled trial specifically addressed to polymyositis (Cherin et al., 2002). This study reported clinical improvement in 71% of patients with significant improvement in muscle power, muscle disability scores, and creatinine kinase levels ($P < 0.01$). All of the 22 patients who received intravenous immunoglobulin were able to significantly reduce the dose of glucocorticoids ($P < 0.05$). In conclusion, in polymyositis, intravenous immunoglobulin can be considered as an alternative therapeutic option in patients who do not respond to conventional first-line treatment (glucocorticoids). Dose and duration of the treatment are as recommended for dermatomyositis (Feasby et al., 2007; Elovaara et al., 2008).
Despite intravenous immunoglobulin demonstrating adequate efficacy and rapid onset of beneficial effects, there are no indications for its use as first-line therapy. The use of intravenous immunoglobulin, in an attempt to replace glucocorticoids as first-choice treatment to avoid steroid-related myopathy in six adult patients with dermatomyositis and in five with polymyositis, did not lead to a significant increase in muscle strength, although creatine kinase levels significantly decreased (Cherin et al., 1994). Only three patients showed significant clinical improvement. The low success rate obtained by intravenous immunoglobulin as first-choice in inflammatory myopathies, compared to their usual efficacy in association with glucocorticoids in chronic refractory diseases, suggests a synergistic action on both cellular and humoral systems (Cherin et al., 1994). More recent studies, in accordance with previous literature, confirm indication of the value of intravenous immunoglobulin as a second-line agent in patients with dermatomyositis and polymyositis (Cherin, 2008; Dalakas, 2010).

2.5 Other indications of intravenous immunoglobulin

Besides the cutaneous and muscle involvement, intravenous immunoglobulin has been evaluated in other clinical manifestations of inflammatory myopathies. A rapid onset of therapeutical effects was substantiated by Marie et al. (2010) in a recent retrospective multicentre study reviewing 73 patients with oesophageal involvement in which intravenous immunoglobulin (1 g/kg daily for two consecutive days each month for at least seven months) produced improvement within two weeks after the first infusion with a clinical resolution or a marked improvement of oesophageal clinical involvement in 65 patients (89%), thus suggesting their use as first-line therapy in life-threatening oesophageal manifestations. This data confirms previous studies in smaller series (Marie et al., 1999; Cherin et al., 2001). Contrasting results have been documented in interstitial lung disease associated with polymyositis and dermatomyositis, in which only a small number cases show benefits from intravenous immunoglobulin (Suzuki et al., 2009).

Intravenous immunoglobulin may also be an alternative option when other drugs are not recommended, especially during pregnancy and in breast-feeding mothers. Pregnancy in association with an inflammatory myopathy is a rare event, therefore any published data is primarily based on case reports or very small groups of patients (Silva et al., 2003; Mosca et al., 2005; Williams et al., 2007). Even in this context, intravenous immunoglobulin has been shown to be very effective in the treatment of inflammatory myopathies, in particular in dermatomyositis (Cherin et al., 2002), and is widely used for various autoimmune conditions during pregnancy. It is also used in the treatment of other pregnancy complications, such as idiopathic thrombocytopenic purpura and recurrent miscarriages, and appears to be safe and well tolerated by pregnant patients (Branch et al., 2001).

2.6 Our experience with intravenous immunoglobulin in polymyositis and dermatomyositis

We report our experience on the use of intravenous immunoglobulin only associated with glucocorticoids in polymyositis and dermatomyositis diagnosed according to the Bohan and Peter criteria (1975). Despite alternative classifications being previously proposed and the fact that this classification presents some limitations it is the most widely used set of criteria in the literature.

	Definition
Diagnosis of polymyositis and dermatomyositis	Bohan and Peter's criteria (1975): Symmetrical weakness, usually progressive, of the limb-girdle muscles Muscle biopsy evidence of myositis Elevation in serum of creatine kinase levels Electromyographic triad of myopathy Characteristic dermatologic features of dermatomyositis
Active disease	Decreased skeletal muscle strength assessed using the Medical Research Council scale (Miller et al., 1992); Elevation of creatine kinase for at least 2 months; Typical electromyographic features (Kimura, 1989; Wilbourn, 1993)
Refractory disease	Inadequate response to steroid and/or at least 2 immunosuppressants given for at least two months; OR Steroid-dependency: flare-up when the steroid dose was reduced to less than 0.25 mg/kg/day; OR Steroid-resistance: non-responsiveness to high-dose steroid treatment (at least 1 mg/kg/day for six weeks)
Relapse	Disease reactivation after a remission lasting six months or more

Table 1. Working definitions used in this chapter.

The data of the ten patients in which we used intravenous immunoglobulin were extrapolated from our series of 74 patients with polymyositis and dermatomyositis, prospectively followed up in our Department.
There were five cases each of polymyositis and dermatomyositis in one male and nine females (all Caucasian) with a median age of onset at 49 years (range 28-63 years). In six patients the disease was particularly aggressive with severe muscle involvement and dysphagia. Associated clinical features were arthritis (four patients), Raynaud's phenomenon (other four), interstitial lung disease (two patients) and cardiovascular involvement (one case). Before treatment serum creatine kinase values were 2326.5 U/l (range 637-5500). ANA and anti-ENA positivity were detected in two cases each. Disease duration prior to treatment was 17 months (range 4-131), and the median follow-up period was 82 months (range 30-170 months). Intravenous immunoglobulin was given on occurrence of refractory (7 patients) or relapsed disease (3 patients), definitions of which are illustrated in Table 1.
Initial therapy was based on oral steroids (prednisone 1mg/kg/daily) for one month and then slowly tapered to 5-10 mg every other week. Intravenous immunoglobulin was infused at 1 g/kg (5g/hour) on two consecutive days each month for six months, followed by three further cycles given every other month. The response to treatment was evaluated as outlined in Table 2.

Complete remission	an increase in strength of at least one Medical Research Council grade and normalisation of the serum creatine kinase levels.
Partial remission	when only one of the above criteria was fulfilled
Relapse	recurrence of active disease after a remission lasting six months or more

Table 2. Parameters employed to evaluate the response to treatment.

After one month of therapy we documented a partial improvement of muscle strength associated with a decrease in creatine kinase levels. At one year follow-up this result was confirmed, with six patients in complete remission and three in partial remission (Figure 1). The last patient dropped out from the study for meningism related to the intravenous immunoglobulin infusion. At long-term follow-up (mean 82 months), we could observe three relapses, two of which in patients with previous relapsing-remitting recurrences (respectively after 31 and 61 months from the beginning of the treatment).
The treatment was well tolerated with a low incidence of mild adverse events (nausea and vomiting) which could be successfully managed by reducing the speed of infusion. All patients reported a good tolerance profile of the intravenous administration of immunoglobulin. In Dalakas' study (1993) of dermatomyositis no adverse events were reported. In the study of Cherin and Herson (1994) no patients stopped infusions because of side effects. Accordingly to the literature, the treatment with intravenous immunoglobulin is generally a safe procedure, when given in a slow infusion rate in well-hydrated patients, and avoiding patients with known risk factors (Katz et al., 2007). Our data, in accordance with the literature, confirms our previous findings (Danieli et al., 2009b) that intravenous immunoglobulin is an effective and safe option as second-line therapy in patients with

refractoriness to steroids or with relapsing-disease. Subjects treated with intravenous immunoglobulin achieve a clinical and functional remission in a high percentage of cases which is maintained at long follow-up period.

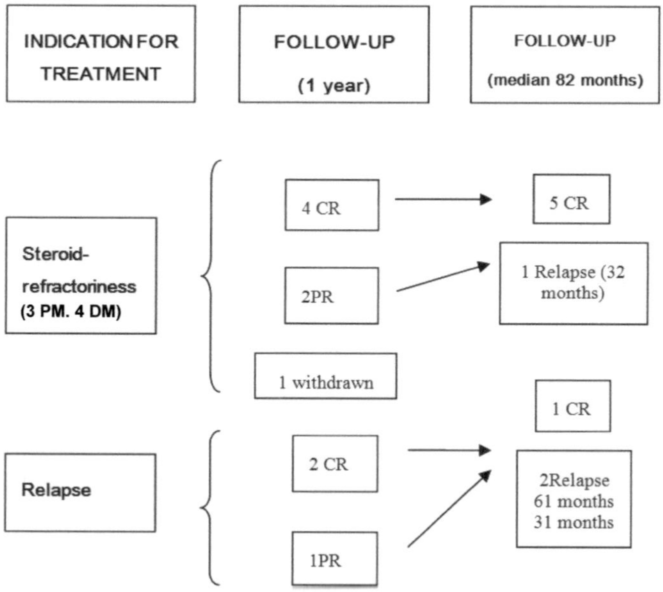

Fig. 1. Outcome and treatment response in 10 patients treated with glucocorticoids and intravenous immunoglobulin.

3. Cyclosporine A and intravenous immunoglobulin in inflammatory myopathies

3.1 Introduction

The use of cyclosporine is widely accepted in organ rejection, other studies emphasizes its importance in the therapy of systemic lupus erythematosus (Moroni et al., 2009) and other immune-mediated disease such as inflammatory myopathies. The following presents our experience with this drug in a large series of patients with polymyositis and dermatomyositis, testing the hypothesis if the add-on of intravenous immunoglobulin could improve the outcome or reduce the rate of side effects usually linked to the immunosuppressant's use. Finally, we report the revision of the literature related to the use of cyclosporine A in polymyositis and dermatomyositis.

Cyclosporine is a pro-drug in which its immune effects are secondary to a relative selective inhibition of T cell activation. In the cytoplasm, cyclosporine A, after binding to its specific cytoplasmic receptor cyclophillin, interferes with calcineurin, a complex of phosphatases crucial for the progression of the events that ultimately lead to the lymphocyte proliferation. During the physiological immune response, the contact between antigen-presenting cells and lymphocytes triggers a strong influx of calcium ions into lymphocytes, with calcineurin activation and subsequent dephosphorylation of a family of proteins called nuclear factor activating T cells (NFAT). The dephosphorylation mediated by calcineurin leads nuclear factor activating T cells (NFAT) to enter the nucleus and promote the synthesis of interleukin-2 that, in turn, activates the lymphocyte proliferation. By interfering in this cascade, cyclosporine may alter the production of the pro-inflammatory cytokines that interplay at different levels among the cellular, immunological and biochemical mediators of inflammation. Cyclosporine A may hamper the pro-inflammatory cytokines that promote the activation, the maintenance of the immune inflammation, and the migration of the lymphocytes to target organs. The main role of cyclosporine A resides thus in the interference with T autoreactive cells, while it has little impact on humoral immunity.

3.2 Our experience with cyclosporine A and intravenous immunoglobulin in inflammatory myopathies

Since 1992, we used three different cyclosporine A-based regimens to treat 24 patients with definite myositis according to the Bohan and Peter criteria (1975). The 24 patients had either dermatomyositis (12 cases) or polymyositis (12 cases); subjects with connective tissue-associated, cancer-associated or inclusion body and those with juvenile myositis were excluded. The disease was newly diagnosed in seven patients, three of them had glucocorticoid refractoriness (Group I). The other 17 patients presented with refractory disease, as indicated by non-responsiveness to high-dose steroid treatment or to methotrexate and/or azathioprine (nine cases, Group II) or the recurrence of a previously quiescent disease (eight cases, Group III). All of the patients had active disease, as confirmed by the parameters of increased median values of creatine kinase levels (in all cases), Medical Research Council grade (in all cases), the electromyographic myogenic changes (in all cases) and the histological characteristics (in 75% of the 18 patients who underwent muscle biopsy). The baseline characteristics of the three groups of patients were homogenous, as shown in the following table.

	Group I Control group (PDN-CsA)	Group II Refractory disease (PDN-IVIg-CsA)	Group III Relapsed disease (PDN-IVIg-CsA)
PM/DM	3/4	4/5	5/3
Men /women	2/5	3/6	1/7
Age of onset (years)	34	48	35
Baseline serum CK levels (U/l)	706	2584	2468
Baseline MRC scale	74.4	73.4	68.8
Disease duration * (months)	14	24	35
Duration of follow-up (months)	40	57	59

* Before the start of indicated treatment.

Table 3. Baseline characteristics of the three groups of patients treated with different cyclosporine A-based regimens. Data are expressed as median. Abbreviation: AZA, azathioprine; CsA, cyclosporine A; CK, creatine kinase; DM, dermatomyositis; IVIg, intravenous immunoglobulin; MRC, Medical Research Council; MTX, methotrexate; PDN, prednisone; PM, polymyositis.

As customary, the treatment was based on oral prednisone, which was started at 1 mg/kg/day and then slowly tapered to an average of 0.25 mg/kg every other day. Initially, oral cyclosporine A was given as 3 mg/kg/day for six months, and then reduced to a maintenance dose of 2 mg/kg/day. Patients were given microemulsion (Sandimmun Neoral ®, Novartis) which has a better bioavailability and more predictable pharmacokinetic properties. In the 17 patients with refractory disease (Group II and III), intravenous immunoglobulin were infused at 1 g/kg (5g/hour) on two consecutive days each month for six months, followed by three further cycles given every other month. In all of the patients, the first treatment period lasted one year during which the patients were re-evaluated every three months. The parameters used to evaluate the response to treatment are outlined in Table 2. The mean follow-up of the entire series as a whole is five years. The responses in the three groups are shown in Figure 2.

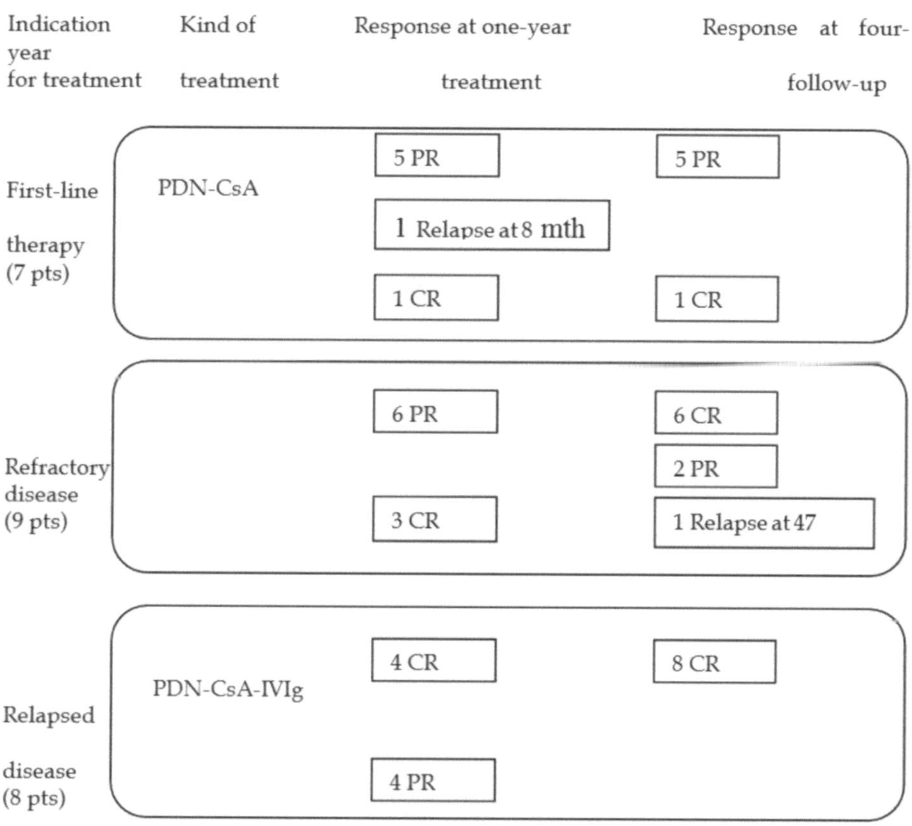

Fig. 2. Response to cyclosporine A associated or not with intravenous immunoglobulin in 24 patients with Polymyositis and dermatomyositis.

At the end of the one-year treatment period, we did not document any significant difference among the three treatment groups. Indeed, five of the patients in group I had a partial response, one was in complete remission and one relapsed eight months after the start of treatment. All of the patients in group II and III had improved. In the following period, positive results were documented almost exclusively in patients treated with cyclosporine A associated with intravenous immunoglobulin (Groups II and III). In group I, one patient was in clinical and functional remission 19 months after the start of treatment; the other five cases were still in partial remission. In Group II, all of the patients improved with a complete remission in six out of nine patients, and one patient was able to maintain a complete remission without any further treatment; only one patient relapsed. In group III all of the patients were in persistent remission after having discontinued all treatment. Globally 82% (14/17) maintain a complete remission at the end of the follow-up period.

The statistical analyses revealed a significant difference at the end of the follow-up period between patients in remission with intravenous immunoglobulin and those treated only with cyclosporine A and prednisone ($P < 0.001$, chi-square analysis). We could not detect any other correlation between the response to treatment in the three groups and other variables such as the kind of myositis (polymyositis or dermatomyositis), the duration of the disease prior to the treatment with intravenous immunoglobulin and cyclosporine A, or the kind of organ involvement.

No new or major side effects leading to the interruption of treatment were recorded during the trial. In 30% of the patients treated with cyclosporine A we documented minor adverse effects consisting of hypertrichosis (three cases) minor gastrointestinal disturbance (nausea or vomiting in two cases), gingival hyperplasia (one case), transient increase in serum creatinine levels (one case).

3.3 Literature review on the use of cyclosporine A in inflammatory myopathies

We revised the English language literature related to the use of cyclosporine A in myositis. Since 1976, reports have been published of more than 100 patients with polymyositis and dermatomyositis treated with cyclosporine A. In early trials, cyclosporine A was given at high doses, ranging from 7.5 to 10 mg/kg/day, in patients with disease unresponsive to glucocorticoids or immunosuppressants. As reported, the disease improved, but unacceptable side effects were documented in the majority of patients. In more recent years, improved knowledge of the drug made it possible to lessen the dosage of cyclosporine A, with a proportional decrease of side effects. Cyclosporine A, usually between 2 and 5 mg/kg/day, allowed for a complete remission in 70% of cases, even in those with refractory disease (Danieli et al., 2002; Dankò & Szegedi, 1991; Qushmaq et al., 2000; Vencovsky et al., 2000). Two retrospective studies of respectively ten (Dankò & Szegedi, 1991) and twelve (Sanchez Román et al., 1995) patients have suggested the efficacy of cyclosporine A as a valid second-line therapy in refractory dermatomyositis. The only randomized controlled trial that has evaluated the impact of cyclosporine A in the treatment of polymyositis and dermatomyositis was carried by Vencovsky et al. (2000). The authors could not document any significant difference between cyclosporine A and methotrexate in terms of efficacy and toxicity evaluated at 6-month. In the majority of the cited reports, a good clinical response was documented within the first weeks of treatment.

The efficacy of cyclosporine A was principally evaluated in the treatment of interstitial lung disease associated with myositis. The two first reports of respectively eight (Maeda et al., 1997) and five (Nawata et al., 1999) patients confirmed its effectiveness, in particularly when used early. Other later reports confirm these data, with a complete or partial remission in more than 50% of the patients (Kameda et al., 2005; Kotani et al., 2008). It is important to remember that most patients typically died of respiratory failure related to interstitial pneumonia.

The usefulness of cyclosporine A in myositis seems to be improved by the association with intravenous immunoglobulin. Saadeh et al. (1995) were the first to describe a patient with dermatomyositis who improved after being treated with cyclosporine A and intravenous immunoglobulin. This preliminary report is in line with our experience, in which 82% of treated patients reached a complete remission. The patients had a particularly severe disease, due to the presence of non-responsiveness to high-dose steroid treatment or a previous relapse. Our data at long-term follow-up reinforces these results, with a highly statistically significant difference detected at the end of the follow-up period when compared to patients treated with prednisone and intravenous immunoglobulin. The association of intravenous immunoglobulin and low-dose cyclosporine A produces improved control of disease activity and keeps the least amount of glucocorticoids.

In literature, no serious side effects are generally described, but 8-15% of patients treated with cyclosporine A develop arterial hypertension, hypertrichosis, tremor and transient renal dysfunction (Qushmaq et al., 2000). Other adverse events linked to the use of cyclosporine A are hyperlipaemia and diabetes. All these events are usually dose related. It is extremely important to keep the dose of cyclosporine A at 3 mg/kg/day to avoid untoward side effects. It is also recommended to avoid cyclosporine A in patients with renal impairment (creatinine clearance <60 ml/min) and/or uncontrolled arterial hypertension, and to carefully monitor the serum creatinine and potassium levels. Revising the literature, we documented that 20% of the patients with inflammatory myopathies treated with cyclosporine A experienced a major side effect such as renal toxicity and arterial hypertension. These percentages are lower in subjects treated with cyclosporine A and intravenous immunoglobulin, with 5% of patients reporting renal dysfunction and none arterial hypertension. Despite these statistics, the conceivable value of intravenous immunoglobulin is that its use makes it possible to reduce the doses of glucocorticoids and cyclosporine A in most patients, thus lowering the rate of side effects linked to use of these drugs.

While treating patients with cyclosporine A it is important to slowly taper the drug to avoid the risk of hyperacute relapse of the disease, as it has been reported in patients with systemic lupus erythematosus (Radhakrishnan et al., 1995). To improve the tolerance to the drug, some authors advocate the single daily administration, that has been demonstrated to be as effective than the bis in die administration but with fewer side effects in patients with organ transplant (Tarantino et al., 2004) and in those with idiopathic nephrotic syndrome (Rasche et al., 2007). Another important issue is how long to treat patients safely with cyclosporine A. We did not document nephrotoxicity even in long term treated patients, perhaps because we used lower doses of the drug (<2- 3mg/kg/day) than usually reported. However, the optimal duration of the treatment is unknown.

In our series cyclosporine A associated with intravenous immunoglobulin was successfully used both to control the disease activity and to keep the doses of glucocorticoids to a minimum. With this combined treatment we documented the best and statistically significant results as compared to steroid-cyclosporine A based treatment. This treatment was beneficial even in subjects with refractory disease and major organ involvement. We did not find any increase in the number or type of side effects. Further randomized trials may confirm the true benefits of various treatments in different subset of polymyositis and dermatomyositis.

4. Mycophenolate mofetil and intravenous immunoglobulin in inflammatory myopathies

4.1 Introduction

Mycophenolate mofetil is an immunosuppressive drug mainly used in the prevention of allograft rejection in renal, cardiac or liver transplantation and in immune-mediated diseases, such as systemic lupus erythematosus, with or without renal involvement (Bomback & Appel, 2010; Mok, 2007), systemic vasculitis (Hoffman, 2010), autoimmune rheumatic diseases (Iaccarino et al., 2007) and myasthenia gravis (Hehir et al., 2010). Mycophenolate mofetil is a prodrug of mycophenolic acid that was developed to enhance its bioavailability. Following oral administration, mycophenolate mofetil is entirely metabolized to mycophenolic acid. With regards to its action, mycophenolate mofetil is a potent selective inhibitor of inosina-5′-monophosphate dehydrogenase. Mycophenolate mofetil blocks the de novo synthesis of guanosine nucleotides, a critical pathway for the DNA synthesis in lymphocytes, acting on T- and B- cell proliferation and interfering on expression of adhesion molecules and on antibody production (reviewed in Ritter & Pirofski, 2009). Thus, mycophenolate mofetil could influence the course of cell- and antibody-mediated diseases.

Despite its use in myositis since 2000, literature supporting the efficacy of mycophenolate mofetil is scarce with only case reports and a few small series. The following describes our experience with patients with polymyositis and dermatomyositis and compares our results with those of previous reports.

4.2 Our experience with mycophenolate mofetil and intravenous immunoglobulin in inflammatory myopathies

In an open study we prospectively followed up nine patients with polymyositis and dermatomyositis, the baseline characteristics are shown in the following table. Our previous positive experiences with intravenous immunoglobulin prompted us to treat them with a combined therapy based on intravenous immunoglobulin serial infusions and oral daily mycophenolate mofetil administration.

In this series, polymyositis and dermatomyositis were diagnosed according to the Bohan and Peter's criteria and the diagnosis was further confirmed by a muscle biopsy in all patients, except one case who declined. Indications for treatment were refractoriness to steroid (three cases) or two immunosuppressants given for at least two months (four cases) and glucocorticoids dependency (two cases). Overall patients received a median of two immunosuppressants (range from one to five) including methotrexate, cyclosporine A, cyclophosphamide, azathioprine and rituximab. The disease had a particularly aggressive course with myogenic damage predominating in the axial muscles in one case (F/49 with dermatomyositis) and cardiopulmonary involvement with cardiac arrhythmias and progressive decrease of lung function in another patient (FM/35 with dermatomyositis). At study entry, all of the patients had active myositis (see Table 1 for definition) with severe muscle involvement with difficult walking and dysphagia and/or dyspnoea. In subjects with dermatomyositis, the skin involvement was characterised by diffuse erythematosus and heliotrope rash. Median serum creatine kinase levels were above the normal range (Median ±SD = 1909±714; normal values < 170 IU/l). The initial oral mycophenolate mofetil dose of 500 mg/day was gradually increased to the definite dosage of 30 mg/kg/day in all of the patients with a subsequent median treatment duration of three years. As previously reported, intravenous immunoglobulin was infused at 1 g/kg (5g/hour) on two consecutive days each month for six months, followed by three further cycles given every other month. Prednisone was used according to our standard regimen. Previous immunosuppressants were withdrawn at the start of the study. Within two months of the start of the treatment an improvement in muscle strength with attenuation of cutaneous findings was observed.

Sex/ Age at the diagnosis (years)	DM/PM (date of diagnosis)	Disease duration prior to IVIg-MMF (months)	Previous ineffective therapies	Indications for IVIg-MMF treatment	Outcome
F/51	PM	204	PDN, IVM, MTX, CSA, CYC, Rituximab	Refractory to immunosuppressants	Partial remission Withdrawn MMF
F/50	DM	120	PDN, IVM, MTX, CSA, AZA	Refractory to immunosuppressants	Complete remission
F/38	PM	16	PDN, IVM, MTX, CSA	Refractory to immunosuppressants	Complete remission Withdrawn MMF
F/65	PM	14	PDN, MTX	Refractory to immunosuppressants	Complete remission
F/49	DM	45	PDN, IVM, MTX, CSA	Glucocorticoid-dependency	Complete remission Withdrawn MMF
F/57	PM	16	PDN, CYC	Glucocorticoid-dependency	Complete remission Withdrawn MMF
F/47	DM	42	PDN, IVM	Refractory to glucocorticoids	Complete remission
M/52	DM	16	PDN, IVM	Refractory to glucocorticoids	Partial remission
F/35	DM	13	PDN, IVM	Refractory to glucocorticoids	Partial remission Withdrawn MMF

Abbreviations: AZA, azathioprine; CSA, Cyclosporine A; CYC, cyclophosphamide; DM, dermatomyositis; IVM, intravenous methyl-prednisolone; IVIg, intravenous immunoglobulin; MMF, mycophenolate mofetil; MTX, methotrexate; PDN, prednisone; PM, polymyositis.

Table 4. Baseline characteristics of nine patients with polymyositis or dermatomyositis treated with intravenous immunoglobulin associated with mycophenolate mofetil.

During the subsequent follow-up period, the treatment with intravenous immunoglobulin and mycophenolate mofetil enabled a significant improvement in the clinical (cutaneous and muscle strength) parameters, with a concomitant reduction of serum muscle enzymes and a progressive decrease and then disappearance of spontaneous pathological activity in the sampled muscles at electromyographic studies performed at month 8 from the start of the treatment. In addition, we documented a significant improvement of Medical Research Council scale and modified Rankin score, the two main parameters employed to evaluate the muscle strength and the degree of disability, respectively. Another important result of this combined treatment was the statistically significant reduction of the daily prednisone dose. At the end of the follow-up period of nearly four years (49 ± 16 months), three of the patients (Table 4) showed a partial response, six were in complete remission. These successful results allowed us to withdraw mycophenolate mofetil in four patients who are now in remission with a low-dose prednisone.

The treatment was well tolerated in all of the patients. The most prevalent complaint was represented by abdominal discomfort at the beginning of the mycophenolate mofetil treatment with a spontaneous resolution over time. In another patient, the administration of intravenous immunoglobulin was associated with mild headache which was subsequently resolved by reducing the infusion rate. Considering our complete series of patients with inflammatory myopathies treated with intravenous immunoglobulin, we detected a relative low prevalence of side effects (Table 5).

Meningism	Withdrawn	1/36 (2%)
Nausea e/o vomiting	Resolution after infusion speed slowing down	7/36 (19%)
Headache	Resolution after paracetamol administration and/or infusion speed slowing down	3/36 (8%)

Table 5. Adverse events observed in our complete series of patients with polymyositis and dermatomyositis treated with intravenous immunoglobulin. Ten patients have been treated only with intravenous immunoglobulin, the other 26 with intravenous immunoglobulin associated with cyclosporine A (17) or mycophenolate mofetil (9).

4.3 Literature review on the use of mycophenolate mofetil in inflammatory myopathies

With regards to the literature on/relating to mycophenolate mofetil in inflammatory myopathies, the experience is still limited, since only case reports or predominantly retrospective small case series have been published. We performed a Medline search of English language from 2000 to 2011 related to the use of mycophenolate mofetil in dermatomyositis and polymyositis in adult patients. We analysed in particular the role of mycophenolate mofetil on muscle involvement. The literature search revealed that 62 subjects (23 polymyositis and 39 dermatomyositis), including ours, have been reported to date. Indications for treatment were mainly refractoriness to glucocorticoids or to immunosuppressants and prior intolerance to previous drugs employed to control the myositis (Danieli et al., 2009a). In two series (Chaudhry et al., 2001; Majithia & Harisdangkul, 2005) mycophenolate mofetil was used as initial immunosuppressive agent. The administration of mycophenolate mofetil, orally at 2 g daily, is linked to clinical improvement and decrease in serum creatine kinase levels in 73% of the subjects with polymyositis and in 77% of those with dermatomyositis. Mycophenolate mofetil is active even in cutaneous manifestations, initially documented by Gelber et al. (2000) in four patients with dermatomyositis refractory to glucocorticoids, hydroxychloroquine and methotrexate. Analysis of these reports appears to confirm our data that the association of intravenous immunoglobulin to mycophenolate mofetil may improve the proportion of patients in remission and reduce the rate of side effects. Indeed, in approximately 30% of the responding patients (6/17 for polymyositis and 7/30 for dermatomyositis) remission was reached by a treatment based on intravenous immunoglobulin and mycophenolate mofetil even in refractory or particularly severe cases. The synergism in the action of intravenous immunoglobulin associated with mycophenolate mofetil is probably linked to the suppression of early stages of the activation and proliferation of lymphocytes. This synergism could even explain the relatively fast response (within one month in our experience) of the disease to the treatment, as it has been known that the onset of action of mycophenolate mofetil is usually delayed. In the literature, serum levels of mycophenolic acid, the active metabolite of mycophenolate mofetil, were not reported, probably as they are not usually performed in clinical practice. However, a recent paper on mycophenolate mofetil in kidney transplantation documented that patients exhibiting a lower rejection rate were those in whom the mycophenolate mofetil dose was not fixed but in accordance to serum mycophenolic acid levels (Le Meur et al., 2007). We cannot exclude that patients who did not respond to mycophenolate mofetil received a lower dose than necessary.

Among the advantages linked to this combined therapy, there is the issue of drug-associated side effects. With regards to glucocorticoids, the majority of patients is able to taper or discontinue the dose of prednisone, thus significantly reducing the rate of side effects linked to its use.

Concerning infective complications, the reported papers show a higher frequency and a greater severity of major side effects in dermatomyositis when compared to polymyositis. In their series of ten patients with dermatomyositis, Rowin et al. (2006) reported an exceedingly high rate of opportunistic infections (30%) that were, however, associated with contributing factors such as interstitial lung disease in two patients and previous treatment with cyclophosphamide in one patient. The same subject received a high mycophenolate mofetil dose (3 g daily). The third patient with opportunistic infection had open skin lesions predisposing her to *Mycobacterium xenopi* abscess of the left thigh. In those patients described in the literature in which mycophenolate mofetil was associated to intravenous immunoglobulin, no infectious complications were documented. It is conceivable that intravenous immunoglobulin enables a reduction in the infective risk in subjects treated with an immunosuppressant. This point is of particular interest since immunodeficiency states are increasingly recognised in patients with immune-mediated diseases and they are due to intrinsic defects linked to the disease itself and/or to the immunosuppressive drugs employed throughout the disease management. Diagnostic strategies have been recently addressed for rheumatic diseases (Samson et al., 2010).

4.4 Other indications for mycophenolate mofetil

A paper of Morath et al. (2006) suggests a cardioprotective role in vivo for mycophenolate mofetil due to its inhibitory effect on the proliferation of fibroblasts and vascular smooth muscle cells. This effect, if documented in larger series of patients, is of great importance, given the high rate of cardiovascular disease associated with inflammatory myopathies. In systemic lupus erythematosus, the data indicating a cardioprotective role of mycophenolate mofetil are, unfortunately, uncertain (Davies et al., 2009). In cardiology, anti-inflammatory effects of intravenous immunoglobulin has been studied in some patients with heart failure, dilated cardiomyopathy, myocarditis, pericardial diseases, neonatal lupus (Nussinovitch & Shoenfeld, 2008).

The choice of the immunosuppressant should be adjusted to the patient's characteristics. For example, mycophenolate mofetil has no, theoretically, mutagenic potential but is teratogenic in rats, rabbits and, probably, in humans. Atypical malformations (microtia or anotia in twelve newborns, external auditory canal atresia in nine and cardiovascular malformations in other six) in fourteen offspring of women exposed to mycophenolate mofetil in early pregnancy have been recently reported (Anderka et al., 2009). The underlying maternal conditions were different, ranging from kidney, liver or heart transplantation (nine patients), lupus nephritis (four cases), and recurrent erythema multiforme (one patient). No correlation between dose of mycophenolate mofetil and severity was noted. Hence when long-term immunosuppression is planned in a woman in child-bearing age, it is important to choose the immunosuppressant accordingly. Azathioprine and cyclosporine A can be safely used during pregnancy whereas mycophenolate mofetil and methotrexate are absolutely contraindicated.

Another relevant issue, especially during economically restrained times, is that of cost. With regards to intravenous immunoglobulin, this point will be addressed in Paragraph 6. As for mycophenolate mofetil, the cost is generally ten times higher than that of other, older, immunosuppressants, such as azathioprine and cyclosporine A. However cost should be balanced against the effectiveness of the drug and its relative safety.

5. Subcutaneous immunoglobulin

5.1 Introduction

The subcutaneous administration of immunoglobulin could be considered as an alternative to the more common intravenous route. Subcutaneous immunoglobulin is a blood product containing immunoglobulin G from normal subjects, initially used in primary immunodeficiency diseases and, more recently, in immune-mediated diseases or neurological conditions. In primary immunodeficiency, subcutaneous immunoglobulin used at replacement dosage, has been demonstrated to be linked to a lower incidence of adverse reactions, with reliable efficacy and improvement of the quality of life of treated subjects. Subcutaneous immunoglobulin has become increasingly popular in recent years, and now, the attention focuses on their possible use as a treatment of immune-mediated disease: we have been the first to publish on a series of seven patients with inflammatory myopathies successfully treated with subcutaneous immunoglobulin (Danieli et al., 2011).

5.2 Proposed mechanism of subcutaneous immunoglobulin in inflammatory myopathies

Like intravenous immunoglobulin, subcutaneous immunoglobulin could have multiple mechanisms, relevant to the pathogenesis of polymyositis and dermatomyositis (Vani et al., 2008; Seite et al., 2008). Subcutaneous immunoglobulin treatment leads to more stable immunoglobulin levels, without peaks which are frequently responsible for side effects. However, since their kinetics is different from that of intravenous immunoglobulin, it is possible that subcutaneous immunoglobulin could act at different levels. Recent studies brought attention to the role of T-regulatory cells in autoimmune diseases, due to their role in suppressing the activation, the proliferation and the cytokine production of self-reactive T cells, thus contributing to the prevention of autoimmune phenomena and to the regulation of the immune homeostasis. Kessell et al. (2007), from the group of Professor Shoenfeld, were the first to demonstrate the direct influence of intravenous immunoglobulin on peripheral CD4+ CD25+ T-regulatory cells by increasing their suppressive function. Moreover, in the mouse model of experimental autoimmune myositis, which resembles human polymyositis in several aspects, the depletion of T-regulatory cells aggravated the disease, whereas the injection of polyclonal T-regulatory cells reduced both the incidence and the severity of the disease (Allenbach et al., 2009). Intravenous immunoglobulin treatment has also been shown to be effective in a mouse model for experimental allergic encephalomyelitis (Ephrem et al., 2008) increasing numbers and function of peripheral CD4+ CD25+ T-regulatory cells. Recent studies have demonstrated that intravenous immunoglobulin induces the expansion of T-regulatory cells and enhances their suppressive functions (Maddur et al., 2010). Even though no data is available on the action of subcutaneous immunoglobulin on T-regulatory cells, it can be hypothesised that in chronic autoimmune disease, such as inflammatory myopathies, the effects on T-regulatory cells exerted by subcutaneous immunoglobulin (von Gunten et al., 2008) could be more relevant due to the accelerated catabolism of pathogenic IgG, than intravenous immunoglobulin (Vani et al., 2008; Seite et al., 2008).

5.3 Our experience with in subcutaneous immunoglobulin inflammatory myopathies

Since 2009, January, we offered the option of subcutaneous immunoglobulin to our patients with idiopathic inflammatory myopathies (polymyositis or dermatomyositis) diagnosed according to the Bohan and Peter's criteria. The disease was considered refractory, resistant or recurrent as shown in Table 1. Patients unable to follow instructions, with known allergic reaction to intravenous immunoglobulin, cancer-associated disease, inclusion body myositis or juvenile myositis, were excluded.

At the start of our study, eight subjects agreed to perform the treatment with subcutaneous immunoglobulin: all the patients were Caucasian females; in all of them, the diagnosis was confirmed by a muscle biopsy, and the histological samples collected were examined by means of light and electron microscopy. Major findings were the changes in fibre size and the myofibers degeneration and regeneration with diffuse or focal inflammatory infiltrates, sometimes confined to the peri- and endomysium but usually interspersed between the individual muscle fibres as well. Perifascicular and perivascular inflammatory infiltrates were the typical findings in dermatomyositis. In all of the patients we performed nerve conduction and concentric needle electromyographic studies according to standard techniques that were repeated when clinically indicated. Fibrillation potentials and recruitment abnormalities were rated using commonly described methods (Wilbourn, 1993) and motor unit potentials were evaluated on the basis of their duration, configuration and amplitude by means of a trigger and delay line using a Nicolet Viking IV. At the start of subcutaneous immunoglobulin treatment, all the patients had active disease, confirmed by increased serum creatine kinase levels and the electromyographic findings. Clinically, they presented diffuse and persistent weakness due to severe muscle involvement with dysphagia in two cases and diffuse skin rash in four further cases.

5.3.1 Treatment regimen

At the beginning of treatment all the patients were taking oral prednisone at the previously assumed dose, maintained for at least one month. After this first period, prednisone was slowly tapered to an average of 0.25 mg/kg every other day. Two patients were treated only with prednisone, whereas the remaining patients were using it in addition to several other immunosuppressants. In particular, one patient was treated with oral cyclosporine A (3 mg/kg/day in two refracted doses), two patients with oral mycophenolate mofetil (at 30 mg/kg/day) and the last three patients with methotrexate (15 mg/week i.m.). During the

first three months of treatment with subcutaneous immunoglobulin, previous immunosuppressants were continued at the initial dose, and then, according to the patient's clinical condition, these were slowly tapered.
Prior to starting treatment with subcutaneous immunoglobulin all patients, apart from one case, were given immunoglobulin by the intravenous route at the dose of 2 g/kg, generally infused at 1 g/kg (5g/hour) on two consecutive days each month for at least six months. Four of them were successfully treated with intravenous immunoglobulin several years earlier. The three cases already in intravenous immunoglobulin treatment switched to the subcutaneous treatment one week after the last intravenous infusion, whereas the other patient directly began subcutaneous weekly infusion.

5.3.2 Treatment with subcutaneous immunoglobulin

At the beginning of the study, when we decided to treat our patients with inflammatory myopathies with subcutaneous immunoglobulin, one problem we encountered was dosage. We consequently decided to give patients the usual intravenous bimonthly dose (2g/kg) fractioned into equal doses given subcutaneously at weekly intervals: so, subcutaneous immunoglobulin (Vivaglobin ® CSL Behring) was infused weekly at the dose of 0.2 g/kg/week, nearly double the dose infused in subjects with primary immunodeficiency diseases (Berger, 2008).
Subcutaneous immunoglobulin administration needs a programmable pump (CRONO super PID), with a syringe capacity of 10, 20, 30 or 50 ml, depending on the producer. The site of administration must change for every infusion, choosing among arms, abdomen or thigh, allowing the administration of no more than 15 ml of the product (2.4 g of subcutaneous immunoglobulin) in the same subcutaneous area, at the infusion rate of 10 ml/h into each site and, accordingly to the patient's tolerance, it could be progressively increased up to 20-22 ml/h, according to the literature (Berger, 2008) and to what is currently advised in Italy. No premedication is required.

5.3.3 Training of the patients

A very important step for enhancing adherence to this kind of home regimen is training which can improve patient's home-infusion experience and increase their acceptance of subcutaneous immunoglobulin. Therefore, all patients received an explicative brochure and were trained to perform home self-administration. Patients were even alerted about the potential problems linked to infusion and consequent management. In particular it is important to explain to them what might occur during infusion and how to minimise their own discomfort. It is essential to provide telephone support, so, a telephone emergency number was supplied to all patients. Best practice is reached by obtaining feedback on the process and its relative possible problems: a telephone follow-up should be conduced to evaluate the infusion experience and verify proper infusion techniques. The first two initial infusions were usually given in Day Hospital regimen with the aid of a physician and a nurse who instructed patients about performing subcutaneous infusion and explained the procedure to them: only when patients and a relative feel confident with the treatment, can further self-infusions be carried out at home.

5.3.4 Results

At 3-month evaluation, almost all patients showed a good response to the treatment, documented by creatine kinase serum levels normalisation, improvement in the Medical research Council scale (a mean of 8 point) and in Rankin modified scores. Only two patients showed a partial response to the subcutaneous immunoglobulin treatment.

Table 6 shows long-term follow-up analyses (a mean of 16.8 months). A marked beneficial clinical and laboratory response was documented in six patients in this series; they were all able to reduce the glucocorticoid dose and three of them were able to suspend the immunosuppressive agent. Even patients with relapsed disease showed a good response to subcutaneous immunoglobulin. Among these patients, the following briefly reports the history of a 69-year-old woman with a 2-year history of polymyositis, previously treated only with prednisone and methotrexate. She had never previously been treated with intravenous immunoglobulin. In her case, indication for the treatment with subcutaneous immunoglobulin was the appearance, after six months of treatment with methotrexate, of an elevated lymphocyte count (lymphocytes=4130 /mmc) with a small clonal NK/T CD3+ CD4+ CD8+ CD56+ cell population (10% of the total circulating lymphocytes) bearing monoclonally the V/β17 chain of TCR (90% of these CD4+ CD8+ cells). Due to the risk of progression to lymphoma linked to the use of methotrexate, we decided to discontinue this drug and to start the subcutaneous immunoglobulin treatment. After six months, with the patient's muscle disease in remission, we documented the lymphocyte count normalisation and the clonal population reduction (70% of the CD4+ CD8+ cells).

Among the partially responding patients is the case of a 39-year-old woman, presenting with long-term dermatomyositis (more than 20 years). From the onset, she showed a very aggressive form of the disease, with diffuse erythematosus and heliotrope rash, severe muscle involvement, characterised by weakness of the proximal and paraspinal muscles with a hanging head and an inability to execute any upward movement, rendering her dependent in performing daily activities. Over the years, she tried different types of therapeutic approaches; including methotrexate, cyclosporine A, high-dose glucocorticoids. The disease was eventually controlled only with serial infusion of intravenous immunoglobulin, which was maintained with increasing intervals for some years. In January 2009, she returned to our attention with a new relapse of the disease. She was immediately treated with high-dose prednisone, subsequently tapered, and intravenous immunoglobulin (2 g/kg) in monthly infusion for six months and then switched onto subcutaneous administration. After an initial positive response, at month 6, she had a flare-up with persistent weakness and elevated serum creatine kinase levels requiring an intravenous immunoglobulin infusion (at the dose of 2 g/kg in two consecutive days) that brought the disease's activity under control. The intravenous immunoglobulin was repeated three months later. In the subsequent follow-up period, while continuing the subcutaneous immunoglobulin, she was able to reduce the prednisone dose and despite this recurrence of disease, she showed a high level of satisfaction with treatment.

One patient, a 74-year-old woman with polymyositis diagnosed on July 2006, had no response to subcutaneous treatment. She was initially treated with methyl-prednisolone (1 g per day for 3 days) followed by a decreasing dose of oral prednisone associated with methotrexate (10 mg/weekly i.m.) with a poor response. In 2008, she presented a recurrence of the disease with reduction in muscle strength and a marked increase in serum creatine kinase levels; we thus decided to start intravenous immunoglobulin at monthly cycles (2 g/kg for each month), obtaining a good response. She subsequently switched to subcutaneous self-administration with clinical stabilisation, but without any laboratory improvement. At the first follow up visit, after one month, we noticed a slight increase of serum creatine kinase levels, despite stability in clinical assessment, tested by the Medical

Sex/ Age at the diagnosis (years)	DM/PM (date of diagnosis)	Disease duration prior to SCIg (months)	Previous ineffective therapies	Indications for SCIg treatment	Outcome
F/54	DM	72	PDN, IVIg, MTX, PP, CSA	Refractory to immunosuppressant	Partial remission. Reduction of immunosuppressant
F/53	DM	223	PDN, MTX, Anti-TNF, MMF, IVIg	Refractory to immunosuppressant	Complete remission. Withdrawn MMF
F/39	DM	167	PDN, MTX, CSA, IVIg	Refractory to immunosuppressant and steroid-dependency	Initial remission, but new flare-up after six months controlled by IVIg
F/47	PM	151	PDN, CYC, IVIg	Recurrence of a previously quiescent disease	Complete remission. Significant reduction of PDN and MMF dosage
F/71	PM	52	PDN, MTX, CSA, MMF, PP, IVIg	Recurrence of a previously quiescent disease	Complete remission. Withdrawn MTX
F/43	DM	10	PDN, MTX, IVIg	Recurrence of a previously quiescent disease	Complete remission. Significative reduction of PDN dosage
F/69	PM	24	PDN, MTX	Contraindication to immunosuppressant	Complete remission. No immunosuppressant consumption
F/74	PM	43	PDN, MTX, IVIg	Recurrence of a previously quiescent disease	Poor response with slight improvement in muscular power and persistant elevation of CPK levels
M/22	OM	144	PDN, MTX, CSA	Refractory to immunosuppressant and steroid-dependency	Complete remission. Withdrawn CSA and significant reduction of PDN dosage

Abbreviations: anti-TNF□, etanercept; CSA, Cyclosporine A; CYC, cyclophosphamide; IVIg, intravenous immunoglobulin; MMF, mycophenolate mofetil; MTX, methotrexate; OM, ocular myositis; PDN, prednisone; PP, plasmapheresis.

Table 6. Baseline characteristics and treatment response in 8 patients treated with glucocorticoids and subcutaneous immunoglobulin.

Research Council scale. Moreover, laboratory tests showed an elevation on liver enzymes that induced a discontinuation of methotrexate and to introduce mycophenolate mofetil, by continuing the subcutaneous immunoglobulin infusion.

In this series, we encountered the case of a 22-year-old-boy affected from infancy by an ocular form of myositis, previously refractory to different immunosuppressive therapies (cyclosporine A and methotrexate) and steroid-dependent. After starting the treatment with subcutaneous immunoglobulin, he was able to discontinue the immunosuppressants and to gradually reduce the prednisone (used for 15 years of his life).

In all of the responding patients, the subcutaneous administration of immunoglobulin was continued one year after remission, associated in most cases with a low-dose prednisone.

5.3.5 Patient satisfaction with subcutaneous immunoglobulin

Satisfaction with the subcutaneous immunoglobulin treatment was high in all patients. At the end of the follow-up period we documented an improvement in our patient's quality of life, the highest scores being for global mental health, measured using the validated Italian version of the Medical Outcome Study Short Form 36 (SF-36) questionnaire, which has two major domains - physical health and mental health indexes - and measures physical activity and restrictions, physical pain, global health status, vitality, social and occupational activities, restrictions and mental health (Apolone & Mosconi, 1998). We investigated patient interest in and satisfaction with the treatment, and the quality of communication provided by the staff, testing the level of agreement with a statement. The most significant items suggested by the patients were the reduction in problems while receiving treatment and the increased freedom in organizing daily activities. Considerable satisfaction was felt with the quality of disease-related information, its usefulness in treatment management and the high level of communication with health professionals.

5.3.6 Side effects with subcutaneous immunoglobulin

In our series, no major side effects were documented. In literature, systemic adverse effects have been reported in less than 1% of subcutaneous infusions, as opposed to 5% of intravenous infusion (Berger, 2008). These only include mild local reactions, including swelling, redness and "burning" sensation in the infusion site that usually resolve spontaneously within 24-48 hours, as reported in literature (Wasserman, 2008). These effects were transient and declined over time, specifically after 8 to 10 weeks. The recording of side effects is subjective and it is possible that very weak reactions were not mentioned by the patients, due to their acceptance of the treatment and to their gradual adaptation to the local phenomena.

The different pharmacokinetic properties between intravenous and subcutaneous immunoglobulin regimens reflect the differences in their adverse effects. Despite not checking the serum IgG levels in our patients, it is conceivable that fractioning the usual monthly intravenous dose into subcutaneous weekly doses facilitated near stable IgG levels. It is likely that the metabolised IgG are constantly being replaced by IgG freshly absorbed from the subcutaneous injection site. Taking this into account, the subcutaneous route administration and the reduced dose given in weekly subcutaneous infusion could lead to a reduction in the risk of systemic reactions and of thromboembolic events. It is noteworthy that various reports described the safe use of subcutaneous immunoglobulin in patients with previous serious systemic adverse reactions to intravenous immunoglobulin (Quinti et al., 2008).

Finally, the global costs of subcutaneous immunoglobulin treatment, are usually 15-25% less than those of intravenous immunoglobulin treatment as later reported (Paragraph 6). Furthermore, the ability to use subcutaneous immunoglobulin in patients with difficult venous access or in those with associated selective IgA deficiency, of course after a tolerability check given the variable individual response of the IgA deficient patients, will in future make subcutaneous immunoglobulin as the first choice.

5.4 Subcutaneous immunoglobulin in other immune-mediated diseases

Although subcutaneous self-infusion of immunoglobulin is currently labelled and increasingly used for replacement therapy in primary immune deficiencies, with documented effectiveness and safety, only a few cases report the use of subcutaneous immunoglobulin for its immunomodulatory and anti-inflammatory properties in chronic inflammatory disease.

In a case report, subcutaneous immunoglobulin was successfully used as an adjuvant treatment in a subject with dermatomyositis (Schleinitz et al., 2008) after 1-year follow-up.

Other experiences with subcutaneous immunoglobulin as a treatment of chronic inflammatory disease were carried out in particular for immune-mediated neurological disorder, as multifocal motor neuropathy or chronic inflammatory demyelinating polyneuropathy.

A preliminary experience was reported by Koller at al. (2006) in three subjects with chronic inflammatory demyelinating polyradiculoneuropathy with relapses, in which the use of subcutaneous immunoglobulin (at the dose of 0.1 g/kg of body weight given once weekly for 6 months), in concomitance with mycophenolate mofetil, lead to a stable disease during the 6-month follow-up period. Subsequently, Harbo et al. (2009) performed a randomized single-blind cross-over study on nine intravenous immunoglobulin responsive patients suffering from multifocal motor neuropathy, directly comparing the subcutaneous and the intravenous route, given in sequence, showing that using equivalent doses, the effectiveness of two treatments is similar in regard to muscular strength. No significant differences between treatments on health-related quality of life occurred, but as suggested by the authors and by Dimberg (2009), who discussed this data the relatively short treatment period may have played down subcutaneous immunoglobulin. In this regard, he performed another study, showing that long-term subcutaneous immunoglobulin therapy is an alternative approach to intravenous immunoglobulin that is desirable for some patients (Dimberg, 2009) in a small case series of six intravenous immunoglobulin responsive patients with multifocal motor neuropathy on long-term subcutaneous immunoglobulin maintenance therapy with dose equivalent to their previous intravenous regimen, followed for two years. Five of them preferred to continue the subcutaneous administration after the trial and another patient chose to apply for this kind of treatment. A case report on a patient with multifocal motor neuropathy positively treated for six months and in maintenance therapy with subcutaneous immunoglobulin was described by an Italian group (Dacci et al., 2010). Similar results were reported by Eftimov et al. (2009); in his single-centre open-label pilot intervention study, ten patients affected by multifocal motor neuropathy treated with intravenous immunoglobulin were included and then they were switched to weekly subcutaneous immunoglobulin. The first group (five patients) started with a subcutaneous dose equivalent to 50% of the intravenous dose, and then, in case of deterioration they received a loading dose of intravenous immunoglobulin and doubling of subcutaneous dose. The second group (five patients) started with a dose equivalent to the intravenous maintenance dose. They demonstrated that in four patients, the subcutaneous immunoglobulin therapy was feasible and safe and maintained strength as well as the intravenous route, while in the latter case a higher dose was needed; he brought attention to the subcutaneous dose as a maintenance treatment, monitoring serum immunoglobulin concentrations. Whereas patients in intravenous treatment show a swinging trend of immunoglobulin levels, with spikes corresponding to the therapy and deep valleys in the interim periods, during subcutaneous immunoglobulin treatment, immunoglobulin levels appeared stable and slightly higher than normal, preventing end- of-dose weaving observed in intravenous treatment. In previous experiences in primary immunodeficiency patients treated with subcutaneous immunoglobulin, it was documented that the mean serum IgG levels are usually higher than those obtained by the intravenous route when using the same total monthly dose (Berger, 2008).

6. Cost of the immunoglobulin treatment

The use of intravenous immunoglobulin is linked to the well known problems of supply and costs. First of all, the decision to use intravenous immunoglobulin for the treatment of myositis should be made in consultation with an expert in neuromuscular disease. Before treatment, it is essential to have a pathologic confirmation by means of a skeletal muscle biopsy for the diagnosis of polymyositis or dermatomyositis. As recommended by Feasby et al. (2007), the muscle specimen must be procured, processed, and interpreted in a specialised laboratory and the final diagnosis must be made by an expert in neuromuscular pathology. Once a diagnosis is obtained, immunoglobulin should be used in accordance with the main international guidelines (Feasby et al., 2007; Elovaara et al., 2008) and local directives.

The preparation of immunoglobulin is a multi-step process that leads to different products as supplied by manufacturers (Gurcan, 2010). In order to discover the real benefits of (intravenous or subcutaneous) immunoglobulin therapy in health-economical terms, analyses must be performed in each country, since economic systems for the provision of healthcare, including pharmacy handling, vary substantially (Gardulf, 2007). Most of these data, unfortunately, are inadequate and the majority of the reports published in the literature are related to the pharmacoeconomic evaluation on the use of intravenous or subcutaneous immunoglobulin in patients with antibody deficiency.

The first ever health-economic evaluation of immunoglobulin therapy has been performed in Sweden (Gardulf, 1995). It showed that the change from in-hospital intravenous immunoglobulin therapy to home-based subcutaneous immunoglobulin treatment saved $US10.100 per patient per year (1993 annual costs). All factors being equal, the use of subcutaneous immunoglobulin self-infusions at home for 80% of the 1300 Swedish patients known to be using immunoglobulin replacement therapy today would lead to a cost reduction of $US 10.504.000 per year for Swedish society. A recent cost analysis in Germany showed that a switch of 60% of the patients on intravenous to subcutaneous immunoglobulin therapy would lead to the German health insurance system saving between €17 million and €77 million each year (Hogy et al., 2005).

In the US, it has also been calculated that the cost of subcutaneous immunoglobulin self-infusions at home is $US 48, compared with $US 164–314 for using intravenous immunoglobulin at home administered by nurses (Radinsky & Bonagura, 2003) and that "it may be expected that cost savings of $US2000–5000 per patient per year" will be the result of home instead of hospital therapy (Berger, 2003).

In Italy the only cost-minimisation analysis has been performed by Matucci et al. (2008) using data from the Tuscany Health Service. It compares the annual direct medical costs (immunoglobulin, premedication, infusion pump, infusion materials, medical staff, ambulatory) of subcutaneous and intravenous immunoglobulin in patients with antibody deficiency observing a difference of € 2,212.98 in favour of subcutaneous immunoglobulin due to lower costs for both medical staff and ambulatory. The Italian experience, in accordance with the literature, substantiates the cost-sparing effect of subcutaneous immunoglobulin home treatment from both patient and medical point of view. It is important to note that the production of intravenous immunoglobulin is more complex than that of subcutaneous immunoglobulin, thus largely rendering the latter a more viable option in regards to overall yield. Moreover, home management lead to a reduction in the costs linked to hospitalisation, substantially reducing the time and the workload necessary for the department to handle the intravenous therapy of patients. Indirect costs that favour the use of subcutaneous immunoglobulin are transportation to hospital and time lost from work (Gaspar et al., 1998).

Another concern regarding the costs of intravenous immunoglobulin therapy is the frequent need of their use as maintenance therapy after the initial remission. Dalakas (2006) documented that the benefits appear lasting an average of six weeks and that for long-term benefits, continued infusions may be required. Genevay et al. documented that low-dose (0,8 g/kg/monthly) treatment with intravenous immunoglobulin can be helpful in maintaining clinical remission after high-dose initial infusions (2g/kg/monthly) in patients with refractory polymyositis (Genevay, 2001).

However, the problem of cost should be balanced with proven effectiveness in otherwise life-threatening situations or as short-term treatment in patients with severe refractory disease.

7. Conclusions

In this chapter we examined the role of immunoglobulin therapy in polymyositis and dermatomyositis. The revision of the literature evidenced the lack of randomised controlled trial, basically due to the rarity of the diseases. Another major problem in evaluating the published reports in polymyositis and dermatomyositis is the lack of international consensus on diagnostic criteria and outcome measures. A consensus on this will significantly improve the analyses of published data. Despite these biases, most of the papers report the efficacy and the safety of intravenous immunoglobulin, when standard therapeutic regimens fail, even in refractory or relapsing cases. Indication for the use of intravenous immunoglobulin is in particular the oesophageal involvement. In other reports intravenous immunoglobulin is used in association with immunosuppressants. In relation to cyclosporine A and mycophenolate mofetil, the add-on of intravenous immunoglobulin enables an increase in the rate of responding patients, with a short- and long-term stable remission and a reduced rate of infective complications. Recently, subcutaneous immunoglobulin has been used in selected autoimmune diseases. We documented the feasibility and the high tolerability of subcutaneous immunoglobulin, with relevant improvement in the clinical and laboratory features. Moreover, subcutaneous immunoglobulin increases patient quality of life giving them the possibility to receive treatment at home. This "self-management" is generally appreciated by most patients, in particular as it renders them independent from healthcare providers and hospitalisation, with a significant improvement in treatment satisfaction. This improvement is mostly associated with flexibility, reduced infusion-related issues and enhanced freedom in organising daily activities. The low rate of side effects which improves quality of life, the possibility to withdraw the immunosuppressants and the steroid sparing effect, make the subcutaneous immunoglobulin a viable option in selected patients with myositis when standard therapeutic regimens fail or when immunosuppressants are contra-indicated.

8. Acknowledgement

We are deeply grateful to Miss Ciara O'Hanharan for her helpful and valuable editing assistance.

9. References

Agmon-Levin, N.; Lian, Z. & Shoenfeld, Y. (2011). Explosion of autoimmune diseases and the mosaic of old and novel factors. Cellular and Molecular Immunology, (February 2011).

Allenbach, Y.; Solly, S.; Grégoire, S.; Dubourg, O.; Salomon, B.; Butler-Browne, G.; Musset, L.; Herson, S.; Klatzmann, D.; Benveniste, O. (2009). Role of regulatory T cells in a new mouse model of experimental autoimmune myositis. , Vol. 174, No.3, pp.989-998

Anderka, M.T.; Lin, A.E.; Abuelo, D.N.; Mitchell, A.A. & Rasmussen, A.A. (2008). Reviewing the evidence for mycophenolate mofetil as a new teratogen: case report and review of the literature. American Journal of Medical genetics part A, Vol. 149 A, No. 6, (May 2009), pp.1241–1248

Anthony, R.M.; Nimmerjahn, F; Ashline, D.J.; Reinhold, V.N.; Paulson, J.C. & Ravetch, J.V. (2008). Recapitulation of IVIG anti-inflammatory activity with a recombinant IgG Fc. Science. Vol.18, No.320, (April 2008), (5874) pp.373-6

Apolone, G. & Mosconi, P. (1998). The Italian sf-36 health survey: translation, validation and norming. Journal of Clinical Epidemiology; Vol. 5, pp.1025-36

Arnson, Y.; Shoenfeld, Y. & Amital, H. (2009). Intravenous immunoglobulin therapy for autoimmune diseases. Autoimmunity, Vol. 42, No.6, pp.553-60

Aschermann, S.; Lux, A.; Baerenwaldt, A.; Biburger, M. & Nimmerjahn, F. (2010) The other side of immunoglobulin G: suppressor of inflammation. Clinical and Experimental Immunology, Vol.160, No.2, pp.161-7

Australian Health Ministers' Conference Criteria for the clinical use of intravenous immunoglobulin in Australia. Available at: http:// www.nba.gov.au/ivig/ pdf/criteria-qrg.pdf

Berger, M. (2003). Subcutaneous immunoglobulin replacement in primary immunodeficiencies. Clinical Immunology, Vol.112, No. 1, (July 2004), pp. 1-7

Berger, M. (2008). Subcutaneous administration of IgG. Immunology and Allergy Clinics of North America, Vol.4, No.4, pp.779-802

Bohan, A. & Peter, J.B. (1975). Polymyositis and dermatomyositis. New England Journal of Medicine, Vol. 292, (February 1975), pp. 344-7 & 403-7

Bomback, A.S.& Appel, G.B. (2010). Updates on the treatment of lupus nephritis. Clinical Journal of the American Society of Nephrology, Vol. 21, No. 12, pp. 2028-35

Branch, D.W.; Porter, T.F.; Paidas, M.J.; Belfort, M.A. & Gonik, B. (2001). Obstetric uses of intravenous immunoglobulin: successes, failures, and promises. Journal of Allergy and Clinical Immunology, Vol. 108, Suppl 4:S133–8

Chaudhry, V.; Cornblath, D.R.; Griffin, J.W.; O'Brien, R. & Drachman, D.B. (2001). Mycophenolate mofetil: a safe and promising immunosuppressant in neuromuscular diseases. Neurology, Vol.56, pp. 94-6

Cherin, P.; Herson, S.; Wechsler, B.; Piette, J.C.; Bletry, O.; Coutellier, A.; Ziza, J.M. & Godeau, P. (1991). Efficacy of intravenous gammaglobulin therapy in chronic refractory polymyositis and dermatomyositis: an open study with 20 adult patients. The American Journal of Medicine, Vol. 9, No. 2, (August 1991), pp.162-8

Cherin, P.; Piette, J.C.; Wechsler, B.; Bletry, O.; Ziza, J.M.; Laraki, R.; Godeau, P. & Herson, S. (1994). Intravenous gamma globulin as first line therapy in polymyositis and dermatomyositis: an open study in 11 adult patients. Journal of Rheumatology, Vol. 21, No. 6, pp. 1092-7

Cherin, P. & Herson, S. (1994). Indications for intravenous gammaglobulin therapy in inflammatory myopathies. Journal of Neurology, Neurosurgery & Psychiatry with Practical Neurology, Vol. 57 (Supplement), (November 1994), pp.50-4

Cherin P. (2000). Intravenous immunoglobulins in the treatment of polymiositis/ dermatomyositis. Annales de Medicine Interne, Vol. 151 Suppl 1, pp. 48-50

Chérin, P. (2008). Current therapy for polymyositis and dermatomyositis. La Revue de Medecine Interne, Vol.29, No.2, pp.9-14

Cherin, P.; Pelletier, S.; Teixeira, A.; Laforet, T.; Genereau, A.; Simon, T.; Maisonobe, B.; Eymard, B. & Herson, S. (2002). Results and long term follow up of intravenous immunoglobulin infusions in chronic, refractory polymyositis: an open study with thirty-five adult patients. Arthritis and Rheumatism, Vol. 46, No. 2, pp. 467–474

Choy, E.H.S. & Isenberg, D.A. (2002). Treatment of dermatomyositis and polymyositis. Rheumatology,Vol. 41, No.1, pp. 7–13

Choy, E.H.S., Hoogendijk JE, Lecky B, Winer JB & Gordon, P. (2011). Immunosuppressant and immunomodulatory treatment for dermatomyositis and polymyositis (Review). Cochrane Database of Systematic Reviews, Issue 3, No. CD003643. DOI: 10.1002/14651858.CD003643, ISSN 1464-780X

Dacci, P.; Riva, N.; Scarlato, M.; Andresen, I.; Schmidt, D.; Comi, G. & Fazio, R. (2010). Subcutaneous immunoglobulin therapy for the treatment of multifocal motor neuropathy: a case report. Neurological Sciences, Vol. 31, No. 6, pp. 829-31

Dalakas, M.C. (1991). Polymyositis, dermatomyositis, and inclusion-body myositis. New England Journal of Medicine, Vol. 325, pp.1487–98

Dalakas, M.C.; Illa, I.; Dambrosia, J.M.; Soueidan, S.A.; Stein, D.P.; Otero, C.; Dinsmore, S.T. & McCrosky, S. (1993). A controlled trial of high-dose intravenous immune globulin infusions as treatment for dermatomyositis. New England Journal of Medicine, Vol.329, pp. 1993-2000

Dalakas, M.C. (1999). Intravenous immunoglobulin in the treatment of autoimmune neuromuscular diseases: present status and practical therapeutic guidelines. Muscle & Nerve , Vol. 22, No. 11, pp. 1479-97

Dalakas, M.C. (2001). Progress in inflammatory myopathies: good but not good enough. Journal of Neurology, Neurosurgery and Psychiatry, Vol. 70, No. 5, pp. 569–73

Dalakas, M.C. (2006 a). Mechanisms of disease: signaling pathways and immunobiology of inflammatory myopathies. Nature Clinical Practice Rheumatology, Vol 2, pp.219–27

Dalakas, M.C. (2006 b). The role of high-dose immune globulin intravenous in the treatment of dermatomyositis. International Immunopharmacology, Vol.6, No. 4, pp. 550-6

Dalakas, M.C. (2010). Immunotherapy of myositis: Issues, concerns and future prospects. Nature Reviews Rheumatology, Vol. 6, No.3, pp.129-37

Damianovich, M.; Blank, M.; Raiter, A.; Hardy, B. & Shoenfeld Y. (2009). Anti-vascular endothelial growth factor (VEGF) specific activity of intravenous immunoglobulin (IVIg). International immunology, Vol.21, No.9, (September 2009) pp.1057-63

Danieli, M.G.; Malcangi, G.; Palmieri, C; Logullo, F.; Salvi, A.; Piani, M. & Danieli, G. (2002). Cyclosporine A and intravenous immunoglobulin treatment in polymyositis/ dermatomyositis. Annals of the Rheumatic Diseases, Vol.61, pp.37-41

Danieli, M.G.; Cappelli, M.; Malcangi, G.; Logullo, F.; Salvi, A. & Danieli, G. (2004). Long-term effectiveness of intravenous immunoglobulin in Churg-Strauss syndrome. Annals of the Rheumatic Diseases, Vol. 63, pp.1649-54

Danieli, M.G.; Calcabrini, L.; Calabrese, V.; Marchetti, A.; Logullo, F. & Gabrielli, A. (2009 a). Intravenous immunoglobulin as add on treatment with mycophenolate mofetil in severe myositis. Autoimmunity Reviews, Vol. 9, No.2, pp.124-7

Danieli, M.G.; Spalletta, C.; Moretti, R.; Calabrese, V.; Marchetti, A.; Gabrielli, A. & Logullo, F. (2009 b). La terapia immunosoppressiva nelle miositi refrattarie. Recenti Progressi in Medicina, Vol.100, No.10, pp.451-7

Danieli, M.G.; Pettinari, L.; Moretti, R.; Logullo, F. & Gabrielli, A. (2011). Subcutaneous immunoglobulin in polymyositis and dermatomyositis: a novel application. Autoimmunity Reviews, Vol.10, pp.144-9

Dankò, K. & Szegedi, G. (1991). Cyclosporin A treatment of dermatomyositis. Arthritis Rheumatism, Vol.34, No.7, (July 1991), pp. 933-4

Davies, R.; Sangle, S.R. & Murru, V. (2009). A randomized controlled trial of mycophenolate mofetil versus placebo on surrogate markers of atherosclerosis in systemic lupus erythematosus. ACR/ARHP Annual Scientific Meeting. Arthritis Rheumatism; Suppl:103A

Dimberg, E.L. (2009). Treatment of multifocal motor neuropathy with immunoglobulin: does route of administration matter? European Journal of Neurology, Vol.16, No.5, (May 2009), pp. 553-4

Eftimov, F.; Vermeulen, M.; de Haan, R.J.; van den Berg, L.H. & van Schaik, I.N. (2009). Subcutaneous immunoglobulin therapy for multifocal motor neuropathy. Journal of Peripheral Nervous System, Vol.14, No.2, (June 2009), pp.93-100

Elovaaraa, I.; Apostolski, S.; Van Doorn, P.; Gilhus, N.E.; Hietaharju, A.; Honkaniemi, J.; Van Schaik, I.N.; Scolding, N.; Soelberg Sørensen, P. & Udd, B. (2008). EFNS guidelines for the use of intravenous immunoglobulin in treatment of neurological diseases. European Journal of Neurology, Vol.15, No.9, (September 2008), pp. 893–908

Ephrem, A.; Chamat, S.; Miquel, C.; Fisson, S.; Mouthon, L.; Caligiuri, G.; Delignat, S.; Elluru, S; Bayry, J.; Lacroix-Desmazes, S.; Cohen, J.L.; Salomon, B.L. & Kazatchkine, M.D. (2008). Expansion of CD4+CD25+ regulatory T cells by intravenous immunoglobulin: a critical factor in controlling experimental autoimmune encephalomyelitis. Blood, Vol.111, No.2, pp.715-22

Feasby, T.; Banwell, B.; Benstead, T.; Bril, V.; Brouwers, M.; Freedman, M.; Hahn, A.; Hume, H.; Freedman, J.; Pi, D. & Wadsworth, L. (2007). Guidelines on the use of intravenous immune globulin for neurologic conditions. Transfusion Medicine Reviews, Vol.21, (April 2007), Suppl.1, pp.57–107

Fernandez-Cruz, E.; Kaveri, S.V.; Peter, H.H.; Durandy, A.; Cantoni, N.; Quinti, I.; Sorensen, R.; Bussel, J.B.; Danieli, M.G.; Winkelmann, A.; Bayry, J.; Käsermann, F.; Späth, P.; Helbert, M.; Salama, A.; Van Schaik, I.N. & Yuki, N. (2009). 6th International Immunoglobulin Symposium: poster presentations. Clinical & Experimental Immunology, Vol. 158, (December 2009), Supplement 1:60-7

Gardulf, A. (2007). Immunoglobulin treatment for primary antibody deficiencies: advantages of the subcutaneous route. BioDrugs, Vol.21, No.2, (January 2007), pp.105-116

Gardulf, A.; Andersen, V.; Björkander, J.; Ericson, D.; Frøland, S.S.; Gustafson, R.; Hammarström, L.; Jacobsen, M.B.; Jonsson, E. & Möller, G. (1995). Subcutaneous immunoglobulin replacement in patients with primary antibody deficiencies: safety and costs. Lancet, Vol.345, (February 1995), pp. 365-9

Gaspar, J.; Gerritsen, B. & Jones, A. (1998). Immunoglobulin replacement treatment by rapid subcutaneous infusions. Archives of Disease in Childhood, Vol.79, No.1, (July 1998), pp.48-51

Gelber, A.C.; Nousari, H.C. & Wigley, F.M. (2000). Mycophenolate mofetil in the treatment of severe skin manifestations of dermatomyositis: a series of 4 cases. Journal of Rheumatology; Vol.27, pp. 1542-5

Gelfand, E.W. (1989). The use of intravenous immune globulin in collagen vascular disorders: a potentially new modality of therapy. The Journal of Allergy and Clinical Immunology, Vol.84, (October 1989), pp.613-5

Genevay, S.; Saudan-Kister, A.; Guerne, P.A.; Hachulla, E. & Levesque, H. (2001). Intravenous gammaglobulins in refractory polymyositis: lower dose for maintenance treatment is effective. Annals of the Rheumatic Diseases, Vol.60, No.6, (June 2001),pp.635-6

Göttfried, I.; Seeber, A.; Anegg, B.; Rieger, A.; Stingl, G. & Volc-Platzer, B. (2000). High dose intravenous immunoglobulin (IVIG) in dermatomyositis: clinical responses and effect on sIL-2R levels. European Journal of Dermatology, Vol.10, No.1, (January-February 2000), pp.29–35

Gürcan, H.M.; Keskin, D.B. & Ahmed, A.R. (2010). Information for healthcare providers on general features of IGIV with emphasis on differences between commercially available products. Autoimmunity Reviews, Vol. 9, No.8, (June 2010), pp.553-9

Hartung, H.P.; Mouthon, L.; Ahmed, R.; Jordan, S.; Laupland, K.B. & Jolles, S. (2009). Clinical applications of intravenous immunoglobulins (IVIG)--beyond immunodeficiencies and neurology. Clinical and Experimental Immunology, Vol.158, (December 2009), Supplement 1: 23–33

Harvey, R.D. III (2005). The patient: emerging clinical applications of intravenous immunoglobulin. Pharmacotherapy, Vol.25, No.11, (November 2005), pp.85S–93S

Hehir, M.K.; Burns, T.M.; Alpers, J.; Conaway, M.R.; Sawa, M. & Sanders, D.B. (2010). Mycophenolate mofetil in AChR-antibody-positive myasthenia gravis: outcomes in 102 patients. Muscle Nerve. Vol. 41, No.5 (May, 2010), pp. 593-8

Hoffman, G.S. (2010). Therapeutic interventions for systemic vasculitis. Journal of American Medical Association; Vol. 304, No.21, (December, 2010) pp. 2413-4

Högy, B.; Keinecke, H.O. & Borte, M. (2005). Pharmacoeconomic evaluation of immunoglobulin treatment in patients with antibody deficiencies from the perspective of the German statutory health insurance. European Journal of Health Economics; Vol. 6, pp. 24-29

Iaccarino, L.; Rampudda, M.; Canova, M.; Della Libera, S.; Sarzi-Puttini, P. & Doria A. (2007). Mycophenolate mofetil: what is its place in the treatment of autoimmune rheumatic diseases? Autoimmunity Reviews; Vol. 6, No.3 (January, 2007) pp. 190-5

Imbach, P.; Barandun, S.; d'Apuzzo, V.; Baumgartner, C.; Hirt, A.; Morell, A.; Rossi, E.; Schoni, M.; Vest, M. & Wagner, H.P. (1981). High-dose intravenous gammaglobulin for idiopathic thrombocytopenic purpura in childhood, Lancet, Vol.1, pp.1228-1231

Kameda, H.; Nagasawa, H.; Ogawa, H.; Sekiguchi, N.; Takei, H.; Tokuhira, M.; Amano, K. & Takeuchi, T.(2005). Combination therapy with corticosteroids, cyclosporin A, and intravenous pulse cyclophosphamide for acute/subacute interstitial pneumonia in patients with dermatomyositis. The Journal of Rheumatology, Vol.32, No.9, pp.1719-26

Katz, U.; Achiron, A.; Sherer, Y. & Shoenfeld, Y. (2007). Safety of intravenous immunoglobulin (IVIG) therapy. Autoimmunity Review, Vol.6, No.4, pp.257-9

Kessel, A.; Ammuri, H.; Peri, R.; Pavlotzky, E.R.; Blank, M.; Shoenfeld, Y. & Toubi, E. (2007). Intravenous immunoglobulin therapy affects T regulatory cells by increasing their suppressive function. The Journal of Immunology, Vol.179, No.8, (October 2007), pp.5571-5

Kimura, J. (1989). Electrodiagnosis in diseases of nerve and muscle: principles and practice. ISBN Philadelphia, F.A. Davis Company, 1989

Kivity, S.; Katz, U.; Daniel, N.; Nussinovitch, U.; Papageorgiou, N. & Shoenfeld, Y. (2010). Evidence for the use of intravenous immunoglobulins—a review of the literature. Clinical Reviews in Allergy and Immunology, Vol.38, No.2-3, (April 2010), pp.201-69

Kotani, T.; Makino, S.; Takeuchi, T.; Kagitani, M.; Shoda, T.; Hata, A.; Tabushi, Y. & Hanafusa, T. (2008). Early intervention with corticosteroids and cyclosporin A and 2-hour postdose blood concentration monitoring improves the prognosis of acute/subacute interstitial pneumonia in dermatomyositis. The Journal of Rheumatology, Vol.35, No.2, pp.254-9

Lang, B.A.; Laxer, R.M.; Murphy, G.; Silverman, E.D. & Roifman, C.M. (1991). Treatment of dermatomyositis with intravenous gammaglobulin. The American Journal of Medicine, Vol.91, No.2, (August 1991), pp.169-72

Le Meur, Y. ; Büchler, M. ; &Thierry, A. (2007). Individualized mycophenolate mofetil dosing based on drug exposure significantly improves patient outcomes after renal transplantation. American Journal of Transplantation; Vol.7, pp.2496-503

Maddur, M.S.; Othy, S.; Hegde, P.; Vani, J.; Lacroix-Desmazes, S.; Bayry, J. & Kaveri, S.V. (2010). Immunomodulation by intravenous immunoglobulin: role of regulatory T cells. Journal of Clinical Immunology, Vol.30, Suppl.1 (May 2010), pp.4-8

Maeda, K.; Kimura, R.; Komuta, K. & Igarashi, T. (1997). Cyclosporine treatment for polymyositis/dermatomyositis: is it possible to rescue the deteriorating cases with interstitial pneumonitis? Scandinavian Journal of Rheumatology, Vol.26, pp.24-9

Majithia, V. & Harisdangkul, V. (2005). Mycophenolate mofetil (CellCept): an alternative therapy for autoimmune inflammatory myopathy. Rheumatology; Vol. 44, pp.386-389

Marie, I.; Menard, J.F.; Hatron, P.Y.; Haculla, E.; Mouthon, L.; Tiev, K.; Ducrotte, P. & Cherin, P. (2010). Intravenous immunoglobulins for steroid-refractory esophageal involvement related to polymyositis and dermatomyositis: A series of 73 patients. Arthritis Care & Research, Vol.62, No.12, (December 2010), pp.1748-1755

Marie, I.; Hachulla, E.; Levesque, H.; Reumont, G.; Ducrotte, P.; Cailleux N.; Atron, P.Y.; Devulder, B. & Courtois, H. (1999). Intravenous immunoglobulins as treatment of life threatening esophageal involvement in polymyositis and dermatomyositis. The Journal of Rheumatology, Vol.26, No.12, (December 1999) pp.2706-9

Marie, I.; Hachulla, E.; Hatron, P.Y.; Hellot, M.F.; Levesque, H,; Devulder, B. & Courtois, H. (2001). Polymyositis and dermatomyositis: short term and long term outcome, and predictive factors of prognosis. The Journal of Rheumatology, Vol.28, No.10, (October 2001), pp.2230-7

Mastaglia, F.L.; Phillips, B.A. & Zilko, P.J. (1998). Immunoglobulin therapy in inflammatory myopathies. Journal of Neurology, Neurosurgery, and Psychiatry, Vol.65, No.1, (July 1998), pp.107-10

Matucci, A.; Ravasio, R.; Voltaggio, A. & Maggi, E. (2008). Analisi di minimizzazione dei costi della terapia con immunoglobuline (Ig) per il trattamento di pazienti con immunodeficienza primaria: confronto tra terapia con Ig sottocute vs endovena. HTA Giornale Italiano di Health Technology Assessment, Vol.1, No.1, 84-8

Miller, F.W.; Leitman, S.F.; Cronin, M.E.; Hicks, J.E. Leff, R.L. Wesley, R.; Fraser, D.D.; Dalakas, M. & Plotz, P.H. (1992). Controlled trial of plasma exchange and leukapheresis in polymyositis and dermatomyositis. The New England Journal of Medicine, Vol.326, No. 21, (May 1992), pp.1380-4

Mimouni, D.; Blank, M.; Payne, AS.; Anhalt, G.J.; Avivi, C.; Barshack, I.; David, M. & Shoenfeld Y. (2010). Efficacy of intravenous immunoglobulin (IVIG) affinity-purified anti-desmoglein anti-idiotypic antibodies in the treatment of an experimental model of pemphigus vulgaris. Clinical and Experimental Immunology, Vol.162, No.3, (December 2010) pp.543-9

Mizuno, K.; Yachie, A., Nagaoki, S.; Wada, H.; Okada, K.; Kawachi, M.; Toma, T.; Konno, A.; Ohta, K.; Kasahara, Y. & Koizumi, S. (2004). Oligoclonal expansion of circulating and tissue-infiltrating CD8+ T cells with killer/effector phenotypes in juvenile dermatomyositis syndrome. Clinical and Experimental Immunology, Vol.137, No.1, (2004 July), pp.187-94

Mok, CC. (2007). Mycophenolate mofetil for non-renal manifestations of systemic lupus erythematosus: a systematic review. Scandinavian Journal of Rheumatology; Vol. 36, No.5. (September-October 2007), pp. 329-337

Morath, C.; Schwenger, V. & Beimler, J.(2006). Antifibrotic actions of mycophenolic acid. Clinical Transplantation, Vol. 20 Suppl, No.17, pp. 25–9

Moroni, G.; Doria, A. & Ponticelli, C. (2009). Cyclosporine A (CsA) in lupus nephritis: assessing the evidence. Nephrology Dialysis Transplantation; Vol.24, No.10, (October 2008), pp.15-20

Mosca, M.; Strigini, F.; Carmignani, A.; D'ascanio, A.; Genazzani, A.R. & Bombardieri, S. (2005). Pregnant patient with dermatomyositis successfully treated with intravenous immunoglobulin therapy. Arthritis and Rheumatism, Vol.53, No.1, (February 2005), pp.119-21

Mouthon, L. (2006) Indications for intravenous immunoglobulins. Presse Medicale, Vol.35, No.2, (April 2006), pp.714-9

Mydlarski, P.R.; Ho, V. & Shear, N.H. (2006). Canadian consensus statement on the use of intravenous immunoglobulin therapy in dermatology. Journal of Cutaneous Medicine and Surgery, 2006; Vol.10, No.5, (September-October 2006), pp.205-21

Nawata, Y.; Kurasawa, K.; Miike, S.; Takabayashi, K.; Watanabe, N. Hiraguri, M.; Kita, Y.; Kavay, M.; Saito, Y. & Iawamoto, I. (1999). Corticosteroid resistant interstitial pneumonitis in dermatomyositis/polymyositis: prediction and treatment with cyclosporine. The Journal of Rheumatology, Vol.26, No.7, (July 1999), pp.1527-33

Nussinovitch, U & Shoenfeld, Y. (2008). Intravenous immunoglobulin and mechanisms in cardiovascular diseases. Autoimmunity Reviews; Vol.7, No.6, pp. 445-52

Quinti, I.; Soresina, A.; Agostini, C.; Spadaro, G.; Matucci, A.; Sfika, I.; Martini, H.; Borghese, F.; Guerra, A.; Alessandra, V.; Vicentini, M.; Plebani, A. & Fiorilli, M. (2008). Prospective study on CVID patients with adverse reactions to intravenous or subcutaneous IgG administration. Journal of Clinical Immunology. Vol.28, No.3, (May 2008), pp.263-7

Qushmaq, K.A.; Chalmers, A. & Esdaile, J.M. (2000). Cyclosporin A in the treatment of refractory adult polymyositis/dermatomyositis: population based experience in 6 patients and literature review. The Journal of Rheumatology, Vol.27, No.12, (December 2000), pp.2855-9

Radhakrishnan, J.; Valeri, A.; Kunis, C. & Appel, G.B. (1995). Use of cyclosporine in lupus nephritis. Contributions to Nephrology, Vol.114, (1995), pp. 59-72

Radinsky, S. & Bonagura, V.R. (2003). Subcutaneous immunoglobulin infusion as an alternative to intravenous immunoglobulin. The Journal of Allergy and Clinical Immunology, 2003; Vol.112, pp.630-3

Rasche, F.M.; Keller, F.; Kunze, G.; Boesler, B. & Czock, D. (2007). Single daily dose of cyclosporine in patients with primary glomerulonephritis and nephrotic syndrome. Clinical Nephrology, Vol.67, No.5, (May 2007), pp.285-292

Ritter, M.L. & Pirofski, L. (2009). Mycophenolate mofetil: effects on cellular immune subsets, infectious complications, and antimicrobial activity. Transplantation Infectious Diseases. Vol.11, No.4, (August, 2009), pp. 290-297

Roifman, C.M.; Schaffer, F.M.; Wahcsmuth, S.E.; Murphy, G. & Gelfand, E.W. (1987) Reversal of chronic polymyositis following intravenous immune serum globulin therapy. Journal of the American Medical Association, Vol.258, No.4, (July 1987), pp.258:513-5

Rowin, J.; Amato, A.A.; Deisher, N.; Curio, J. & Meriggiali, M.N. (2006). Mycophenolate mofetil in dermatomyositis: is it safe? Neurology; Vol. 66, pp. 1245-7

Saadeh, C.; Bridges, W.; Burwick, F. (1995). Dermatomyositis: remission induced with combined oral cyclosporine and high-dose intravenous immune globulin. Southern Medical Journal, Vol.88; pp. 866-70

Samson, M.; Audia, S.; Lakomy, D.; Bonnotte, B; Tavernier, C. & Ornetti, P. (2010). Diagnostic strategies for patients with hypogammaglobulinemia in rheumatology. Joint Bone Spine doi: 10.1016/j.jbspin.2010.09.016

Schleinitz, N.; Jean, E.; Benarous, L.; Mazodier, K.; Figarella-Branger, D. & Bernit, E. (2008). Subcutaneous immunoglobulin administration: an alternative to intravenous infusion as adjuvant treatment for dermatomyositis? Clinical Rheumatology, Vol.27, No.8, pp.1067-8

Schwartz-Albiez, R.; Monteiro.; RC.; Rodriguez.; M.; Binder.; C.J. & Shoenfeld, Y. (2009). Natural antibodies, intravenous immunoglobulin and their role in autoimmunity, cancer and inflammation. Clinical and Experimental Immunology, Vol.158, Supplement.1, (December 2009), pp.43-50

Seite, J.F.; Shoenfeld, Y.; Youinou, P. & Hillion, S. (2008). What is the contents of the magic draft IVIg? Autoimmunity Reviews, Vol.7, No.6, pp.435-9

Silva, C.A.; Sultan, S.M. & Isenberg, D.A. (2003). Pregnancy outcome in adult-onset idiopathic inflammatory myopathy. Rheumatology (Oxford), Vol.42, pp.1168–72

Suzuki, Y.; Hayakawa, H.; Miwa, S.; Shirai, M.; Fujii, M.; Gemma, H.; Suda, T. & Chida, K. (2009). Intravenous immunoglobulin therapy for refractory interstitial lung disease associated with polymyositis/dermatomyositis. Lung, Vol.187, No.3, (May-Jun 2009), pp.201-6

Tarantino, A.; Passerini, P. & Campise, M. (2004). Is cyclosporine in renal-transplant recipients more effective when given twice a day than in a single daily dose? Transplantation, Vol.78, pp.675-80

UK Department of Health. Clinical guidelines for immunoglobulin use, 2nd Edition. (2009). Available at: http://www.dh.gov.uk /en/Publicationsandstatistics/ Publications /PublicationsPolicyAnd Guidance/DH_085235

Vani, J.; Elluru, S.; Negi, V.S.; Lacroix-Desmazes, S.; Kazatchkine, M.D.; Bayary, J. & Kaveri, S.V. (2008). Role of natural antibodies in immune homeostasis: IVIg perspective. Autoimmunity Reviews, Vol.7, No.6, pp.440-4

Vencovsky, J.; Jarosova, K.; Machacek, S.; Studynkova, J.; Kafkova, J. & Bartunkova, J. (2000). Cyclosporine A versus methotrexate in the treatment of polymyositis and dermatomyositis. Scandinavian Journal of Rheumatology, Vol.29, pp. 95-102

von Gunten, S. & Simon, H.U. (2008). Natural anti-Siglec autoantibodies mediate potential immunoregulatory mechanisms: implications for the clinical use of intravenous immunoglobulins (IVIg). Autoimmunity Reviews, Vol.7, No.6, pp.453-6

Wasserman, R.L. (2008). Common infusion-related reaction to subcoutaneous immunoglobulin therapy: manging patient expectations. Patient prefer adherence, Vol.2,. No.2, pp.163-6

Wilbourn, A.J. (1993). The electrodiagnostic examination with myopathies. Journal of Clinical Neurophysiology, Vol.10, pp.132-48

Williams, L.; Chang, P.Y.; Park, E.; Gorson, K.C. & Bayer-Zwirello. L. (2007). Successful treatment of dermatomyositis during pregnancy with intravenous immunoglobulin monotherapy. Obstetrics and Gynecology, Vol. 109, No.2, pp.561-3

11

Pregnancy in Myositis: Challenges and Pitfalls

Codrina Mihaela Ancuta[1,2], Eugen Ancuta[3] and Rodica Marieta Chirieac[1]
[1]Department of Rheumatology;
[2]Gr.T.Popa Center for Biomedical Research – European Center for Translational Research; "Gr.T.Popa" University of Medicine and Pharmacy;
[3]Research Department, "Cuza-Voda" Hospital Iasi
Romania

1. Introduction

Over the last decade, a lot of papers have been published by scientists and clinicians in order to disseminate their knowledge about major steps accomplished in the research of autoimmune disorders and pregnancy.

While pregnancy is delayed until later age in the majority of western countries and the incidence of autoimmune disorders, particularly rheumatic conditions, is increasing specifically in women of 25 to 40 years, patient's selection for a safe pregnancy becomes a very important concern.

It is essential to define a multidimensional concept that focus on how disease and its treatment affect pregnancy in autoimmune disorders. Based on values, goals and preferences of patients, physicians seem to be more critical in making decisions. Moreover, given the necessity to outline every physician's role in the management of pregnancy and autoimmune conditions there was a strong progress toward an interdisciplinary approach comprising rheumatologists, obstetricians, endocrinologists, immunopathologists, geneticians and neonatologists.

It was suggested formerly that women diagnosed with autoimmune diseases should avoid pregnancy due to excessive maternal and fetal risk, as autoimmunity can be reflected virtually on every aspect of reproduction (Borchers et al., 2010; Doria et al., 2006; Gordon, 2004; Peaceman & Ramsey-Goldman, 2008). Nevertheless, recent advances in the immunopathogenesis, assessment, monitoring and specific treatment options in patients with systemic autoimmune rheumatic disorders have resulted not only in optimal disease control, improved survival as well as quality of life, but also have been reflected in better pregnancy outcomes.

As patients with autoimmune rheumatic disorders are predominantly young women at childbearing potential (between 20 and 40 years), pregnancy is a major issue with prospective interest regarding the influence of both disease and therapy on pregnancy and, conversely, the effect of pregnancy on disease outcomes (Marker-Herman & Fisher Betz, 2010; Mecacci et al, 2007).

The physiological adaptation of the immune system to pregnancy (Th2-type response) potentially affects the course of the immune-mediated rheumatic conditions; equally, autoimmunity may compromise the fetal outcomes (Adams Waldorf & Nelson, 2008;

Borchers et al., 2010; Marker-Herman & Fisher Betz, 2010). Besides, systemic autoimmune conditions may be induced as a result of maternal hormonal changes and aberrant function of the immune system during pregnancy (autoimmune rheumatic disorders associated with pregnancy) or as a consequence of materno-fetal microchimerism recognized as the long-term persistence of a small number of cells from a genetically distinct organism (autoimmune rheumatic disorders in post-partum period) (Adams Waldorf & Nelson, 2008; Gordon, 2004; Scott, 2002).

Over the last decades, most epidemiological studies have focused on pregnancy in systemic lupus erythematosus, anti-phospholipid syndrome and rheumatoid arthritis, with special emphasis on a greater risk of relatively poor fetal outcome than in the general population, particularly with increased disease activity before conception and early in pregnancy (Doria et al., 2004; Doria et al., 2006; Gayed & Gordon, 2007; Mecacci et al., 2007). Pregnancy can also occur in patients with rare autoimmune rheumatic diseases, specifically systemic sclerosis, polymyositis/dermatomyositis, systemic vasculitis (Wegener's granulomatosis, Churg-Strauss syndrome, polyarteritis nodosa, microscopic polyangiitis, Takayasu arteritis) and Behçet disease (Doria et al., 2004; Doria et al., 2006).

The association of myositis with pregnancy is rarely described, mainly related to average age of onset of the illness that is past reproductive age; besides, the paucity of data prevent any real assumption concerning the effects of pregnancy on idiopathic inflammatory myopathies, chiefly represented by polymyositis (PM) and dermatomyositis (DM), whether these patients find it harder to conceive or if the outcome of pregnancy is adversely affected by the myositis (Doria et al., 2004; Doria et al., 2006; Linardaki et al., 2010).

Polymyositis and dermatomyositis are heterogenous conditions characterized by a broad clinical spectrum including proximal skeletal muscle weakness, skin lesions and systemic organ involvement, particularly interstitial lung disease, biochemical and histopathological background of varying degrees of muscle inflammation. Although the exact etiology is still controversial, there is now strong evidence that autoimmunity plays a central role in both entities; endomysial autoaggressive CD8+T cells are essentially involved in PM, while perivascular B cells and TCD4+ cells in DM (Aleksza et al., 2005). Because of their clinical and laboratory similarities the term "PM/DM" will further apply when referring to both disease subtypes.

The prevalence of PM/DM is 2.4 -10.7/100.000 cases, women being affected more often than males (Chopra et al., 2008, Silva et al., 2003). There is a bimodal age distribution, with peaks between 10-15 years (juvenile PM/DM) and 30-60 years (adult PM/DM) (Chopra et al., 2008). Furthermore, in over 85% of patients, the disease starts after childbearing age (de Man & Hazes, 2009), only 14% of cases presenting during reproductive period (Andreoli et al., 2010; Tincani et al., 2006). As a consequence, pregnancy in this group of myositis is uncommon (Linardaki et al., 2011).

Current concepts on immunology of normal pregnancy and specific intervention of myositis, effects of pregnancy on PM/DM and vice-versa, therapeutic options for PM/DM during pregnancy, fertility *versus* contraception in PM/DM will be further highlighted.

1.1 Immunology of normal pregnancy

Pregnancy is defined as a specific status of high levels of sex hormones and permanent cross-talk between mother and fetus, two major processes being essentially involved in physiological adaptation to pregnancy: (i) the modification of maternal immune system with subsequent conversion of cytokine profile and (ii) the changes of hormonal milieu throughout the course of gestation (Adams Waldorf & Nelson, 2008; Borchers et al., 2010; Gordon C, 2004).

1.1.1 Immune system and cytokines in normal pregnancy

Crucial modification of the innate immune system generally occurs during normal pregnancy aiming to attain immune tolerance toward paternal antigens expressed by fetal cells (considered as a semi-allogenic graft) (Kelling & Oswald, 2009; Tincani et al., 2006; Zen et al., 2010); furthermore, both local (feto-maternal interface) and systemic changes are directly guided by increasing levels of sex steroids (Kelling & Oswald, 2009; Zen et al., 2010). The cytokine network in pregnancy is conflicting even before any debate of concurrent rheumatic disease (Kelling & Oswald, 2009). It is widely accepted that maternal immune system modulates the cytokine pattern, promoting increased Th2-type cytokines production and decreased Th1-type response with subsequent Th2 polarisation that is crucial for a positive pregnancy outcome (Tincani et al., 2006; Zen et al., 2010). Moreover, it is actually well known that not only cytokine concentrations, but also soluble cytokine receptors change throughout the stages of normal pregnancy (Zen et al., 2010).

As a matter of fact, Th2-type background comprises key mediators with anti-inflammatory properties such as IL-4 and IL-10, IL-3, IL-5, IL-13 and Gm-CSF, classically accepted to enhance humoral immunity and to induce antibody production, being also involved in advancing placental growth and preventing fetal rejection (Raghupathy & Kalinka, 2008; Tincani et al, 2006; Zen et al., 2010). On the other hand, Th1-type cytokines such as TNF-α, IFN-γ, TNF-β, IL-1β, IL-6 and IL-2 secreted by Th1 cells are involved in cell-mediated immunity and inflammatory reactions and appear to have a primary role in early pregnancy, including embryo implantation and placental development (Raghupathy & Kalinka, 2008; Zen et al., 2010). In particular, although serum level of most Th1 cytokines significantly decreases in the third trimester, TNF-α level seems to remain stable in addition to increase in soluble TNF-α receptor, acting in order to protect from adverse outcomes such as preeclampsia, intrauterine growth retardation and pathological labor (Zen et al., 2010).

1.1.2 Hormones in normal pregnancy

Profound changes of the hormonal state take place during pregnancy (Østensen et al., 2011). Therefore, the Th1/Th2 shift is the result of a progressive increase in progesterone and estrogens levels during pregnancy driven by feto-placental unit, with a peak level accomplished in the third trimester of gestation (Kelling & Oswald, 2009; Zen et al., 2010).

Clearly, there have been described major differences in estrogen control on pro- and anti-inflammatory pathways in different immune-inflammatory cells (particularly T-cells, B-cells and activated monocytes). Thus, at high levels commonly encountered during gestation (3 to 8 times to baseline), estrogens seem mainly to suppress Th1-cytokines, particularly TNF-α, and to stimulate Th2-mediated immunological responses as well as antibody production (Cutulo et al., 2008; Cutulo et al., 2008; Tincani et al., 2006). On the other hand, the dynamics of progesterone, a potent immunomodulator hormone primarily secreted by placenta during the first 6-8 weeks of gestation, shows a spectacular increase (4 to 6 times), while deoxycorticosterone, one of its metabolites, reaches 1000 times higher concentration than in non-pregnant state; furthermore, progesterone inhibits Th1-type cytokine synthesis from T cells and induces Th2 cytokine, leading to a stimulation of humoral immunity (Zen et al., 2010).

Interestingly, temporary aberrant levels of free steroid hormones (glucocorticoids), gonadotrophin-releasing hormone (GnRH) and prolactin may also play a role in pregnancy and postpartum period, inducing changes of the immunocompetent cells (Kelling & Oswald, 2009; Zen et al., 2010). In addition, prolactin up-regulates Th-1-derived cytokines, including IL-12, IL-1, IL-6 and IFN-γ, modulating equally immune and inflammatory responses (Zen et al., 2010).

1.2 PM/DM in pregnancy

It is now much better established that the particular hormonal, biochemical and immunological interference in pregnancy may shape the course of autoimmune rheumatic diseases, including PM/DM (Cutulo et al., 2008; Cutulo et al., 2008). Furthermore, the mutual impact between the immune system and endocrine axis could explain why both of them may be affected by autoimmune diseases (Zen et al., 2010). As a result, the previous accepted Th2-Th1 paradigm is still considered the background of the disease flare during pregnancy and the improvement after delivery in Th2-mediated systemic autoimmune diseases. Several studies strongly support the link between the underlying pathological process and the course of such illness during gestation (Cutulo et al., 2008; Cutulo et al., 2008): Th1 predominant diseases like rheumatoid arthritis usually improve, with potential exacerbation after delivery (Cutulo et al., 2008; Cutulo et al., 2008; Váncsa et al., 2007); conversely, Th2-mediated disorders like systemic lupus erythematosus tend to remain relatively unchanged or, primarily, to worsen (Tincani et al., 2006).

Furthermore, the relationship between pregnancy and pathophysiological mechanisms of PM/DM is also unclear (Váncsa et al., 2007), due to extremely limited data. Cytokines and chemokines are essential players in the initiation and progression of the PM/DM, current evidence promoting the predominance of Th1-mediated immunity in different myositis subsets (Aleksza et al., 2005; de Paepe et al., 2009; Szodoray et al., 2010). It has been recently suggested, particularly for patients diagnosed with DM, that the onset of the disease may be triggered by the raise in serum estrogen concentration with subsequent effects on TNF-α synthesis as described in early pregnancy (Linardaki et al., 2011). The central role of TNF-α cytokine in the pathogenesis of DM is largely accepted; not only up-regulation of TNF-α expression in inflammatory and endothelial cells from muscle specimens and high soluble type 1 and 2 TNF-receptors, but also over-expression of TNF-α in regenerating muscle fibers have been identified (Aleksza et al., 2005; de Paepe et al., 2009; Linardaki et al., 2011).

Moreover, aberrant immunologic response caused by the presence of fetal cells in the maternal circulation and/or certain viral infections (Coxsackie viruses, Parvoviruses, Enteroviruses, Retroviruses, in particular Human T-lymphotropic virus and HIV) with subsequent impairment of humoral immune responses have also been proposed for the pathogenesis of pregnancy-associated DM (Linardaki et al., 2011).

Unfortunately, only a small number of reports on pregnancy outcomes in women with rare autoimmune rheumatic disorders such as PM/DM are yet available. The spectrum of possible adverse effects in pregnant women with myositis varies largely from intrauterine growth retardation and preterm delivery to increase frequency of fetal loss (spontaneous abortion, miscarriage, fetal death), and, finally, even to autoimmune disease in offspring (Borchers et al., 2010; Mecacci et al., 2007).

On the other hand, given the relationship between PM/DM and pregnancy three specific categories can be individualized: (i) flare-up/exacerbation of preexisting disease during gestation, (ii) onset of new PM/DM throughout the course of pregnancy, and (iii) postpartum flare or onset of myositis (Silva et al., 2003).

Fetal and maternal prognosis in patients diagnosed with myositis will be further discussed based on disease subsets (juvenile *versus* adult PM/DM), disease onset (pre-existing *versus* new-onset pregnancy-associated) and disease status (inactive *versus* active type).

2. Effects of PM/DM on pregnancy outcomes

As a matter of fact, pregnancy complicating myositis is a rare event, as the average age of onset for the disease is past reproductive age (Doria et al., 2006). However, similar to other autoimmune rheumatic diseases, it should be considered as a high-risk population if previous pregnancy complications, underlying systemic manifestation of myositis in target organs and flare of rheumatic illness are present (Borchers et al., 2010; Doria et al., 2006).
Overall, the course of pregnancy and fetal prognosis are considered to reflect the level of maternal disease status, paralleling the activity of myositis (Linardaki et al., 2011; Silva et al., 2003); the more active the myositis during the pregnancy, the greater the chance of fetal loss (Linardaki et al., 2011).

2.1 Pre-existing PM/DM

Better pregnancy outcomes in childhood onset versus adult PM/DM.
Since the majority of pregnancies reported in juvenile subset of PM/DM developed in an inactive phase of the disease, fetal outcome is favorable (de Man & Hazes, 2009; Silva et al., 2003) Moreover, up to 70% of cases presented with full term birth. Although perinatal pathology was defined, major adverse events including fetal death and abortion were rarely observed (de Man & Hazes, 2009; Tincani et al., 2006).
On the other hand, in patients with adult onset disease before pregnancy, fetal prognosis is worse, only half of women presenting full term deliveries (de Man & Hazes, 2009; Silva et al., 2003; Tincani et al., 2006).
Better pregnancy outcomes in inactive versus active PM/DM.
Pregnancy occurring during quiescent phase of pre-existing disease, controlled with or without low dose corticosteroids, is characterized by minimal fetal risk (Váncsa et al., 2007). Indeed, despite the fact that women with myositis who get pregnant must be considered as having a relatively high risk of developing complications, the outcome is better when the disease is inactive (Andreoli et al., 2010; Chopra et al., 2008; de Man & Hazes, 2009; Silva et al., 2003; Tincani et al., 2006). Furthermore, if the disease is maintaining inactive during pregnancy, excellent fetal outcomes with high percentage of normal deliveries have been mentioned (Andreoli et al, 2010; de Man & Hazes, 2009; Silva et al., 2003; Tincani et al., 2006; Váncsa et al., 2007). Since optimal pregnancy success can be anticipated if the diseases in remission before conception (Silva et al., 2003; Váncsa et al., 2007), up to 55% cases present with perinatal morbidity and mortality, mainly fetal growth restriction (Chopra et al, 2008).
Conversely, pregnancy in active PM/DM should be considered at high-risk for both the mother and the baby meaning risk for intrauterine retardation, high rate of pregnancy loss (death) or prematurity (Clowse, 2010; de Man & Hazes, 2009; Mecacci et al, 2007; Silva et al., 2003; Váncsa et al., 2007).
As it appear that the major risk is related to active disease, significant differences in pregnancy course and outcomes in active versus inactive PM/DM subsets have been suggested by most authors: rates of full term birth (72% versus 47%, respectively), intrauterine fetal death (43% versus 13.6%, respectively) and intrauterine growth

retardation/premature delivery (33% versus 13.6%, respectively) (Chopra et al, 2008; de Man & Hazes, 2009; Silva et al., 2003; Tincani et al, 2006; Váncsa et al., 2007). However, some papers advanced the idea that the proportion of fetal loss is quite similar in active versus inactive myositis, supporting the key role of monitoring in order to detect pregnancy complications (Silva et al., 2003).

Worse pregnancy outcomes in PM/DM exacerbation during pregnancy.

About a quarter of childhood onset PM/DM subset and up to 16% of adult PM/DM (de Man & Hazes, 2009) flared-up during pregnancy; the exacerbation of pre-existent disease account also for a significantly worse pregnancy outcome (Tincani et al., 2006). On the other hand, no sign of autoimmune disease has been observed in offspring (Tincani et al., 2006).

2.2 New-onset PM/DM

Worse pregnancy outcomes in new-onset versus pre-existing PM/DM

PM/DM starting during pregnancy or new-onset disease is a rare event, commonly reported in the first trimester of gestation (de Man & Hazes, 2009; Tincani et al, 2006; Váncsa et al., 2007). The risk of both maternal and fetal pathology is particularly high, over 50% fetal death (spontaneous abortion, intrauterine death, fetal loss) and high rate of prematurity being classically seen (Váncsa et al., 2007; de Man & Hazes, 2009).

Worse pregnancy outcome in PM/DM starting during early versus late pregnancy

It is now evident that pregnancy outcome is particularly poor with disease onset early in the gestation compared to the second or third trimester, when the fetal prognosis is usually good (Tincani et al, 2006; Váncsa et al., 2007; Chopra et al, 2008; de Man & Hazes, 2009). More recent cases had a good outcome, probably because active new-onset disease during pregnancy could be controlled by increasing corticosteroids, remissive agents, even therapeutic abortion in life-threatening cases to decrease the maternal mortality (Váncsa et al., 2007).

3. Effects of pregnancy on PM/DM outcomes

Although PM/DM does not seem to be particularly influenced by pregnancy, four main types could be identified based on clinical course in relation to gestation: (i) inactive-stable disease, (ii) relapsing disease, (iii) new-onset disease and (iv) either postpartum onset or flare of the disease (de Man & Hazes, 2009; Váncsa et al., 2007). The evolution of myositis is considered to be stable, if the patient remains free of clinical and laboratory disease activity during gestation, while a relapse is defined as disease exacerbation or reactivation because of the increase in serum muscle enzymes (creatine kinase and/or lactic dehydrogenase), typical clinical signs of proximal muscle involvement (weakness, pain) with or without characteristic skin signs (heliotrope rash, Gottron's papules). Consequently, maternal prognosis appears to be directly linked to disease course in pregnancy (de Man & Hazes, 2009; Silva et al., 2003; Tincani et al, 2006; Váncsa et al., 2007).

No increase in disease activity has been noted in nearly 90% of the pregnant women with adult PM/DM subset (de Man & Hazes, 2009; Váncsa et al., 2007). Moreover, the chance of juvenile disease to remain stable during gestation varies between 60% and 75%, positive maternal outcomes being typically documented (de Man & Hazes, 2009; Tincani et al, 2006; Váncsa et al., 2007). Finally, the overall relapse rate on corticosteroid therapy is 16% during pregnancy in the inactive phase of the myositis (Váncsa et al., 2007).

Although new-onset myositis during pregnancy is uncommon, patients typically develop very active therapy-resistant disease, with subsequent interference of both pregnancy and

labor (de Man & Hazes, 2009; Tincani et al, 2006; Váncsa et al., 2007) and worse maternal prognosis.
Furthermore, postpartum onset PM/DM have been recognized in several cases, suggesting that the post-partum period (1 to 3 months) may be a trigger for the development of myositis as a consequence of exposure to fetal antigens (Silva et al., 2003).
A summary of fetal and maternal outcomes based on PM/DM subset and disease activity is shown in Table 1.
Interestingly, recurrence in subsequent pregnancies is rarely seen (Pasrija et al., 2005); variable maternal and fetus outcomes in the same women but with different pregnancies could support the intervention of autoimmune pathology and consequently utero-placental involvement, even when disease is in remission (Chopra et al, 2008).

Disease subset	Fetal prognosis	Maternal prognosis
Pre-existing inactive PM/DM Juvenile subset Adult subset	 Favorable Moderate to Negative	 Low risk for disease flare-up Low to moderate risk for flare-up
Pre-existing active PM/DM Juvenile subset Adult subset	 Negative Negative	 Negative outcomes Negative outcomes
New-onset PM/DM during pregnancy	Negative	High risk for worse outcomes
Flare-up of preexisting PM/DM	Negative	High risk for worse outcomes
Post-partum onset PM/DM or flare	Not applicable	Moderate risk for worse outcomes

Table 1. Maternal and fetal outcome based on disease subset and activity.

4. Treatment options for PM/DM in pregnancy

Management of PM/DM in pregnancy is often a challenge even face to advancing knowledge in the immunopathogenesis of myositis and pregnancy. Main concerns are related to anti-rheumatic drugs use taking into account the teratogenic potential, adverse outcomes on fetal growth and development, as well as potential harmful effects on the offspring (Motta et al., 2008; Østensen, 2004; Østensen et al., 2005; Østensen et al., 2008; Østensen et al, 2011). Moreover, special considerations should be made on their effect on disease activity and maternal side effects.
The most important reasons for treatment of PM/DM during gestation are: (i) to prevent a disease flare-up, (ii) to control disease activity and (iii) to assure a good pregnancy outcome (Chopra et al, 2008; Lockshin, 2006; Østensen, 2004; Østensen et al., 2005; Østensen et al., 2008; Østensen et al., 2011).
As in non-pregnant PM/DM, the available medication for treating myositis in pregnancy can be divided in two main categories: (i) *first-line therapy* meaning steroids and (ii) *second-line therapy* meaning Disease Modifying Anti-Rheumatic Drugs (DMARDs) and intravenous immunoglobulins (IVIG) (Chopra et al, 2008; Østensen et al., 2004; Pasrija et al., 2005).
Extensive critical reviews of the current evidence and consensus regarding the use of anti-rheumatic drugs in pregnancy and lactation have already been published (Keeling &

Oswald, 2009; Østensen, 2004; Østensen et al., 2008; Saar et al., 2006). Even if the differences between various stages of gestation and between experimental and human pregnancies are not listed, clinical experience has shown that certain drugs, if properly monitored, can be maintained throughout gestation, resulting in better fetal outcome and better control of the disease in postpartum period (Keeling & Oswald, 2009; Motta et al., 2008; Østensen, 2004; Østensen et al., 2008). Pros and contra for their use in pregnant women diagnosed with PM/DM will be further discussed and summarized in table 2.

4.1 Corticosteroids

As for other autoimmune rheumatic disorders, patients with myositis require aggressive short-term corticosteroids to promptly suppress disease activity (Kelling & Oswald, 2009; Østensen, 2004; Østensen et al., 2005; Østensen et al., 2008; Østensen et al., 2011). While medium to high doses of prednisone and prednisolone are widely accepted as first-line therapy in pregnant women with myositis, dexamethasone and betamethasone are commonly reserved for fetal treatment (Kelling & Oswald, 2009; Linardaki et al., 2011; Østensen, 2004; Østensen et al., 2005; Østensen et al., 2008; Østensen et al, 2011).

Drug	FDA category*	Concerns	Clinical signification	Breastfeeding
Corticosteroids	C	Cleft palate Premature rupture of membranes Gestational diabetes mellitus Hypertension (conflicting reports)	Safe < 10 mg/day Caution > 20 mg/day	Safe; delaying feed by 4 hours with > 20 mg daily
(Hydroxy)-chloroquine	C	Fetal eye-ear effects (theoretical) No increased risk of malformations	Commonly used in pregnancy in autoimmune rheumatic disorders	Safe; small amount in breast milk (2%)
Azathioprine	D	Intrauterine growth restriction Prematurity	Commonly used, possible safe	Probable safe
Intravenous immune-globulins	C		Few case reports	Probable safe
Methotrexate	X	Teratogenicity, malformations, abortion	Discontinue 3-4 months prior to conception	Excreted in breast milk; not safe

*FDA category C (risk cannot be ruled out); D (positive evidence of risk); X (contraindicated in pregnancy)

Table 2. Anti-rheumatic drugs and their Food and Drug Administration (FDA) classifications in pregnancy and lactation in women with PM/DM.

Corticosteroids are essentially used in pregnancy myositis for dual reason, to control disease and to support pulmonary fetal maturity, but they are Food and Drug Adminstration (FDA) category C (Kelling & Oswald, 2009; Pasrija et al., 2005). It is well known that systemic steroids cross the placenta and the amounts vary according to steroid type, prednisolones crossing in low concentrations while dexamethasone and betamethasone in larger ones (Kelling & Oswald, 2009). Since placental enzymes such as 11-beta-hydroxylases partially inactivate all corticosteroids, with further decrease in steroid concentration in the fetal blood to 5-10% of the administered dose, the fetal risk appears to be very low at or below 15 mg/day (Linardaki et al., 2011; Østensen, 2004; Østensen et al., 2005; Østensen et al., 2008; Østensen et al., 2011, Silva et al., 2003;). Conversely, long-term use of medium to high doses, particularly during late pregnancy, may result in toxicity (Linardaki et al., 2011). Infrequently reported side effects consist of significant increase in cleft palate with first trimester exposure, high risk of premature rupture of membranes and preterm deliveries with more than 20 mg prednisone daily in late pregnancy, growth retardation, gestational diabetes, neonatal cataracts, adrenal suppression in neonates and high risk for infection (Kelling & Oswald, 2009; Linardaki et al., 2011; Østensen, 2004; Østensen et al., 2005; Østensen et al., 2008; Østensen et al., 2011).

The risk–benefit ratio must be considered on a case-by-case basis. Those patients on steroids at the time of delivery require additional stress doses indicated for labor and delivery to prevent acute adrenal insufficiency (Østensen, 2004; Østensen et al., 2008; Silva et al., 2003;). Although small amounts of steroids are also excreted in milk, breastfeeding is considered safe; doses over 20 mg daily should delay the next breastfeed with at least 4 hours (Kelling & Oswald, 2009).

4.2 Conventional DMARDs

Severe active potentially life-threatening cases of new-onset PM/DM and flare-up of pre-existing PM/DM are perhaps the only indications for the use of chemotherapeutic agents for the management of myositis during pregnancy (Østensen, 2004; Østensen et al., 2005; Østensen et al., 2008; Østensen et al., 2011; Silva et al., 2003). Immunosuppressives should be added if corticosteroids are not able to control the disease or as steroid-sparing drugs; the clinical use of these medications differs according to their FDA categories (Kelling & Oswald, 2009).

Azathioprine, an anti-neoplastic agent considered FDA category D for pregnancy, is safe during gestation and has been administered in pregnant women with myositis at 1.5-2 mg/kg/day. Case reports have shown increased rates of intrauterine growth restriction and prematurity, occasionally suppression of the fetal bone marrow (Linardaki et al., 2011; Østensen, 2004; Pasrija et al., 2005).

Cloroquine and **hydroxychloroquine** are antimalarials commonly used for DM patients; although they are FDA category C, the major concern includes theoretical risks of fetal oculo-toxicity or oto-toxicity and developmental abnormalities as both drugs crosses the placenta and accumulates preferentially in melanin-containing structures such as fetal uveal tract and inner ear (Kelling & Oswald, 2009; Østensen, 2004; Østensen et al., 2005; Østensen et al., 2008; Pasrija et al., 2005). Despite small amounts of excretion in breast milk (up to 2%), it is safe in breastfeeding (Kelling & Oswald, 2009).

Methotrexate and **cyclophosphamide** are contraindicated during pregnancy and lactation because of potential teratogenicity, mutagenicity and embryotoxicity (Kelling & Oswald, 2009;

Østensen, 2004; Pasrija et al., 2005; Saar et al., 2006). **Methotrexate**, a FDA category X drug, should be prescribed in fertile women only under safe contraception. Moreover, since active metabolites persist for about two months after discontinuation of therapy, conception should be delayed up to three months after withdrawal, while folate supplementation should be continued throughout gestation. Although indicated in the management of different forms of myositis, **cyclophosphamide** is a human teratogen; safe contraception is necessary in with women with childbearing potential and conception should be delayed until three months after drug discontinuation (Østensen, 2004; Pasrija et al., 2005).

4.3 Intravenous Immunoglubulin G

Finally, the intravenous administration of high doses of IgG (IVIG) seems to be an attractive alternative for pregnancy-associated DM given its efficacy, corticosteroid-sparing effect and the reduced risk of steroid-related side effects (Linardaki et al., 2011; Pasrija et al., 2005). While the benefits of IVIG are widely accepted in a variety of autoimmune disorders including DM in adults, uncontrolled observations suggest that it may also be effective in up to 70% of patients with PM (Linardaki et al., 2011).

Although the exact mechanism of action of IVIG in DM is not accurately defined, it is believed to be linked to suppression of pathogenic cytokines, modulation of pathogenic autoantibodies and Fc receptor blockade, with subsequent adjustment of T cell function. Additionally, the complications of IVIG therapy are relatively mild and consist primarily of non-anaphylactic reactions, such as fever, chills and back pain, aseptic meningitis in up to 10% of patients, acute tubular necrosis basically in patients with preexisting renal disease and, rarely, thrombo-embolic events due to increased serum viscosity (Linardaki et al., 2011).

Interestingly, the benefits of IVIG have been considered in a small number of DM presenting during pregnancy (Linardaki et al., 2011); IVIG given either as monotherapy or in combination with corticosteroids resulted in disease remission in all cases, with no maternal or fetal complications and positive fetal outcomes (Linardaki et al., 2011). However, there are still unanswered questions regarding the optimal therapeutic protocol (safest effective dose, frequency of administration, discontinuation before or maintenance after delivery) (de Man & Hazes, 2009; Linardaki et al., 2011).

Generally, a good fetal outcome can be expected if the maternal disease remains inactive during pregnancy (Chopra et al, 2008). Besides, it appears that the disease activity in active either pre-existing or new-onset cases could be controlled by increasing the corticosteroid dose (Chopra et al, 2008, Váncsa et al., 2007) and/or by adding remissive drugs such as azathioprine and hydroxicloroquine. Moreover, intravenous immunoglobulins should be considered in non-responders or, as recently suggested, monthly in order to prevent abortion (Váncsa et al., 2007, Linardaki et al., 2011). Therapeutic abortion has to be considered in life-threatening cases to decrease the maternal mortality (Linardaki et al., 2011), while the expected postpartum disease flare may be avoided by restarting medications soon after delivery.

5. Fertility and contraception in PM/DM

It is actually widely recognized that fertility is generally maintained in patients with rheumatic autoimmune conditions (Clowse, 2010). Furthermore, the rate of nulliparity among women with myositis is comparable with the general population (about 12%) (Silva et al., 2003). Although it has been suggested that fertility rates are significantly different before and after the onset of PM/DM, the late age of onset and the use of contraceptives exclude a specific evaluation of the influence of the disease on fertility (Costa et al., 2008; Clowse, 2010).

Contraception is an important issue in all autoimmune rheumatologic disorders since active disease and potential use of teratogenic anti-rheumatic drugs may result in adverse pregnancy outcomes (Costa et al., 2008; Clowse, 2010).

Three main contraceptive options are available, being applicable also in women diagnosed with PM/DM, including

i. *barrier methods* (condoms, diaphragm, with or without spermicides),
ii. *progestin-only methods* (daily pills, every 3-months injections, a 3-year implant, emergency contraception) and
iii. (progesterone-containing) *intrauterine devices* (IUDs) (Clowse, 2010).

It is widely accepted that progesterone, either systemic or locally released, does not worsen the rheumatologic illness as they do not increase immune activity or the risk for thrombosis. Furthermore, emergency contraception with levonorgestrel which is prescribed to prevent conception following unprotected intercourse and is responsible for the inhibition of ovulation, prevention of fertilization and prevention of implantation by modifying the endometrium, is known to be safe for patients with autoimmune rheumatic disorders. In addition, local effects described in progesterone-containing IUD comprise induction of atrophy of the uterine lining, impairment transport of sexual cell and decreased the frequency of ovulation, being also safe in autoimmune rheumatic pathology (Costa et al., 2008; Clowse, 2010).

Finally, it is well known that the combination of oestrogen and progestatives is commonly used to reduce certain side effects related to progesterone administration; as a consequence, a high oestradiol level (nearly 200 pg ml^{-1}) is constantly maintained, advancing thrombosis in susceptible individuals (Clowse, 2010). Therefore, oestrogen-based contraception is thought to be risky in systemic lupus erythematosus, with no evidence for PM/DM (Costa et al., 2008; Clowse, 2010).

6. Recommendations for pregnancy in PM/DM

Several general recommendations targeting maternal, fetal and neonatal complications have been already proposed for more prevalent autoimmune rheumatic disorders and seem to be suitable also for rare condition such as PM/DM (Andreoli et al., 2010; ; Doria et al., 2004; Kumar et al., 2010; Lockshin, 2006; Ruiz-Irastorza & Khamashta, 2008, 2010; Saar et al., 2006; Váncsa et al., 2007).

The most important points to remember are summarized in table 3 and include the following (Doria et al., 2004; Lockshin, 2006; Ruiz-Irastorza & Khamashta, 2008, 2010; Saar et al., 2006):

- every pregnancy in PM/DM should be regarded as a high-risk case, based on adverse fetal outcomes, maternal disease flares and drugs with potential teratogenic risk;
- all women should undergo counseling before conception, being informed for their specific risk to become pregnant (assess for risk factors, stratify risk as low/high, discuss potential adverse fetal effects);

- appropriate pre-conceptional diagnostic procedures are obligatory, particularly if pregnancy related pathology has been detected previously; specific contraindications including severe organ dysfunction such as cardiopulmonary pathology should be identified, while full antibody profile should be assessed;
- pregnancies should be planned when myositis is in remission or is considered as low disease activity for a period of at least 3 to 6 months before pregnancy;
- women with a high-risk profile should be strictly monitored during gestation (visits should be more frequent as pregnancy advances, classically every 4 weeks until delivery) and postpartum (at least one visit 12 weeks thereafter) by a multidisciplinary team including rheumatologist, obstetrician and neonatologists is mandatory; uterine and umbilical artery Doppler and fetal echocardiography should be planned at every visit;
- adequate aggressive management (high doses corticosteroids and/or immunomodulators and immunosuppressors) should be recommended during flare-up and new-onset PM/DM as active disease can be more harmful for fetus than drugs and particularly severe prognosis is recognized.

	Recommendation for myositis and pregnancy
1	Consider every pregnancy in PM/DM as a high-risk pregnancy • adverse fetal outcomes • maternal disease flare • drugs with potential teratogenic risk
2	Pre-pregnancy councelling of patients with myositis
3	Obligatory pre-conceptional diagnostic procedures • diagnose severe organ dysfunction
4	Plan pregnancy in quiescent PM/DM • inactive or remission disease
5	Monitor during gestation and postpartum • every 4 weeks until delivery and at least one visit 12 weeks in postpartum • multidisciplinary team: rheumatologist-obstetrician-neonatologists
6	Indicate aggressive management during flare-up and new-onset PM/DM • potential harmful for fetus than drugs and particularly severe prognosis is recognized

Table 3. Recommendation for PM/DM pregnancy.

7. Conclusions

Pregnancy in women suffering from PM/DM is a rare event, requiring special attention since considered as a high-risk pregnancy. Adverse fetal outcome (fetal loss, premature delivery, intrauterine growth restriction, neonatal autoimmune disease), maternal disease flares or new-onset disease during gestation and the use of anti-rheumatic drugs with potential teratogenic risk are the mainstay to declare high-risk profile for myositis pregnant women.

Furthermore, suitable pre-conceptional diagnostic proceedings and recognition of specific risk factors for unfavorable outcomes, close monitoring of disease activity and fetal prognosis with specific interdisciplinary (rheumatologist, obstetrician, neonate) intervention is mandatory.

Optimal pregnancy outcome can be anticipated in patients with pre-existing quiescent disease, while new-onset myositis and flare-up during pregnancy promotes significantly adverse pregnancy outcomes.

Finally, professional supervision warrants for a reliable pregnancy for the majority of women diagnosed with PM/DM.

8. References

Adams Waldorf, K.M. & Nelson, L.J. (2008). Autoimmune disease during pregnancy and the microchimerism legacy of pregnancy. *Immunol Invest,* Vol.37, No.5, pp. 631–644, ISSN 0882-0139

Aleksza, M.; Szegedi, A., Antal-Szalma´s, P., Irinyi, P., Gergely, L., Ponyi, A., Hunyadi, J., Sipka, S., Zeher, M., Szegedi, G. & Danko, K. (2005). Altered cytokine expression of peripheral blood lymphocytes in polymyositis and dermatomyositis. *Ann Rheum Dis,* Vol.64, pp. 1485–1489, ISSN (printed) 0003-4967

Andreoli, L.; Bazzani, C., Taraborelli, M., Reggia, R., Lojacono, A., Brucato, A., Meroni, P.L. & Tincani, A. (2010). Pregnancy in autoimmune rheumatic diseases: The importance of counselling for old and new challenges. *Autoimmunity Reviews,* Vol.10, pp. 51–54, ISSN 1568-9972

Borchers, A.T.; Naguwa, S.M., Keen, C.L. & Gershwin, M.E. (2010). The implications of autoimmunity and pregnancy. *J Autoimmun* (2010 May), Vol.34, No.3, pp. J287-J299, ISSN 0896-8411

Chopra, S.; Suri, V., Bagga, R., Thami, M.R., Sharma, A. & Bambery, P. (2008). Autoimmune Inflammatory Myopathy in Pregnancy. *Chopra et al, 2008 J Med,* Vol.10, No.1, pp. 17, ISSN 1934-1997

Clowse, M.E.B. (2010). Managing contraception and pregnancy in the rheumatologic diseases. *Best Practice & Research Clinical Rheumatology,* Vol.24, pp. 373–385, ISSN: 1521-6942

Costa, M. & Colia, D. (2008). Treating infertility in autoimmune patients. *Rheumatology,* Vol.47, pp. iii38–iii41, online ISSN 1462-0332, print ISSN 1462-0324

Cutulo, M.; Matucci-Cerinic, M., Lockshin, M. & Østensen, M, (2008). Introduction: new trends in pregnancy and rheumatic diseases. *Rheumatology,* Vol.47, Suppl. No.3, pp. iii1-iii2, online ISSN 1462-0332, print ISSN 1462-0324

Cutolo, M.; Capellino, S. & Straub, R.H. (2008). Oestrogens in rheumatic diseases: friend or foe?. *Oxford Journals Medicine Rheumatology* , Vol.47, Suppl No.3, pp. iii2-iii5, online ISSN 1462-0332, print ISSN 1462-0324

Doria, A.; Iaccarino, L., Ghirardello, A., Briani, C., Zampieri, S., Tarricone, E. & Gambari, P.F. (2004). Pregnancy in rare autoimmune rheumatic diseases: UCTD, MCTD, myositis, systemic vasculitis and Beçhet disease. *Lupus,* Vol.13, No.9, pp. 690-5, online ISSN 1477-0962, print ISSN 0961-2033

Doria, A.; Iaccarino, L., Ghirardello, A., Arienti, S., Zampieri, S., Rampudda, M.E., Tincani, A. & Todesco, S. (2006). Rare autoimmune rheumatic illnesses during pregnancy. Systemic sclerosis, polymyositis /dermatomyositis and vasculitis. *Z Rheumatol,* Vol.65, No.3, pp. 200-208, ISSN 0340-1855

Gayed, M. & Gordon C. (2007). Pregnancy and rheumatic diseases. *Rheumatology,* Vol.46, No.7, pp. 1634–1640, online ISSN 1462-0332, print ISSN 1462-0324

Gordon, C. (2004). Pregnancy and autoimmune diseases. *Best Pract Res Clin Rheumatol* (2004 Jun), Vol.18, No.3, pp. 359-379, ISSN 1521-6942

de Man, Y.A. & Hazes, J.M.W. (updated March 2009). Pregnancy in rheumatic diseases: an overview. In: *Oxford Textbook of Rheumatology (2004) 3rd edition,* De Man & Hazes, 2009, D.A., Woo, P., Glass, D. & Breedveld, F.C, pp. 117-125, Oxford University Press, Oxford, UK

de Paepe, B.; Creus, K.K. & de Bleecker, J.L. (2009). Role of cytokines and chemokines in idiopathic inflammatory myopathies. *Curr Opin Rheumatol* (2009 Nov), Vol.21, No.6, pp. 610-616, ISSN 1040-8711

Keeling, S.O. & Oswald, A.E. (2009). Pregnancy and rheumatic disease: "by the book" or "by the doc". *Clin Rheumatol,* Vol.28, pp. 1–9, online ISSN 1434-9949, print ISSN 0770-3198

Kumar, S.; Suri, V. & Wanchu, A. (2010). Pregnancy and rheumatic disorders. *Indian Journal of Rheumatology* (March 2010), Vol.5, No.1, pp. 35–41, ISSN 0973-3698.

Linardaki, G.; Cherouvim, E., Goni, G. & Boki, K.A. (2011). Intravenous immunoglobulin treatment for pregnancy-associated Dermatomyositis. *Rheumatol Int,* Vol.31, pp. 113–115, ISSN: 0172-8172

Lockshin, M.D. (2006). Treating rheumatic diseases in pregnancy: dos and don'ts. *Ann Rheum Dis,* Vol.65, Suppl No.III, pp. iii58–iii60, ISSN (printed) 0003-4967

Märker-Hermann, E. & Fischer-Betz, R. (2010). Rheumatic diseases and pregnancy. *Curr Opin Obstet Gynecol* (Dec 2010), Vol.22, No.6, pp. 458-65, ISSN 1040-872X, Online ISSN 1473-656X

Mecacci, F.; Pieralli, A., Bianchi, B. & Paidas, M.J. (2007). The Impact of Autoimmune Disorders and Adverse Pregnancy Outcome. *Seminars in Perinatology,* Vol. 31, No.4, pp. 223-226, ISSN: 0146-0005

Motta, M.; Tincani, A., Meroni, P.L. & Cimaz, R. (2008). Follow-up of children exposed antenatally to immunosuppressive drugs. *Rheumatology,* Vol.47, pp. iii32–iii34, online ISSN 1462-0332, print ISSN 1462-0324

Østensen, M. (2004). Disease specific problems related to drug therapy in pregnancy. *Lupus.* Vol.13, pp. 746-750, online ISSN: 1477-0962, print ISSN: 0961-2033

Østensen, M.; Förger, F., Nelson, J.L., Schuhmacher, A., Hebisch, G. & Villiger, P.M. (2005). Pregnancy in patients with rheumatic disease: anti-inflammatory cytokines increase in pregnancy and decrease post partum. *Ann Rheum Dis,* 2005 June, Vol.64, No.6, pp. 839–844, ISSN (printed) 0003-4967

Østensen, M.; Lockshin, M., Doria, A., Valesini, G., Meroni, P., Gordon, C., Brucato, A. & Tincani, A. (2008). Update on safety during pregnancy of biological agents and some immunosuppressive anti-rheumatic drugs. *Rheumatology,* Vol.47, Suppl. No.3, pp. iii28–iii31, online ISSN 1462-0332, print ISSN 1462-0324

Østensen, M.; Brucato, A., Carp, H., Chambers, C., Dolhain, R.J.E.M., Doria, A., Förger, F., Gordon, C., Hahn, S., Khamashta, M., Lockshin, M.D., Matucci-Cerinic, M., Meroni, P., Nelson, J.L., Parke, A., Petri M., Raio, L., Ruiz-Irastorza, R., Silva et al., 2003 C.S., Tincani, A., Villiger, P.M., Wunder, D. & Cutolo, M. (2011). Pregnancy and reproduction in autoimmune rheumatic diseases. *Rheumatology,* Vol.50, No.4, pp. 657-664 online ISSN 1462-0332, print ISSN 1462-0324

Pasrija, S.; Rana, R., Sardana, K. & Trivedi, S.S. (2005). A case of autoimmune myopathy in pregnancy. *Indian J Med Sci.* (Mar 2005), Vol.59, No.3, pp. 109-112, ISSN 0019-5359

Peaceman, A. & Ramsey-Goldman, R. (2008). Autoimmune Connective Tissue Disease in Pregnancy. *Glob. libr. women's med.*, ISSN 1756-2228

Raghupathy, R. & Kalinka, J. (2008). Cytokine imbalance in pregnancy complications and its modulation. *Front Biosci,* Vol.13, pp. 985-994, ISSN: 1093-4715

Ruiz-Irastorza, G. & Khamashta, M.A. (2008). Lupus and pregnancy: ten questions and some answers. *Lupus,* Vol.17, pp. 416-420, Print ISSN 0961-2033, Online ISSN 1477-0962

Ruiz-Irastorza, G. & Khamashta, M.A., American College of Rheumatology Patient Education Task Force. (2010). Pregnancy And Rheumatic Disease, updated Oct 2010, pp. 1-4

Saar, P.; Hermann, W. & Iler-Ladner, M. (2006). Connective tissue diseases and pregnancy. *Rheumatology,* Vol.45, pp. iii30–iii32, online ISSN 1462-0332, print ISSN 1462-0324

Scott, J.R. (2002). Risks to the children born to mothers with autoimmune diseases. *Lupus,* Vol.11, pp. 655-660, Print ISSN 0961-2033, Online ISSN 1477-0962

Silva, C.A.; Sultan, S.M. & De Man & Hazes, 2009, D.A. (2003). Pregnancy outcome in adult-onset idiopathic inflammatory myopathy. *Rheumatology (Oxford)* (Oct 2003), Vol.42, No.10, pp. 1168-1172, online ISSN 1462-0332, print ISSN 1462-0324

Szodoray, P.; Alex, P., Knowlton, N., Centola, M., Dozmorov, I., Csipo, I., Nagy, A.T., Constantin, T., Ponyi, A., Nakken, B. & Danko, K. (2010). Idiopathic inflammatory myopathies, signified by distinctive peripheral cytokines, chemokines and the TNF family members B-cell activating factor and a proliferation inducing ligand. *Rheumatology (Oxford), oct 2010,* Vol. 49, No.10, pp. 1867-1877, online ISSN 1462-0332, print ISSN 1462-0324

Tincani, A.; Nuzzo, M., Motta, M. & Lojacono, A. (2006). Autoimmune diseases and pregnancy. *Haematologica reports* (September 2006), Vol. 2, No.10, pp. 56-60, ISSN: 1824-9337

Váncsa, A.; Ponyi, A., Constantin, T., Zeher, M. & Dankó, K. (2007). Pregnancy outcome in idiopathic inflammatory myopathy. *Rheumatol Int.* (Mar 2007), Vol.27, No.5, pp. 435-439, ISSN: 0172-8172

Zen, M.; Ghirardello, A., Iaccarino, L., Tonon, M., Campana, C., Arienti, S., Rampudda, M., Canova, M. & Doria, A. (2010). Hormones, immune response, and pregnancy in healthy women and SLE patients. *Swiss Med Wkly*, Vol.140, No.13-14, pp. 187-201, ISSN: 1424-3997